Health Care: Advanced Practice Nursing

Health Care: Advanced Practice Nursing

Editor: Eric MacGregor

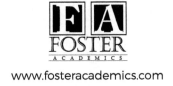

www.fosteracademics.com

www.fosteracademics.com

Cataloging-in-Publication Data

Health care : advanced practice nursing / edited by Eric MacGregor.
    p. cm.
Includes bibliographical references and index.
ISBN 978-1-64646-616-0
1. Nursing. 2. Nurse practitioners. 3. Medical care. 4. Nursing--Practice. 5. Nursing services. I. MacGregor, Eric.
RT42 .H43 2023
610.73--dc23

Foster Academics,
118-35 Queens Blvd., Suite 400,
Forest Hills, NY 11375, USA

ISBN 978-1-64646-616-0 (Hardback)

Contents

Permissions

List of Contributors

Index

Preface

I am honored to present to you this unique book which encompasses the most up-to-date data in the field. I was extremely pleased to get this opportunity of editing the work of experts from across the globe. I have also written papers in this field and researched the various aspects revolving around the progress of the discipline. I have tried to unify my knowledge along with that of stalwarts from every corner of the world, to produce a text which not only benefits the readers but also facilitates the growth of the field.

Healthcare focuses on improving the health of a patient through the prevention, diagnosis and treatment of a condition or a disease. Healthcare is provided by various professionals including doctors, nurses, physicians, therapists and lab technicians. Nursing is a healthcare profession that involves the care of individuals and their families to assist them in the process of recovering from an illness and achieve optimal quality of life. Advanced practice nursing is a type of nursing with advanced interventions that shape clinical healthcare outcomes for individuals, families and diverse populations. The key role of advanced practice nursing is to prescribe medication, as well as diagnose and treat minor illnesses and injuries. This book includes some of the vital pieces of work being conducted across the world, on various topics related to advanced practice nursing in healthcare. It is meant for students and professionals who are looking for an elaborate reference text on this branch of nursing.

Finally, I would like to thank all the contributing authors for their valuable time and contributions. This book would not have been possible without their efforts. I would also like to thank my friends and family for their constant support.

Editor

Care Needs of Patients at the End of Life With a Noncancer Diagnosis Who Live at Home

Jiwon LEE[1] • Younghye PARK[2] • Kyounjoo LIM[3] • Ari LEE[1]
Hanul LEE[1] • Jong-Eun LEE[4]*

ABSTRACT

Background: As the population ages, the prevalence of various chronic diseases increases. Palliative care for patients at the end of life with a noncancer diagnosis is currently limited because of the difficulties of demarcating the boundaries of the end-of-life care period and of determining the various care needs of patients at the end of life.

Purpose: This study aimed to investigate the levels of importance and difficulty of the multidimensional care needs for patients with a noncancer diagnosis during various end-of-life stages.

Methods: This study is a retrospective survey. Home healthcare nurse specialists (HHNS) reviewed medical and nursing records and responded to a structured questionnaire. The caring experiences of HHNS with 115 patients, who were 40 years or older, had received home care nursing throughout the stable (between the onset of the end-of-life stage and 1 week before death) and near-death (1 week before death) stages at Seoul St. Mary's Hospital in Korea, and had died between September 1, 2014, and December 31, 2015, were analyzed.

Results: The care needs of "coordination among family or relatives" and "support for fundamental needs" were more important in the stable stage than in the near-death stage. The care need of "loss, grief care" was more important in the near-death stage than in the stable stage. The care need of "physical symptoms management" was the most difficult to meet in both stages. Lower Palliative Performance Scale score was associated with a higher level of care need, particularly in the "management of physical symptoms" and "psychological support" realms in the stable stage and in the "coordination among family or relatives" realm in both stages.

Conclusions: End-of-life stage and initial score on the Palliative Performance Scale were found to have a significant influence on the multidimensional care needs of patients with a noncancer diagnosis. Thus, healthcare professionals should assess patient care needs according to disease trajectory to provide continuous and holistic care.

KEY WORDS:
end-of-life care, care needs, chronic illness, home care nursing.

Introduction

The main cause of death per 100,000 population in South Korea is cancer (150.9), followed by cardiovascular disease (52.4) and cerebrovascular disease (48.2; Statistics Korea, 2015). Among the top 10 causes of death, mortality from cancer accounted for 28.6%, whereas mortality from chronic diseases, including cardiovascular disease, cerebrovascular disease, pneumonia, diabetes, respiratory disease, liver disorder, and hypertensive diseases, accounted for 34.5%, indicating a higher rate of death due to noncancer chronic diseases (Statistics Korea, 2015). In addition, the rising average age of healthcare consumers means that the prevalence of various chronic diseases is increasing. Therefore, professional care for patients with chronic diseases other than cancer is becoming more important (Reinhard & Young, 2009).

Patients at the end of life with a noncancer diagnosis have needs that are complex and difficult to solve, and these patients tend to complain of various problems and symptoms (Stiel et al., 2014). Compared with patients with cancer, patients with a noncancer diagnosis are older, have multiple disabilities that affect daily life and cognitive function, and require a longer period of care (Ikezaki & Ikegami, 2011). In addition, they frequently have acute clinical symptoms and associated diseases, are more dependent, and appear to have more invasive interventions that require hospitalization (K. S. Lau et al., 2010). In a German study, patients with a noncancer diagnosis complained of neurological symptoms, psychological problems, and insomnia (Stiel et al., 2015). These observations indicate that patients with a noncancer diagnosis may experience a higher symptomatic burden during the end of life than patients with cancer, which may present care needs in multidimensional areas. Unmet palliative care needs have been shown to negatively affect the overall quality of life (QoL) of patients (Bužgová & Sikorová, 2015). However, in noncancer diseases, diagnosis and assessment of disease progression may be difficult because of the relative difficulty of assessing the complicated needs of patients with a noncancer diagnosis, as compared with patients

---

[1]*MSN, RN, Doctoral Candidate, College of Nursing, The Catholic University of Korea, Seoul, Republic of Korea •* [2]*MSN, RN, Team Manager in Home Care, Seoul St. Mary's Hospital, College of Medicine, The Catholic University of Korea, Seoul, Republic of Korea •* [3]*MSN, RN, Assistant Professor, Department of Nursing, Kyungbuk College, Yeongju-si, Republic of Korea •* [4]*PhD, RN, Associate Professor, College of Nursing, The Catholic University of Korea, Seoul, Republic of Korea*

with cancer. Therefore, it is difficult to determine the boundaries of the end-of-life care period (McIlfatrick, 2007). For this reason, needs assessments for patients at the end of life with a noncancer diagnosis and palliative care are relatively limited, and related resources, care services, and an overall social support system are lacking (Burt, Shipman, Richardson, Ream, & Addington-Hall, 2010; Fitzsimons et al., 2007; Kralik & Anderson, 2008; Stiel et al., 2015). Previous studies have reported that patients with a noncancer diagnosis do not receive effective symptom management or sufficient care, although they experience many end-of-life symptoms (Burt et al., 2010). However, 69%–82% of older adults reportedly desire palliative care regardless of diagnosis (Murtagh et al., 2014). Thus, appropriate and continuous palliative care to improve the QoL of patients at the end of life is essential, and the values and multidimensional care needs of patients must be understood in advance (Ben Natan, Garfinkel, & Shachar, 2010). Shimanouchi (2007) recommended that healthcare providers consider the specific care needs of each patient based on end-of-life stage and defined the four stages as beginning, stable, near-death, and afterdeath. Palliative care must be provided according to different illness trajectories for patients with a noncancer diagnosis, who experience a gradual disease process and unpredictable conditions that may rapidly deteriorate (Kralik & Anderson, 2008).

The initial assessment of a patient's condition is critical to the provision of patient-centered care. The Palliative Performance Scale (PPS) is a functional performance instrument in which a PPS level lower than 40% typically signifies low functional status, nutritional impairment, and impaired cognition (Wharton, Manu, & Vitale, 2015). The initial PPS level is a significant predictor of survival (F. Lau et al., 2009). The PPS level may be used to identify significant differences in the severity of various symptoms, with prior findings associating increasingly severe levels of fatigue, anorexia, and dyspnea with a decreasing PPS level (Kamal, Nipp, Bull, Stinson, & Abernethy, 2015). In addition, PPS level may be used to identify differences in mortality rate and is particularly effective in predicting the prognoses of patients with a noncancer diagnosis (Harrold et al., 2005); it is therefore necessary to identify care needs based on the PPS.

The purpose of this study was to assess the physical, psychological, social, and spiritual care needs of patients with chronic diseases other than cancer who received home care, based on end-of-life stage and PPS level, from the perspective of home healthcare nurse specialists (HHNS). In addition, this study aimed to identify the importance of patient-centered needs and the inherent difficulties in the care process. These findings will contribute to the improvement of the overall quality of palliative care by addressing unmet end-of-life care needs effectively.

Methods

Study Design

This retrospective survey, conducted from the perspective of HHNS, was designed to assess the care needs of patients

with a noncancer diagnosis who received nursing care at home during end of life and who later died. The HHNS who participated in this study were all qualified hospice and palliative care professionals who were employed by Seoul St. Mary's Hospital. Forty-nine HHNS responded to the structured questionnaire by reviewing the medical and nursing records of their patients.

Participants

The inclusion criteria for patients, based on Kim, Lee, and Shimanouchi (2014), were (a) aged 40 years or older; (b) received continuous home care nursing throughout the stable and final death stages; (c) died between September 1, 2014, and December 31, 2015; and (d) diagnosed with a noncancerous disease such as cerebrovascular, cardiovascular, nervous, pulmonary, musculoskeletal, digestive, and urogenital disorders. Baseline data were obtained from 115 patients for this analysis. According to Shimanouchi (2007), end-of-life stages comprise the beginning, stable, near-death, and afterdeath stages. The beginning stage represents the first week after starting home care, the stable stage is defined as the second week after home care until 1 week before patient death, and the near-death stage is the week immediately before patient death (Kim et al., 2014; Lee & Kim, 2012). In this study, the stable and near-death stages were used to assess care needs according to differences between these two stages. The HHNS determined the periods for the stable and near-death stages for each patient based on date-of-death information in patient records.

Instruments

The demographic characteristics of the patients were obtained from medical and nursing records and included gender, age, diagnosis, PPS level, vision, hearing, type of primary caregiver, age of primary caregiver, and duration of home care nursing. Primary caregiver refers to the family member who took principal care of the patient. The PPS (Victoria Hospice, 2001) is an indicator that predicts the survival of patients with life-threatening illnesses. It consists of five areas, including ambulation, activity level and evidence of disease, self-care, oral intake, and level of consciousness. The PPS level ranges from 0% (death) to 100% (normal function), and PPS scores are in 10% increments only. An increased level indicates a better level of health functioning in the patient. The PPS was categorized as severely ill, terminal state (10%–20%), disabled state (30%–40%), and moderate state (50%–100%) in this study based on Harrold et al. (2005). The PPS level was measured before patients enter the end-of-life period and was used to assess terminally ill patients' functional status from nursing records.

End-of-life care needs were assessed according to the stages developed by Shimanouchi (2007). This tool was initially developed based on literature reviews and a preliminary survey intended for patients with a noncancer diagnosis who received home care during the terminal stage. This tool was validated in a prior study (Kim et al., 2014), with a Cronbach's α of .97. Eight areas comprising 51 items were addressed with regard, respectively, to level of importance and difficulty: support for fundamental needs (11 items), management of physical symptoms (eight items), psychological support (four items), spiritual care (five items), death management (six items), coordination among family or relatives (five items), loss/grief care (four items), and coordination among care team members (eight items). Each item was scored on a 5-point Likert scale in which 0 indicated "not at all important/difficult" and 4 indicated "very important/difficult." A higher score indicates increased levels of both importance and difficulty.

Data Collection

This study was conducted with the approval of the institutional review board (IRB) of Seoul St. Mary's Hospital in Korea on December 23, 2015 (IRB protocol no. KC15RISE0945). The HHNS in charge of each patient had provided direct care to the patients while they were alive. The 49 HHNS provided written consent, and the research team conducted training on how to fill out the questionnaires for each stage. The HHNS were asked to fill out demographic characteristics, medical state, and PPS information using patient medical records and patient end-of-life care needs based on their recollection of the situation during the stable and near-death stages of each patient. To minimize recall bias, the research team recommended that the HHNS rely as much as possible on nursing records when filling out information on patient end-of-life care needs. Data were collected from January 1 to March 31, 2016.

Data Analysis

The collected data were analyzed using IBM SPSS Statistics Version 20.0 (IBM, Armonk, NY, USA), and two-tailed tests were performed with a threshold for statistical significance of .05. The general characteristics of the patients with chronic diseases other than cancer were analyzed using frequency, percentage, mean, and standard deviation. Changes in care needs across end-of-life stages were analyzed via paired t tests. The importance of care needs relative to the PPS was compared via a one-way analysis of variance, dividing the stable and near-death stages into eight categories. Scheffé's test was used as a post hoc test.

Results

General Characteristics

Most of the 115 patients were women (65.2%), and the mean age was 83.79 (± 9.67) years. The most common patient diagnosis was cerebrovascular disease (32.5%), followed by cardiovascular disease (13.2%) and pulmonary disease (12.3%). Patients had various chronic diseases (e.g., cerebrovascular,

cardiovascular, lung, liver, kidney, nervous system, and musculoskeletal system diseases), and the average number of comorbidities was 2. Regarding functional state, as assessed by the PPS, the PPS 30%–40% group constituted 50.4% of the study population. Patients with normal vision and hearing constituted 48.7% and 36.5%, respectively, of the study population. In total, 30.7% of the patients had a daughter-in-law or son as their primary caregiver, whereas 29.7% had a spouse as their primary caregiver. The average age of primary caregivers was 61.97 (± 13.58) years. The patients received home care for an average of 1.68 (± 0.73) years (Table 1).

Level of Importance of Care Needs by End-of-Life Stage

The area and item that had the highest importance level were the "coordination among family or relatives" area, with a score of 3.13 (± 0.72), and the "caregiver's health status" item, with a score of 3.38 (± 0.74) in the stable stage. The area and item that had the highest importance level were the "management of physical symptoms" area, with a score of

TABLE 1.
Participant Characteristics (N = 115)

Variable	n	%
Gender		
Female	75	65.2
Male	40	34.8
Age (years; *M* and *SD*)	83.79	9.67
Primary diagnosis[a]		
Cerebrovascular disease	37	32.5
Cardiovascular disease	15	13.2
Pulmonary disease	14	12.3
Other	48	42.0
PPS level[a] (*M* and *SD*)	41.95	15.97
10%–20%	13	11.5
30%–40%	57	50.4
≥ 50%	43	38.1
Vision		
Normal	56	48.7
Abnormal	59	51.3
Hearing		
Normal	42	36.5
Abnormal	73	63.5
Primary caregiver[a] (*n* = 101)		
Spouse	30	29.7
Daughter	23	22.8
Son/daughter-in-law	31	30.7
Others	17	16.8
Age of primary caregiver (years; *M* and *SD*)	61.97	13.58
Duration of home care nursing (years; *M* and *SD*)	1.68	0.73

Note. Age ranged from 52 to 103 years, Palliative Performance Scale (PPS) level is from 10 to 80, age of primary caregivers ranged from 20 to 89 years, and duration of home care nursing ranged from 1 month to 12 years.
[a]Missing data.

TABLE 2.
Care Needs in End-of-Life Care by Stage (N = 115)

Area	Level of Importance			
	Stable		Near-death	
	Mean	SD	Mean	SD
1. Support for fundamental needs**	3.06	0.64	2.81	0.83
• Daily life pattern/preferences in daily life**	3.08	0.92	2.56	1.26
• Fall risks	3.36	0.89	–	–
• Personal hygiene*	3.09	0.88	2.88	0.90
• Self-care capacity, ADL, and IADL status**	3.05	0.96	2.49	1.31
• Existence of dementia/problematic behaviors	3.00	1.01	–	–
• Body activity	2.92	0.91	–	–
• Problems in defecation/urination	3.32	0.75	3.19	0.80
• Defecation control	3.18	0.83	–	–
• Sleep states, use of sleeping pills	3.05	0.86	2.98	0.94
• Understand methods of medicine**†	2.98	0.92	2.45	1.17
• Understand side effect**††	2.90	0.94	2.27	1.20
2. Management of physical symptoms††	3.05	0.68	3.10	0.72
• Dyspnea*††	3.06	1.11	3.44	0.84
• Symptomatic problems with digestive systems†	3.10	0.94	3.17	0.91
• Dysphagia††	3.12	1.07	3.35	0.89
• Fever or signs of infection†	3.04	1.02	3.12	1.04
• Fluid in–out balance/food intake and nutritional states	3.22	0.80	3.17	0.94
• Skin trouble	3.23	0.83	3.25	0.88
• Causes of fatigue and other physical sufferings	2.95	0.94	2.94	1.03
• Pain control	3.03	0.93	2.97	1.08
3. Psychological support	2.92	0.83	2.88	0.90
• Confirming patient's wishes or demands on treatments and care	2.94	0.96	2.85	1.00
• Patient's facial expressions, few words, negative attitudes	2.78	0.91	2.78	0.99
• Confirming family's wishes or demands on treatments and service	3.01	0.91	2.94	0.96
• Family's facial expressions, few words, negative attitudes	2.84	0.95	2.73	1.08
4. Spiritual care	2.76	0.76	2.69	0.90
• Confirming patient's needs, concerns, things left behind	2.65	1.00	2.75	1.03
• Belief or faith	2.70	0.95	2.74	1.03
• Living will	2.85	1.09	2.61	1.14
• Loneliness caused by losing personal relations	2.76	0.92	2.63	1.08
• Sufferings or spiritual pain caused by feelings of meaninglessness**†	2.98	0.81	2.50	1.17
5. Death management†	3.00	0.77	3.03	0.88
• Patient's/family's understanding about disease process and changes	3.16	0.76	3.15	0.91
• Patient's will to stay home until the end of life†	3.26	0.76	3.18	0.89
• Fear and anxiety toward death and disease aggravation	3.04	0.97	3.03	1.12
• Wishes of the disease and of prolonging life with medical measures††	2.94	1.07	2.72	1.26
• Confirming where to die	2.97	0.96	3.04	1.04
• Delivering messages between patient and family†	3.01	0.97	2.94	1.07

		Level of Difficulty					
		Stable		Near-death			
t	p	Mean	SD	Mean	SD	t	p
3.109	.002	2.11	0.92	2.09	1.07	0.266	.791
2.792	.007	2.48	1.00	2.47	1.28	0.103	.918
–	–	2.26	1.37	–	–	–	–
2.213	.030	2.19	1.25	2.11	1.24	0.662	.510
3.296	.002	2.42	1.24	2.24	1.39	0.968	.337
–	–	2.21	1.14	–	–	–	–
–	–	2.39	1.11	–	–	–	–
1.494	.139	2.42	1.20	2.42	1.25	0.000	1.000
–	–	2.27	1.24	–	–	–	–
0.663	.510	2.12	1.12	2.07	1.28	0.344	.732
3.135	.003	1.82	1.25	1.39	1.26	2.631	.011
3.501	.001	1.76	1.23	1.25	1.21	3.018	.004
−0.691	.491	2.29	0.96	2.53	1.00	3.277	.001
2.405	.020	2.11	1.22	2.74	1.33	3.042	.004
−0.505	.616	2.17	1.10	2.49	1.38	2.121	.038
1.545	.129	2.21	1.29	2.83	1.29	4.223	< .001
−0.726	.471	1.96	1.28	2.32	1.37	2.353	.022
0.424	.672	2.38	1.18	2.56	1.29	1.560	.123
−0.261	.795	2.44	1.36	2.51	1.35	−0.668	.506
0.159	.874	2.38	1.11	2.43	1.21	−0.375	.709
0.490	.626	2.18	1.33	2.30	1.30	−0.871	.387
0.484	.629	1.93	1.06	1.93	1.17	−0.039	.969
0.814	.418	1.74	1.18	1.85	1.28	−0.739	.462
0.000	1.000	1.83	1.12	1.81	1.30	0.100	.921
0.767	.445	1.98	1.19	1.90	1.22	0.711	.479
1.013	.314	1.94	1.23	1.83	1.24	0.894	.374
1.009	.316	1.78	1.00	1.67	1.15	1.181	.241
1.097	.277	1.60	1.06	1.59	1.27	0.159	.874
−0.504	.616	1.51	1.17	1.41	1.30	0.854	.396
1.881	.067	1.66	1.24	1.46	1.27	1.598	.118
0.758	.452	1.89	1.11	1.76	1.37	0.684	.497
3.157	.003	2.04	1.27	1.60	1.30	2.358	.023
−0.496	.621	1.95	1.04	1.80	1.16	2.367	.020
0.130	.897	1.97	1.09	1.86	1.21	1.196	.235
0.973	.334	1.84	1.28	1.61	1.45	2.205	.030
0.136	.892	2.14	1.17	2.01	1.35	1.199	.234
1.608	.115	2.00	1.29	1.53	1.32	3.454	.001
−0.743	.460	1.50	1.18	1.43	1.37	0.608	.545
1.062	.292	1.91	1.21	1.68	1.33	2.428	.017

TABLE 2.

Care Needs in End-of-Life Care by Stage (N = 115), Continued

Area	Level of Importance			
	Stable		Near-death	
	Mean	SD	Mean	SD
6. Coordination among family or relatives*	3.13	0.72	3.04	0.80
• Consensus development between patient and family, and their coordination ability of different opinions	2.90	0.98	2.81	1.04
• Care participation and motivation of the family members	3.00	0.99	2.88	1.04
• Roles of a main care giver and a decision maker in the family and their care coordination capacity	2.99	0.99	2.99	1.03
• Knowledge and skills of caregiver*	3.23	0.76	3.08	0.90
• Caregiver's health status*	3.38	0.74	3.24	0.88
7. Loss, grief care*	2.93	0.76	3.10	0.89
• Information sharing about judgment and decision making	3.01	0.87	–	–
• Anxiety and psychological states	2.93	0.83	3.04	0.96
• Time for the family	2.90	0.87	–	–
• Family's agreement about death management	–	–	3.13	0.93
8. Coordination among care team members	3.03	0.68	3.08	0.74
• Access to see a doctor*	2.98	1.13	2.65	1.18
• Mutual recognition about care between patient, family, and professionals	3.10	0.80	3.06	0.92
• Family's care capacity	3.25	0.84	3.24	0.91
• Emergency calls*	3.15	0.86	3.33	0.92
• Economic burden of home care	2.98	0.96	2.81	1.18
• Need of staff meetings	2.52	1.21	2.45	1.26
• Patient/family comprehension about medical treatments	3.07	0.82	3.06	0.91
• Patient/family comprehension about medical equipment and how to deal with troubles with them[†]	3.10	0.87	3.06	0.99

Note. ADL = activities of daily living; IADL = instrumental activities of daily living. An en dash "–" means these variables were not measured in the each stage. The significant importance of the care needs: *$p < .05$, **$p < .01$. The significant difficulty of the care needs: [†]$p < .05$, [††]$p < .01$.

3.10 (± 0.72), and the "dyspnea" item, with a score of 3.44 (± 0.84) in the near-death stage.

The importance of the "support for fundamental needs" area had a score of 3.06 (± 0.64) in the stable stage, which was significantly increased compared with 2.81 (± 0.83) in the near-death stage ($p = .002$). The importance of the "coordination among family or relatives" area had a score of 3.13 (± 0.72) in the stable stage, which was significantly increased compared with 3.04 (± 0.80) in the near-death stage ($p = .042$). In contrast, the importance of the "loss, grief care" area had a score of 3.10 (± 0.89) in the near-death stage, which was significantly increased compared with 2.93 (± 0.76) in the stable stage ($p = .021$; Table 2).

Level of Difficulty of Care Needs by End-of-Life Stage

The area "management of physical symptoms" exhibited the highest level of difficulty in both stages: 2.29 (± 0.96) in the

stable stage and 2.53 (± 1.00) in the near-death stage. The item "daily life pattern/preferences in daily life" in the stable stage had a score of 2.48 (± 1.00), whereas the item "dysphagia" in the near-death stage had a score of 2.83 (± 1.29), indicating that these items had the highest difficulty at each stage.

The "death management" area had a score of 1.95 (± 1.04) in the stable stage, which was significantly increased compared with 1.80 (± 1.16) in the near-death stage ($p = .020$). In contrast, the difficulty in the "management of physical symptoms" area had a score of 2.53 (± 1.00) in the near-death stage, which was significantly higher compared with 2.29 (± 0.96) in the stable stage ($p = .001$; Table 2).

Differences Between the Levels of Importance and Difficulty by End-of-Life Stage

The high levels of importance and difficulty of care needs indicate that they are critical. However, these needs are

TABLE 2.
Care Needs in End-of-Life Care by Stage (N = 115)

| | | Level of Difficulty | | | | | |
| | | Stable | | Near-death | | | |
t	p	Mean	SD	Mean	SD	t	p
2.058	.042	2.00	1.06	1.90	1.08	1.224	.224
1.408	.163	1.84	1.22	1.70	1.27	1.351	.181
1.920	.058	1.82	1.18	1.72	1.23	0.970	.335
0.000	1.000	1.87	1.20	1.87	1.33	0.000	1.000
2.203	.030	1.95	1.14	1.89	1.11	0.592	.555
2.120	.037	2.17	1.30	2.05	1.30	1.292	.200
2.359	.021	1.87	0.99	1.89	1.23	−0.239	.812
–	–	1.85	1.11	–	–	–	–
1.157	.251	2.06	1.10	2.13	1.24	−0.648	.519
–	–	1.77	1.06	–	–	–	–
–	–	–	–	1.76	1.36	–	–
−0.924	.357	1.83	0.94	1.71	1.09	1.912	.059
2.234	.031	1.93	1.08	1.83	1.27	0.636	.528
0.647	.519	1.82	1.14	1.67	1.27	1.502	.136
0.123	.902	1.95	1.14	1.76	1.31	1.896	.061
2.181	.032	1.68	1.24	1.65	1.40	0.336	.738
1.589	.118	1.61	1.31	1.50	1.33	1.030	.308
0.812	.423	1.69	1.20	1.53	1.32	1.717	.096
0.168	.867	1.98	1.18	1.84	1.31	1.372	.174
0.504	.616	1.86	1.25	1.65	1.24	2.024	.047

not easily met. The total mean score was used as a cutoff point to determine care needs with high levels of importance and difficulty at each stage. In the stable stage, the total mean scores for importance and difficulty were 2.98 (± 0.60) and 1.97 (± 0.79), respectively. In the near-death stage, the mean scores for importance and difficulty were 2.99 (± 0.62) and 2.00 (± 0.83), respectively.

In the stable stage, the "support for fundamental needs" area included eight items that were identified as important and difficult-to-solve problems: "daily life pattern/preferences in daily life"; "fall risks"; "personal hygiene"; "self-care capacity, activities of daily living (ADL) and instrumental activities of daily living (IADL) status"; "existence of dementia/problematic behaviors"; "problems in defecation/urination"; "defecation control"; and "sleep states, use of sleeping pills." The "management of physical symptoms" area included six items that were identified as important and difficult-to-solve problems: "dyspnea," "symptomatic problems with digestive systems," "dysphagia," "fluid in-out balance/food in-take and

nutritional states," "skin trouble," and "pain control." Both the "confirming family's wishes or demands on treatments and service" item within the "psychological support" area and the "sufferings or spiritual pain caused by feelings of meaningless-ness" item within the "spiritual care" area represented important problems that were difficult to solve. In the "death management" area, the "patient's/family's understanding about disease process and changes" and "fear and anxiety towards death and disease aggravation" items were recognized as being both important and difficult. In the "coordination among family or relatives" area, the "caregiver's health status" item indicated its importance and difficulty. The "patient/family comprehension about medical treatments" item within the "coordination among care team members" area indicated importance and difficulty.

In the near-death stage, within the "support for funda-mental needs" area, the "problems in defecation/urination" item indicated importance and difficulty. The "management of physical symptoms" area included six items identified as important and difficult to solve: "dyspnea," "symptomatic

TABLE 3.
Differences in the Importance of Care Needs by Patient PPS Levels (N = 115)

| | Stable | | | | | | | Near-death | | | | | |
| | PPS 10%–20% | | PPS 30%–40% | | PPS ≥ 50% | | | PPS 10%–20% | | PPS 30%–40% | | PPS ≥ 50% | |
Area	Mean	SD	Mean	SD	Mean	SD	p	Mean	SD	Mean	SD	Mean	SD	p
1. Support for fundamental needs	3.38	0.73[c]	3.08	0.55[d]	2.95	0.69	.099	2.86	0.95[c]	2.81	0.84[d]	2.80	0.82	.970
2. Management of physical Symptoms	3.42	0.50[a]	3.05	0.65	2.90	0.73[b]	.050	3.23	0.60	3.06	0.72	3.06	0.73	.730
3. Psychological support	3.28	0.87	2.98	0.80	2.67	0.80	.035	2.96	1.11	2.97	0.85	2.73	0.89	.432
4. Spiritual care	3.21	0.82	2.79	0.81	2.55	0.68	.057	2.99	0.91	2.71	0.97	2.57	0.82	.441
5. Death management	3.34	0.66	2.93	0.79	2.78	0.81	.091	3.43	0.62	2.99	0.91	2.90	0.90	.170
6. Coordination among family or relatives	3.65	0.73[a]	3.13	0.63	2.98	0.76[b,e]	.014	3.63	0.60[a]	3.09	0.73	2.74	0.83[b,e]	.001
7. Loss, grief care	3.32	0.98	2.90	0.75	2.75	0.75[f]	.107	3.65	0.58	3.03	0.93	3.01	0.85[f]	.104
8. Coordination among care team members	3.40	0.69	3.07	0.68	2.88	0.63	.057	3.43	0.52	3.07	0.67	3.02	0.84	.246

Note. PPS= Palliative Performance Scale.
[a,b]Scheffé's test: difference in care needs by PPS group within stable and near-death stages. [c]Difference in the importance of care needs by stages within the PPS 10%–20% group, $p = .047$. [d]Difference in the importance of care needs by stages within the PPS 30%–40% group, $p = .025$. [e,f]Difference in the importance of care needs by stages within the PPS ≥ 50% group, $p = .007$ and $p = .019$.

problems with digestive systems," "dysphagia," "fever or signs of infection," "fluid in-out balance/food in-take and nutritional states," and "skin trouble." In addition, the "fear and anxiety toward death and disease aggravation" item in the "death management" area, the "caregiver's health status" item in the "coordination among family or relatives" area, and the "anxiety and psychological states" item in the "loss, grief care" area were identified as important and difficult to solve (Table 2).

Importance of Care Needs by PPS Level

The PPS levels were categorized into three groups: 10%–20%, 30%–40%, and 50% and higher. There were significant differences among the three groups in the "management of physical symptoms" ($p = .050$), "psychological support" ($p = .035$), and "coordination among family or relatives" ($p = .014$) areas in the stable stage. In the near-death stage, there was a significant difference only in the "coordination among family or relatives" area ($p = .001$).

Within the PPS 10%–20% ($p = .047$) and 30%–40% ($p = .025$) groups, the importance of "support for fundamental needs" was significantly increased in the stable stage compared with the near-death stage. Within the PPS 50% group, the importance of "coordination among family or relatives" was significantly increased in the stable stage compared with the near-death stage ($p = .007$), whereas the importance of "loss, grief care" was significantly increased in

the near-death stage compared with the stable stage ($p = .019$; Table 3).

Discussion

This study assessed the levels of importance and the difficulties in meeting the care needs of patients at the end of life with a noncancer diagnosis based on end-of-life stages and PPS. The "coordination among family or relatives" area was the most important care need in the stable stage, with a higher score compared with the near-death stage. Deterioration of the physical condition in patients with a noncancer diagnosis may decrease independence and impose a burden on family caregivers (Fitzsimons et al., 2007). Collins and Swartz (2011) found that one third of family caregivers reported a high care burden and that most experienced insomnia and depression; half of the family caregivers had more than one physical illness. The role of informal caregivers directly affected their physical and psychological health, and they could not afford to take care of themselves because of a lack of time (Ranmuthugala, Nepal, Brown, & Percival, 2009). Therefore, policies for community-based long-term care must support the needs of primary caregivers, and healthcare providers should try to facilitate the well-being of family caregivers (Ranmuthugala et al., 2009; Reinhard & Young, 2009). In addition, informational needs were important. The "knowledge and skills of caregiver" item in the "coordination among family or relatives" area showed higher importance in the stable stage than in the near-death stage. Heyland et al. (2006) reported that family caregivers and patients wanted to thoroughly understand the disease medical state, treatment, and process. Moreover, caregivers wanted to receive help through various information sources related to making difficult treatment decisions. The caregivers needed skills, abilities, and knowledge regarding patient care at home. However, most felt that training was inadequate (Collins & Swartz, 2011). Thus, healthcare providers should educate informal caregivers about the knowledge and skills necessary to efficiently care for patients with a noncancer diagnosis from the early stage of a disease onward. Educating caregivers regarding the various signs of the process of dying is necessary to help them cope with death and allow their participation in the treatment plan and decision making during the end-of-life period.

Within the "spiritual care" area, the "sufferings or spiritual pain caused by feelings of meaninglessness" item increased in both importance and difficulty during the stable stage compared with the near-death stage. These findings indicate that patients experience spiritual suffering because of the helplessness and meaninglessness of life with disease. Patients want to find their roles in life independently and have autonomy even during the dying process (Ben Natan et al., 2010). Therefore, psychological and spiritual support is necessary to elevate the self-esteem of patients from the stable stage onward.

In the "death management" area, the "delivering messages between patient and family" and "wishes of the disease and of prolonging life with medical measures" items were more difficult to solve in the stable stage compared with the near-death stage. Thus, early mediation of different opinions through open communication between healthcare professionals, patients, and family is crucial because the importance of care needs may differ according to individual perspectives (Ang, Zhang, & Lim, 2016; Ben Natan, 2008; Heyland et al., 2006). Furthermore, it is critical to provide personal care that maximizes the self-determination of patients depending on patient-centered needs and preferences through communication. Moreover, the "patient's will to stay home until the end-of-life" item was important and more difficult to solve in the stable stage compared with the near-death stage. Increasingly, many individuals prefer to receive home-based end-of-life care and die at home (Gomes, Calanzani, Gysels, Hall, & Higginson, 2013). Thus, HHNS should identify in advance whether a patient wants to stay at home at the end of life and, if the answer is affirmative, should plan for the patient's death at home.

In the near-death stage, the "loss, grief care" area had the highest importance, which was more important compared with in the stable stage. Specifically, the "anxiety and psychological states" item was important and difficult to solve. Moreover, the "fear and anxiety toward death and disease aggravation" item was highly important and difficult to solve in both stages. Patients with a noncancer diagnosis had anxiety because it was difficult to accurately determine the prognosis from uncertain illness trajectories. Thus, nurses should help patients and families plan for a good death at the end of life by

providing care that is centered on emotional communications and relationships (Murray, Kendall, Boyd, Worth, & Benton, 2004). In particular, patients want someone to listen to their fears (Ben Natan, 2008; Ben Natan et al., 2010; Heyland et al., 2006). Thus, it is also necessary to provide psychological support to alleviate the potential fear and anxiety of the patient and family.

The area that exhibited the most difficult care needs was the "management of physical symptoms," which increased in difficulty from the stable stage. Specifically, the "dyspnea" item had the highest importance and highest increased difficulty, whereas the "dysphagia" item was associated with the highest difficulty in the near-death stage. Patients with a noncancer diagnosis who struggled with diseases were bedridden for long periods because of worsening physical symptoms in the near-death stage. Thus, healthcare professionals should focus on relieving worsening physical symptoms rather than support for basic needs of daily life during the terminal stage. A study that investigated symptoms in patients at the end of life showed that the condition of patients with a noncancer diagnosis was marked by long-term, gradual, and rapid deterioration (Kralik & Anderson, 2008). However, patients with a noncancer diagnosis received less symptom care and fewer care resources, which were not sufficient to satisfy end-of-life needs compared with patients with cancer (Burt et al., 2010). Thus, various care approaches should be prepared to address unpredictable, long-term diseases during the end-of-life period (Kralik & Anderson, 2008).

In general, the average importance of care needs increased as the initial level of the PPS decreased in overall areas. This means that worsening of the functional health of patients with chronic illness was associated with increased care needs. Thus, it is necessary to set up a specific plan, including end-of-life care, pain and symptom management, ethical issues, grief and bereavement, and preparation for the dying process, through an accurate assessment of the PPS (Wharton et al., 2015). In the stable stage, the PPS 10%–20% group, which had a severely low performance state, exhibited increased care needs in the "management of physical symptoms" area compared with the above 50% PPS group, which had a moderate performance state. As the PPS decreases, patients spend more time in bed because of limitations in activities due to decreased mobility. Moreover, they could not perform self-care and had nutrition deficits due to poor dietary intake, thus increasing the risk of various diseases. According to Kamal et al. (2015), the bothersome symptoms of patients with a noncancer diagnosis changed and symptom severity increased as PPS decreased. Thus, it would be very effective if appropriate and timely care could be provided by anticipating the severity and deterioration of patients' various symptoms through an assessment of the PPS (Kamal et al., 2015). In the "psychological support" area, the average of importance gradually increased as the PPS decreased in the stable stage. The most unfulfilled care needs that terminal patients felt were "respect and support from health professionals" and "autonomy," followed by "physical symptoms," "social area," and "meaning of life and reconciliation." Moreover, these unsatisfied needs decreased the overall QoL of the patients (Bužgová & Sikorová, 2015). Thus, home care should focus on relationships to achieve the integration and dignity of patients and family members through a holistic approach. In addition, nurses should continue to provide integrated care that addresses comprehensively the physical, functional, social, and emotional aspects through an accurate clinical assessment of these patients while focused on long-term care (Reinhard & Young, 2009).

With respect to limitations, this study utilized a retrospective design. Thus, recall bias may affect the information provided by HHNS. Therefore, prospective further studies are needed to directly assess the care needs of patients in depth during end-of-life stages. A previous study showed that patients may have different symptoms and care needs depending on the chronic disease diagnosis and comorbidities (K. S. Lau et al., 2010). However, this study did not identify differences in care needs based on disease type because of the small sample size, which made disease classification difficult. Thus, we recommend that further research investigate the multidimensional care needs according to disease type and comorbidities from a larger sample of patients at the end of life with noncancer diagnoses who live at home.

Conclusions

This study used end-of-life stage and PPS score to assess the levels of importance and difficulty of the multidimensional care needs of patients with a noncancer diagnosis who received end-of-life care at home. HHNS must clearly assess the functional health state and care needs of these patients at the end of life and then comprehensively provide patient-centered palliative care based on this assessment. It would be helpful to identify ways to effectively treat care needs that are of high importance and difficulty in the end-of-life stages to ensure the QoL of patients with a noncancer diagnosis who receive home care and of their informal caregivers.

Acknowledgments

This study was supported by a grant from the Korea Health Technology R&D Project through the Korea Health Industry Development Institute, funded by the Ministry of Health and Welfare, Republic of Korea (Grant number HI15C0828).

References

Ang, G. C., Zhang, D., & Lim, K. H. (2016). Differences in attitudes to end-of-life care among patients, relatives and healthcare professionals. *Singapore Medical Journal*, *57*(1), 22–28. https://doi.org/10.11622/smedj.2016008

Ben Natan, M. (2008). Perceptions of nurses, families, and residents in nursing homes concerning residents' needs. *International Journal of Nursing Practice*, *14*(3), 195–199. https://doi.org/10.1111/j.1440-172X.2008.00687.x

Ben Natan, M., Garfinkel, D., & Shachar, I. (2010). End-of-life needs as perceived by terminally ill older adult patients, family and staff. *European Journal of Oncology Nursing*, *14*(4), 299–303. https://doi.org/10.1016/j.ejon.2010.05.002

Burt, J., Shipman, C., Richardson, A., Ream, E., & Addington-Hall, J. (2010). The experiences of older adults in the community dying from cancer and non-cancer causes: A national survey of bereaved relatives. *Age and Ageing*, *39*(1), 86–91. https://doi.org/10.1093/ageing/afp212

Bužgová, R., & Sikorová, L. (2015). Association between quality of life, demographic characteristics, physical symptoms, and unmet needs in inpatients receiving end-of-life care. *Journal of Hospice and Palliative Nursing*, *17*(4), 325–332. https://doi.org/10.1097/NJH.0000000000000170

Collins, L. G., & Swartz, K. (2011). Caregiver care. *American Family Physician*, *83*(11), 1309–1317.

Fitzsimons, D., Mullan, D., Wilson, J. S., Conway, B., Corcoran, B., Dempster, M., … Fogarty, D. (2007). The challenge of patients' unmet palliative care needs in the final stages of chronic illness. *Palliative Medicine*, *21*(4), 313–322. https://doi.org/10.1177/0269216307077711

Gomes, B., Calanzani, N., Gysels, M., Hall, S., & Higginson, I. J. (2013). Heterogeneity and changes in preferences for dying at home: A systematic review. *BMC Palliative Care*, *12*, 7. https://doi.org/10.1186/1472-684x-12-7

Harrold, J., Rickerson, E., Carroll, J. T., McGrath, J., Morales, K., Kapo, J., & Casarett, D. (2005). Is the palliative performance scale a useful predictor of mortality in a heterogeneous hospice population? *Journal of Palliative Medicine*, *8*(3), 503–509. https://doi.org/10.1089/jpm.2005.8.503

Heyland, D. K., Dodek, P., Rocker, G., Groll, D., Gafni, A., Pichora, D., … Lam, M. (2006). What matters most in end-of-life care: Perceptions of seriously ill patients and their family members. *CMAJ: Canadian Medical Association Journal*, *174*(5), 627–633. https://doi.org/10.1503/cmaj.050626

Ikezaki, S., & Ikegami, N. (2011). Predictors of dying at home for patients receiving nursing services in Japan: A retrospective study comparing cancer and non-cancer deaths. *BMC Palliative Care*, *10*, 3. https://doi.org/10.1186/1472-684x-10-3

Kamal, A. H., Nipp, R. D., Bull, J., Stinson, C. S., & Abernethy, A. P. (2015). Symptom burden and performance status among community-dwelling patients with serious illness. *Journal of Palliative Medicine*, *18*(6), 542–544. https://doi.org/10.1089/jpm.2014.0381

Kim, S. L., Lee, J. E., & Shimanouchi, S. (2014). Needs for end-of-life care by home care nurses among non-cancer patients in Korea and Japan. *International Journal of Nursing Practice*, *20*(4), 339–345. https://doi.org/10.1111/ijn.12156

Kralik, D., & Anderson, B. (2008). Differences in home-based palliative care service utilisation of people with cancer and non-cancer conditions. *Journal of Clinical Nursing, 17*(11c), 429–435. https://doi.org/10.1111/j.1365-2702.2008.02580.x

Lau, F., Maida, V., Downing, M., Lesperance, M., Karlson, N., & Kuziemsky, C. (2009). Use of the Palliative Performance Scale (PPS) for end-of-life prognostication in a palliative medicine consultation service. *Journal of Pain and Symptom Management, 37*(6), 965–972. https://doi.org/10.1016/j.jpainsymman.2008.08.003

Lau, K. S., Tse, D. M., Tsan Chen, T. W., Lam, P. T., Lam, W. M., & Chan, K. S. (2010). Comparing noncancer and cancer deaths in Hong Kong: A retrospective review. *Journal of Pain and Symptom Management, 40*(5), 704–714. https://doi.org/10.1016/j.jpainsymman.2010.02.023

Lee, J. E., & Kim, S. L. (2012). Physical and psychospiritual care need by end-of-life stages among non-cancer patient at home: Based on the importance and difficulty of care need. *Journal of Korean Academy of Community Health Nursing, 23*(2), 127–133. https://doi.org/10.12799/jkachn.2012.23.2.127

McIlfatrick, S. (2007). Assessing palliative care needs: Views of patients, informal carers and healthcare professionals. *Journal of Advanced Nursing, 57*(1), 77–86. https://doi.org/10.1111/j.1365-2648.2006.04062.x

Murray, S. A., Kendall, M., Boyd, K., Worth, A., & Benton, T. F. (2004). Exploring the spiritual needs of people dying of lung cancer or heart failure: A prospective qualitative interview study of patients and their carers. *Palliative Medicine, 18*(1), 39–45. https://doi.org/10.1191/0269216304pm837oa

Murtagh, F. E., Bausewein, C., Verne, J., Groeneveld, E. I., Kaloki, Y. E., & Higginson, I. J. (2014). How many people need palliative care? A study developing and comparing methods for population-based estimates. *Palliative Medicine, 28*(1), 49–58. https://doi.org/10.1177/0269216313489367

Ranmuthugala, G., Nepal, B., Brown, L., & Percival, R. (2009). Impact of home based long term care on informal carers. *Australian Family Physician, 38*(8), 618–620.

Reinhard, S. C., & Young, H. M. (2009). The nursing workforce in long-term care. *Nursing Clinics of North America, 44*(2), 161–168. https://doi.org/10.1016/j.cnur.2009.02.006

Shimanouchi, S. (2007). *Nursing strategies from the current situation of home care in Japan and research trends.* Paper session presented at the meeting of the 1st Korea-Japan Joint Conference on Community Health Nursing, Seoul, South Korea.

Statistics Korea. (2015). *Causes of death statistics in 2014.* Retrieved from http://kostat.go.kr/portal/eng/pressReleases/1/index.board?bmode=read&aSeq=349053 and aSeq=349053

Stiel, S., Heckel, M., Seifert, A., Frauendorf, T., Hanke, R. M., & Ostgathe, C. (2015). Comparison of terminally ill cancer-vs. non-cancer patients in specialized palliative home care in Germany—A single service analysis. *BMC Palliative Care, 14*, 34. https://doi.org/10.1186/s12904-015-0033-z

Stiel, S., Matthies, D. M., Seuß, D., Walsh, D., Lindena, G., & Ostgathe, C. (2014). Symptoms and problem clusters in cancer and non-cancer patients in specialized palliative care—Is there a difference? *Journal of Pain and Symptom Management, 48*(1), 26–35. https://doi.org/10.1016/j.jpainsymman.2013.08.018

Victoria Hospice. (2001). *Clinical tools—Palliative Performance Scale (PPS, version 2).* Retrieved from http://www.victoriahospice.org/health-professionals/clinical-tools

Wharton, T., Manu, E., & Vitale, C. A. (2015). Enhancing provider knowledge and patient screening for palliative care needs in chronic multimorbid patients receiving home-based primary care. *American Journal of Hospice and Palliative Medicine, 32*(1), 78–83. https://doi.org/10.1177/1049909113514475

The Nutritional and Social Contexts of Celiac Disease in Women

Julián RODRÍGUEZ-ALMAGRO[1]* • David RODRÍGUEZ-ALMAGRO[2] • MCarmen SOLANO-RUIZ[3]
José SILES-GONZÁLEZ[3] • Antonio HERNÁNDEZ-MARTINEZ[4]

ABSTRACT

Background: Previous studies have confirmed that women who are diagnosed with celiac disease report a lower quality of life than men who are diagnosed with the same illness.

Purpose: This article describes the life experiences of women with celiac disease, especially those who adhere to a lifelong gluten-free diet.

Methods: A phenomenological design based on the Giorgi method was used. Twenty-two women who were diagnosed with celiac disease and were between 16 and 75 years old completed the semistructured interviews.

Results: The results showed that celiac disease has differing effects on the lives of women sufferers. The general feeling of being a woman with celiac disease was described as an effort toward achieving a normalized life. Four categories emerged from the results: feelings at diagnosis, limitations in daily life, social perceptions of the illness, and personal meanings of celiac disease.

Conclusions/Implications for Practice: This study shows that celiac disease and its treatment reduce mental and social quality of life in women. Organizations and public institutions should carry out public awareness campaigns targeting celiac disease and promote quality of life in sufferers of celiac disease in general.

KEY WORDS:
chronic disease, celiac disease, illness experience, phenomenology research, qualitative research.

Introduction

Celiac disease (CD) is a common chronic illness that is caused by an inflammatory response to gluten proteins. Gluten causes atrophy of the villi in the small intestine of patients with CD, which may lead to the malabsorption of nutrients (Elli et al., 2015).

Although the prevalence of CD is 1% globally, there are large variations between countries (Lebwohl, Ludvigsson, & Green, 2015). This was confirmed in a recent multicenter study in Europe, which showed a prevalence that varies between 2% in Finland and 0.3% in Germany (Mustalahti et al., 2010) as well as percentages of 1%–2% in the adult population of Western Europe (West et al., 2003). Recent studies have shown that, in North America and Europe, the number of new cases of CD found in a determined period in a given population is rising (West, Fleming, Tata, Card, & Crooks, 2014).

All epidemiological studies have repeatedly documented a global predominance of CD in women, with a female-to-male ratio of 2.5:1–3:1 (Zingone, West, et al., 2015).

The only treatment for CD is a strict, lifelong gluten-free diet (GFD; Pulido et al., 2013). No foods or medicines containing wheat, rye, or barley gluten or their derivatives may be consumed, as even small amounts of gluten may be harmful.

Although conceptually simple, these changes in diet are substantial and have a profound effect on a patient's life. Untreated CD is associated with complications, including an increased risk of mortality, most of which may be avoided by following a strict GFD. However, there are many barriers, including the availability, cost, and safety of gluten-free foods, and gluten cross-contamination. The GFD may be restrictive in social situations, leading to poor quality of life and, ultimately, nonadherence (Kaukinen, Makharia, Gibson, & Murray, 2015).

As the number of patients with CD increases worldwide, clinicians need to be aware of the challenges that patients face. Heightened awareness among physicians, dietitians, and other providers is critical to maximizing successful treatment, improving outcomes, and reducing healthcare costs and disease burden. Routine follow-up is necessary to reinforce the need for a GFD, provide social and emotional support, and achieve mucosal healing, leading to a reduced risk of complications. Unfortunately, there is a wide variation in follow-up practices (See, Kaukinen, Makharia, Gibson, & Murray, 2015).

When an individual is diagnosed with CD, he or she must face important life changes. The perception of being afflicted with a chronic illness and the need to follow a restrictive,

[1]PhD, RN, Nurse, Department of Emergency, University General Hospital of Ciudad Real, Ciudad Real, Spain • [2]MSc, RN, Nurse, Department of Emergency, University General Hospital of Ciudad Real, Ciudad Real, Spain • [3]PhD, RN, Professor, Department of Nursing, School of Health Sciences, University of Alicante, Alicante, Spain • [4]PhD, RN, Nurse Midwife, Nurse Midwife Teaching Unit, General Hospital Mancha-Centro, Alcázar de San Juan, Ciudad Real, Spain.

demanding, and permanent diet, together with periodic medical checks and the possibility of finding out that other family members are affected, mean that the illness has a significant psychosocial impact (A. Lee & Newman, 2003).

As a general rule, after establishing a GFD, the patient with CD will experience a significant improvement in symptoms in a matter of days or weeks (Autodore, Verma, & Gupta, 2012). However, permanently changing dietary habits in an adult poses many problems (Touchy & Jett, 2016), and despite strictly following the diet, many adults never reach the same subjective level of health as the general population (Mulders-Jones, Mitchison, Girosi, & Hay, 2017).

Prior research (Jacobsson, Hallert, Milberg, & Friedrichsen, 2012) shows that the disadvantages related to having CD and following a GFD are more pronounced in women than in men. This suggests that the signs of general malaise should not be attributed to CD itself but rather to complications in adjusting to the nature of the illness (Roos, Kärner, & Hallert, 2009).

Previous studies confirm that women who are diagnosed with CD report a lower quality of life than men who are diagnosed with the same illness (Jacobsson et al., 2012) because of restrictions in day-to-day life (Hallert, Sandlund, & Broqvist, 2003) and in their social lives (Hallert et al., 2002). These previous findings suggest that there are gender-related indications that should be taken into account to understand the difference between men and women with CD.

Recent studies have shown gender differences (Sverker, Östlund, Hallert, & Hensing, 2009) by studying the day-to-day dilemmas of men and women with CD. Although the general patterns are similar, men and women report different social situations in relation to buying and preparing food (Mathew, Gucciardi, De Melo, & Barata, 2012).

Few studies have focused on describing the perceptions of CD in women, and it seems important to explore and uncover these experiences in greater detail to improve support for women in relation to this illness throughout their lives and to provide them with valid strategies for supporting their lifelong, strict GFD.

Therefore, the aim of this study was to describe the life experiences of women with CD, especially those who adhere to a lifelong GFD.

Methods

A study was carried out using a qualitative methodology and semistructured interviews with women with CD. A qualitative methodology is especially useful in understanding a phenomenon from the point of view of those affected by exploring their beliefs, expectations, and feelings and in explaining the reasons underlying their behaviors and attitudes.

Purposive sampling was conducted by (Guetterman, 2015) interviewing adult women with CD who had contacted the research team after having seen appeals that were made between January and April 2016 through celiac associations in Spain and in celiac groups on social networks.

The only criterion for inclusion was to be a female sufferer of CD between 16 and 75 years old. Duration since diagnosis, an important factor affecting adaptation to disease, was not considered in recruiting participants. Convenience sampling was used and was carried out until data saturation had been achieved (Leung, 2015).

Semistructured interviews were conducted. Sociodemographic data collected included age and time since diagnosis with CD. A semistructured script was followed, and interviews were transcribed in their entirety. All of the participants signed informed consent and took part voluntarily. The anonymity of participants and the confidentiality of the information provided were maintained throughout the study and in subsequent public presentations of results. Furthermore, all of the requirements established in the Helsinki Declaration were followed, thus guaranteeing against future ethical problems that could arise from the research.

The participants were identified by codes to safeguard their anonymity, and their statements were identified by the letter E (for "entrevista" [interview]) followed by a sequential number from 1 to 22.

All of the interviews began with an open question (Applebaum, 2012) that invited the participants to relate their experiences living with CD and to focus on the problem: "What is it like for you living with celiac disease?" The interviewees were encouraged to relate their experiences with the illness freely, and the interviewer followed the script freely to encourage the interviewees (Kim & Oh, 2016).

The interviews were analyzed manually based on the Giorgi method, an approach that aims to describe the meanings of a phenomenon from the perspective of the life experiences of a person (Giorgi, 1997) through essential topics. This method facilitated a description of the experiences of women living with CD by categorizing all of the findings into units of meaning based on the philosophy of Edmund Husserl and Merleau-Ponty, an approach that is sufficiently generic to be applied to any science (Applebaum, 2012).

The text of the interviews was therefore analyzed in the following manner (Giorgi, 1997; Jacobsson et al., 2012):

Transcription: The interviews were read while the tapes were listened to in order to obtain an initial superficial interpretation. This step offered ideas on the meaning of the whole and how to proceed with a deeper analysis.

Elaboration of units of general meaning: The interviews were read once again, but this time with the aim of identifying the smallest parts, the units of meaning, within the perspective of the phenomenon of being a woman living with CD.

To avoid theoretical explanations, the data were kept to the most specific level possible. One unit of meaning may be part of a sentence or a paragraph.

Elaboration of units of meaning relevant to the theme of the investigation: Taking as a reference the units of general meaning identified in the previous step, the researchers selected the units of meaning that related to the research theme. When the themes were repeated in the units of meaning, the researchers sought convergences and divergences and categorized themes accordingly. The repetition of themes indicated that it was possible to obtain the essence or meaning of the phenomenon studied.

Verification of the relevant units of meaning: After the units of meaning relevant to the investigation had been identified, the researchers established criteria that grouped the units of meaning into categories reflecting common aspects or characteristics. These categories constituted a new element that allowed a set of relevant units of meaning to be named under one epigraph, theme, or issue.

The process of selection created unit groups, each reflecting a distinct meaning. From these groups, the themes, which show the meaning of experiencing or living a specific phenomenon, were identified and interpreted. The general structure, that is, a new group, was synthesized in a representation of the phenomenon of being a woman living with CD.

During the process, the criteria that were used to ensure methodological rigor in terms of credibility, auditability, and transferability were taken into account (Cornejo Cancino & Salas Guzmán, 2011).

Credibility refers to the level of confidence in the truth, value, or believability of a study's findings. Credibility is shown through strategies such as data and method triangulation (use of multiple sources of data and/or methods), repeated contact with participants, peer debriefing (sharing questions about the research process and/or findings with a peer who provides additional perspective on analysis and interpretation), and member checking (returning findings to participants to determine if the findings reflect their experiences; Polit & Hungler, 2000).

Auditability refers to the documentation, or paper trail, of the researcher's thinking, decisions, and methods related to the study. Field notes, memoranda, transcripts, and the researcher's reflexive journal or diary allow the reader to follow the researcher's decision making (Polit & Hungler, 2000).

The transferability of research findings refers to the degree to which the findings of a study fit beyond its specific context. Fittingness refers to whether the findings have meaning for another group or may be applied in another context. An accurate and rich description of research findings shows fittingness or transferability by providing adequate information to evaluate the data analysis (Polit & Hungler, 2000).

Ethical Considerations

The study design was reviewed and approved by the appropriate institutional ethics review board (no. 12/2013). Participants provided oral and written consent to participate.

Results

The median age of the participants was 31.68 years, and all were undergoing treatment with a GFD. The rigorous review of the interviews allowed the researchers to identify four categories representing the experience of being a woman with CD: feelings at diagnosis, limitations on day-to-day life, social perceptions of the illness, and personal meanings of CD.

Feelings at Diagnosis

Participants reported a lack of information at diagnosis. They expressed feelings of fear and anger toward the unknown, which represented their first true awareness of their illness. However, they concurrently expressed feelings of relief about knowing their condition and perceived that, with a lot of training, they would be able to coexist with their illness:

> *I felt a mixture of anger at what was happening to me and at the little information they gave me at the time, and that I couldn't lead a normal life because of food.* (E2)

> *When they first tell you, it really shocks you, and you don't know if that is what is really happening to you. He told us about the risks and told my mother that I could die, and that's not easy…a mother being told that her daughter could die. Thankfully that is difficult when you know the illness, and my mother and I have been calmer since then.* (E1)

Limitations in Daily Life

The interviews reflected participant experience; regularly following a GFD affects social life. Some were reluctant to go to parties or restaurants because they were unsure of the ingredients of dishes and were also concerned about the possible contamination of cutlery. Social life was perceived as less enjoyable when it revolved around eating with others outside the home, and participants largely viewed eating at home with others as less problematic.

> *Sometimes you even feel embarrassed to order something gluten-free. You just shut up and drink your Coca Cola.* (E7)

Social Perceptions of the Illness

Participants in this study and previous studies reported social situations involving negative emotions in relation to gluten-free food and a GFD (A. R. Lee, Ng, Diamond, Ciaccio, & Green, 2012).

> *It is an illness that isn't viewed the same as others, like diabetes.* (E14)

On a trip to Istanbul I ended up only eating salads for fear of eating something with gluten and doing myself harm. (E4)

Personal Meanings of Celiac Disease

Participants tended to manage their GFD better and thus show reduced anxiety and fear, over time, in this study as well as in previous studies (DiMatteo, Haskard-Zolnierek, & Martin, 2012). However, if levels of anxiety and fear do not decline with time, it may indicate that patients need more confidence in their diet control strategies (Black & Orfila, 2011; DiMatteo et al., 2012).

Society should be made aware about CD. (E11)

In restaurants, there is a lack of training and awareness, and they should consider separating foods, work areas, utensils, and so on. (E12)

Discussion

The results of this study indicate that CD manifests in many different ways in the life of women sufferers. Some of the participants reported that CD had very little effect on daily life, whereas others experienced the illness as a burden. However, all agreed on one issue, which was the normalization of their lives. This is consistent with other studies, which show that most chronically ill people exhibit the desire to achieve a semblance of normality in their lives (Jacobsson et al., 2012). Women with CD who have a stronger sense of security and control tend to have a greater sense of normalcy.

Previous research (Ludvigsson, Reutfors, Ösby, Ekbom, & Montgomery, 2007; Smith & Gerdes, 2012) provide data related to the association between GFDs and negative emotions, including anxiety and depression, which was found in this study. Psychosocial factors may have a stronger effect on health-related quality of life than the CD itself (Sainsbury, Mullan, & Sharpe, 2013). Patients, especially female patients, with CD have higher rates of anxiety and depression than the general population (Arigo, Anskis, & Smyth, 2012; Smith & Gerdes, 2012; Zingone, Swift, et al., 2015).

As in previous studies (See et al., 2015), this study showed that insufficient education about GFD increased the risks of poor adherence and frustration and increased healthcare costs because of patients seeking medical care for ongoing symptoms and/or complications.

Moreover, the participants expressed concern about the future in terms of both their professional and personal lives. This may indicate that many of the feelings expressed by the participants (loneliness, having no one to talk to, and the feeling that nobody cared) may be more prominent in women with CD than in their male counterparts (Roos, Hellström, Hallert, & Wilhelmsson, 2013).

Although the requirement for a strict GFD generally affected the social interactions of sufferers of CD, this effect is greater in women, as shown in this study and previous studies (Rose & Howard, 2014; Zarkadas et al., 2013).

Conclusions

This study shows that CD and its treatment reduce mental and social quality of life in women. Greater awareness of CD as a worldwide public health problem is needed (Catassi & Cobellis, 2007), and more support is needed to help patients with CD cope with the illness and its treatment. Finally, organizations and public institutions should carry out CD-related public awareness campaigns and help promote quality of life in sufferers of CD in general and in women in particular.

All of the participants discussed the importance of raising awareness in nurseries and schools and on television to promote greater public understanding of CD.

As treatment continues and GFDs are increasingly managed correctly, patients with CD gradually become less anxious and fearful about their disease and its impact on their lives. In addition, they concurrently generate valid coping strategies that correspond to an increase in well-being and a valid sense of release for effective daily operations.

This study is limited to a specific population of patients (women with CD). Thus, the findings are not generalizable to other populations because of the methods used. The researchers aimed to gain in-depth knowledge about the experiences of each participant. The findings are important to understand the disease process of women with CD and should be assessed by health science research professionals.

Acknowledgments

We would like to thank all of the interviewees for their participation in this study and for sharing their experiences with celiac disease. This study would not have been possible without them.

References

Applebaum, M. (2012). Phenomenological psychological research as science. *Journal of Phenomenological Psychology, 43*(1), 36–72. https://doi.org/10.1163/156916212X632952

Arigo, D., Anskis, A. M., & Smyth, J. M. (2012). Psychiatric comorbidities in women with celiac disease. *Chronic Illness*, *8*(1), 45–55. https://doi.org/10.1177/1742395311417639

Autodore, J., Verma, R., & Gupta, K. (2012). Celiac disease and its treatment. *Topics in Clinical Nutrition*, *27*(3), 270–276. https://doi.org/10.1097/TIN.0b013e3182625b05

Black, J. L., & Orfila, C. (2011). Impact of coeliac disease on dietary habits and quality of life. *Journal of Human Nutrition and Dietetics*, *24*(6), 582–587. https://doi.org/10.1111/j.1365-277X.2011.01170.x

Catassi, C., & Cobellis, G. (2007). Coeliac disease epidemiology is alive and kicking, especially in the developing world. *Digestive and Liver Disease*, *39*(10), 908–910. https://doi.org/10.1016/j.dld.2007.07.159

Cornejo Cancino, M., & Salas Guzmán, N. (2011). Methodological rigor and quality: A challenge to qualitative social research. *Psycho-perspectives Individual and Society (Psicoperspectivas. Individuo Y Sociedad)*, *10*(2),12–34. https://doi.org/10.5027/psicoperspectivas-Vol10-Issue2-fulltext-144 (Original work published in Spanish)

DiMatteo, M. R., Haskard-Zolnierek, K. B., & Martin, L. R. (2012). Improving patient adherence: A three-factor model to guide practice. *Health Psychology Review*, *6*(1), 74–91. https://doi.org/10.1080/17437199.2010.537592

Elli, L., Branchi, F., Tomba, C., Villalta, D., Norsa, L., Ferretti, F., ... Bardella, M. T. (2015). Diagnosis of gluten related disorders: Celiac disease, wheat allergy and non-celiac gluten sensitivity. *World Journal of Gastroenterology*, *21*(23), 7110–7119. https://doi.org/10.3748/wjg.v21.i23.7110

Giorgi, A. (1997). The theory, practice, and evaluation of the phenomenological method as a qualitative research procedure. *Journal of Phenomenological Psychology*, *28*(2), 235–260. https://doi.org/10.1163/156916297X00103

Guetterman, T. C. (2015). Descriptions of sampling practices within five approaches to qualitative research in education and the health sciences. *Forum Qualitative Sozialforschung/ Forum: Qualitative Social Research*, *16*(2), Art. 25. https://doi.org/10.17169/fqs-16.2.2290

Hallert, C., Grännö, C., Hultén, S., Midhagen, G., Ström, M., Svensson, H., & Valdimarsson, T. (2002). Living with coeliac disease: Controlled study of the burden of illness. *Scandinavian Journal of Gastroenterology*, *37*(1), 39–42. https://doi.org/10.1080/003655202753387338

Hallert, C., Sandlund, O., & Broqvist, M. (2003). Perceptions of health-related quality of life of men and women living with coeliac disease. *Scandinavian Journal of Caring Sciences*, *17*(3), 301–307. https://doi.org/10.1046/j.1471-6712.2003.00228.x

Jacobsson, L. R., Hallert, C., Milberg, A., & Friedrichsen, M. (2012). Coeliac disease—Women's experiences in everyday life. *Journal of Clinical Nursing*, *21*(23–24), 3442–3450. https://doi.org/10.1111/j.1365-2702.2012.04279.x

Kim, M., & Oh, S. (2016). Assimilating to hierarchical culture: A grounded theory study on communication among clinical nurses. *PLoS One*, *11*(6), e0156305. https://doi.org/10.1371/journal.pone.0156305

Lebwohl, B., Ludvigsson, J. F., & Green, P. H. (2015). Celiac disease and non-celiac gluten sensitivity. *British Medical Journal*, *351*, h4347. https://doi.org/10.1136/bmj.h4347

Lee, A., & Newman, J. M. (2003). Celiac diet: Its impact on quality of life. *Journal of the Academy of Nutrition and Dietetics*, *103*(11), 1533–1535. https://doi.org/10.1016/j.jada.2003.08.027

Lee, A. R., Ng, D. L., Diamond, B., Ciaccio, E. J., & Green, P. H. R. (2012). Living with coeliac disease: Survey results from the USA. *Journal of Human Nutrition and Dietetics*, *25*(3), 233–238. https://doi.org/10.1111/j.1365-277X.2012.01236.x

Leung, L. (2015). Validity, reliability, and generalizability in qualitative research. *Journal of Family Medicine and Primary Care*, *4*(3), 324–327. https://doi.org/10.4103/2249-4863.161306

Ludvigsson, J. F., Reutfors, J., Osby, U., Ekbom, A., & Montgomery, S. M. (2007). Coeliac disease and risk of mood disorders—A general population-based cohort study. *Journal of Affective Disorders*, *99*(1–3), 117–126. https://doi.org/10.1016/j.jad.2006.08.032

Mathew, R., Gucciardi, E., De Melo, M., & Barata, P. (2012). Self-management experiences among men and women with type 2 diabetes mellitus: A qualitative analysis. *BMC Family Practice*, *13*, 122. https://doi.org/10.1186/1471-2296-13-122

Mulders-Jones, B., Mitchison, D., Girosi, F., & Hay, P. (2017). Socioeconomic correlates of eating disorder symptoms in an Australian population-based sample. *PLoS One*, *12*(1), e0170603. https://doi.org/10.1371/journal.pone.0170603

Mustalahti, K., Catassi, C., Reunanen, A., Fabiani, E., Heier, M., McMillan, S., ... Mäki, M.; Coeliac EU Cluster, Project Epidemiology. (2010). The prevalence of celiac disease in Europe: Results of a centralized, international mass screening project. *Annals of Medicine*, *42*(8), 587–595. https://doi.org/10.3109/07853890.2010.505931

Polit, D. F., & Hungler, B. P. (2000). *Scientific research in health sciences: Principles and methods* (6th ed.). México City, Mexico: McGraw-Hill Interamericana. (Original work published in Spanish)

Pulido, O., Zarkadas, M., Dubois, S., MacIsaac, K., Cantin, I., La Vieille, S., ... Rashid, M. (2013). Clinical features and symptom recovery on a gluten-free diet in Canadian adults with celiac disease. *Canadian Journal of Gastroenterology*, *27*(8), 449–453.

Roos, S., Hellström, I., Hallert, C., & Wilhelmsson, S. (2013). Everyday life for women with celiac disease. *Gastroenterology Nursing*, *36*(4), 266–273. https://doi.org/10.1097/SGA.0b013e31829ed98d

Roos, S., Kärner, A., & Hallert, C. (2009). Gastrointestinal symptoms and well-being of adults living on a gluten-free diet: A case for nursing in celiac disease. *Gastroenterology Nursing*, *32*(3), 196–201. https://doi.org/10.1097/SGA.0b013e3181a85e7b

Rose, C., & Howard, R. (2014). Living with coeliac disease: A grounded theory study. *Journal of Human Nutrition and Dietetics*, *27*(1), 30–40. https://doi.org/10.1111/jhn.12062

Sainsbury, K., Mullan, B., & Sharpe, L. (2013). Reduced quality of life in coeliac disease is more strongly associated with depression than gastrointestinal symptoms. *Journal of Psychosomatic Research*, *75*(2), 135–141. https://doi.org/10.1016/j.jpsychores.2013.05.011

See, J. A., Kaukinen, K., Makharia, G. K., Gibson, P. R., & Murray, J. A. (2015). Practical insights into gluten-free diets. *Nature Reviews. Gastroenterology & Hepatology*, *12*(10), 580–591. https://doi.org/10.1038/nrgastro.2015.156

Smith, D. F., & Gerdes, L. U. (2012). Meta-analysis on anxiety and depression in adult celiac disease. *Acta Psychiatrica Scandinavica*, *125*(3), 189–193. https://doi.org/10.1111/j.1600-0447.2011.01795.x

Sverker, A., Östlund, G., Hallert, C., & Hensing, G. (2009). 'I lose all these hours...'—Exploring gender and consequences of dilemmas experienced in everyday life with coeliac disease. *Scandinavian Journal of Caring Sciences*, *23*(2), 342–352. https://doi.org/10.1111/j.1471-6712.2008.00628.x

Touchy, T. A., & Jett, K. F. (2016). *Gerontological nursing & healthy aging* (5th ed.). St. Louis, MO: Elsevier.

West, J., Fleming, K. M., Tata, L. J., Card, T. R., & Crooks, C. J. (2014). Incidence and prevalence of celiac disease and dermatitis herpetiformis in the UK over two decades: Population-based study. *The American Journal of Gastroenterology, 109*(5), 757–768. https://doi.org/10.1038/ajg.2014.55

West, J., Logan, R. F., Hill, P. G., Lloyd, A., Lewis, S., Hubbard, R., … Khaw, K. T. (2003). Seroprevalence, correlates, and characteristics of undetected coeliac disease in England. *Gut, 52*(7), 960–965.

Zarkadas, M., Dubois, S., MacIsaac, K., Cantin, I., Rashid, M., Roberts, K. C., … Pulido, O. M. (2013). Living with coeliac disease and a gluten-free diet: A Canadian perspective. *Journal of Human Nutrition and Dietetics, 26*(1), 10–23. https://doi.org/10.1111/j.1365-277X.2012.01288.x

Zingone, F., Swift, G. L., Card, T. R., Sanders, D. S., Ludvigsson, J. F., & Bai, J. C. (2015). Psychological morbidity of celiac disease: A review of the literature. *United European Gastroenterology Journal, 3*(2), 136–145. https://doi.org/10.1177/2050640614560786

Zingone, F., West, J., Auricchio, R., Maria Bevilacqua, R., Bile, G., Borgheresi, P., … Ciacci, C. (2015). Incidence and distribution of coeliac disease in Campania (Italy): 2011–2013. *United European Gastroenterology Journal, 3*(2), 182–189. https://doi.org/10.1177/2050640615571021

Patients With Type 2 Diabetes Mellitus: Obstacles in Coping

Özlem FİDAN[1]* • Şenay TAKMAK[1] • Arife Şanlialp ZEYREK[1] • Asiye KARTAL[2]

ABSTRACT

Background: Diabetes mellitus is a major global threat to public health. Reducing the daily obstacles of coping with the disease for patients with diabetes may improve management.

Purpose: The aim of this study was to investigate daily obstacles to coping with Type 2 diabetes mellitus (T2DM) and related factors.

Methods: A descriptive and cross-sectional design was used. Data were collected from 186 patients with T2DM who were hospitalized in an endocrinology clinic in Turkey. The Hospital Anxiety and Depression Scale and the Diabetes Obstacles Questionnaire were used to collect data. Multiple linear regression analysis was performed to explore the predictors of obstacles to coping in patients with T2DM.

Results: The highest mean score was achieved on the obstacles to coping with diabetes (2.57 ± 3.78) among the subscales of the Diabetes Obstacles Questionnaire. After regression analysis, level of treatment compliance was identified as the most significant predictor (β = .289, p < .001). Anxiety, depression, smoking status, and highest level of education were also identified as significant predictors.

Conclusions: On the basis of these results, nurses should plan and implement interventions to improve treatment compliance and assist patients to overcome obstacles to disease management. Moreover, patient anxiety, depression, and lifestyle behaviors should be addressed.

KEY WORDS:
affecting factors, nursing, obstacles encountered, patients, type 2 diabetes mellitus.

Introduction

Diabetes is considered one of the most important health problems of the 21st century. Diabetes and its complications are currently among the leading causes of death in many countries. In 2017, 424.9 million people aged 20–79 years and 451 million people aged 18–99 years were living with diabetes. By 2, 045, 629 million people aged 20–79 years and 693 million people aged 18–99 years are expected to suffer from diabetes worldwide (Cho et al., 2018).

In a study performed on 26,499 individuals aged 20 years and older in Turkey, it was determined that the incidence of diabetes has reached 13.7%, the rate of increase for diabetes is 90%, and the incidence of impaired glucose tolerance has reached 7.9% (Satman et al., 2013). On the basis of these estimates, Turkey will be among the top 10 highest populations of persons with diabetes worldwide in 2035 (International Diabetes Federation, 2015).

It is important to prevent complications of diabetes to decrease the burden of this disease on individuals and society (Turkish Ministry of Health, Public Health Institution, 2014). Patients with diabetes must monitor and manage their disease to prevent complications. However, patients often face obstacles to successful monitoring that may hinder optimal disease management (Boussageon, Gueyffier, & Cornu, 2014; Song & Kim, 2009). Decreasing disease symptoms, emergency admissions, and hospitalizations; reducing disease-related physiological and psychological effects; preventing dependence on caregivers; and enhancing quality of life may be achieved through effective and sustainable disease management (Demirağ, 2009; Haskett, 2006). If obstacles to self-management are not identified, noncompliance with recommended self-care treatments and complications such as hypoglycemia and impairment in health and quality of life may result (Munshı et al., 2013). Reducing obstacles to coping with disease in patients with diabetes may improve management efficacy and health-related outcomes.

Wilkinson, Whitehead, and Ritchie (2014) reported that communication, education, personal factors, provider issues, and support were identified as inhibiting diabetes management. Nam, Chesla, Stotts, Kroon, and Janson (2011) noted that the commitment, health beliefs, attitudes, and knowledge of patients; financial resources; concomitant diseases; social support; and the attitudes, beliefs, and knowledge of clinicians regarding diabetes were factors inhibiting diabetes management. In a pilot study by Harwood, Bunn, Caton, and Simmons (2013), psychological problems, family problems, nonsupportive environment, communication problems,

[1]MSN, RN, *Institute of Health Sciences, Pamukkale University, Denizli, Turkey* • [2]*PhD, RN, Associate Professor, Faculty of Health Sciences, Department of Nursing, Pamukkale University, Denizli, Turkey.*

physical and psychiatric diseases, educational problems, and problems associated with access to healthcare services were identified as factors inhibiting diabetes management. In Laranjo et al. (2015), related factors included diet, physical exercise, and glycemic control. Finally, Booth, Lowis, Dean, Hunter, and McKinley (2013) divided these factors into six categories, including difficulty in changing habits, negative perception toward a "new" or recommended regimen, social conditions, lack of knowledge and understanding, lack of motivation, and obstacles regarding making lifestyle changes.

Risk of anxiety and depression was found to be high in patients with Type 2 diabetes mellitus (T2DM; Gemeay et al., 2015; Meurs et al., 2016; Sayın, Sayın, Bursalı, & İpek, 2019). Depression and anxiety in patients with T2DM were found to adversely affect treatment compliance and prognosis (Roy & Lloyd, 2012). Depression not only is a common co-morbidity in patients with diabetes but also may be an obstacle to coping with the disease in daily life (Chen, Ruppert, Charron-Prochownik, Noullet, & Zgibor, 2011).

Although the coping skills of patients with T2DM have been closely associated with compliance to treatment, this issue has not been a focus of attention (Rätsep, Kalda, Oja, & Lember, 2006). In the literature, several obstacles to diabetes management have been defined in different populations (Booth et al., 2013; Byers, Garth, Manley, & Chlebowy, 2016; Harwood et al., 2013; Laranjo et al., 2015). The obstacles to coping with diabetes in Turkey have not yet been studied. Moreover, although the effects of self-perceptions and disease on daily life have been described, the effects of specific sociodemographic and disease characteristics on disease care in daily life have not yet been examined. Only one previous Turkish study (Pilv, Rätsep, Oona, & Kalda, 2012) has used the Diabetes Obstacles Questionnaire (DOQ) that was used in this study. Another significant difference of this study is the investigation of the respective effects of anxiety and depression on obstacles to disease management. Identification of the obstacles to coping with diabetes is expected to improve metabolic control and self-management of diabetes and enhance the quality of diabetes care. Identification of these obstacles is also expected to shed light on advanced studies for the treatment of patients with T2DM (Nam et al., 2011). Therefore, on the basis of the above, the obstacles to coping in daily life experienced by patients with T2DM and the factors associated with these obstacles were examined in this study.

Methods

Study Design

The aim of this descriptive and cross-sectional study was to investigate the obstacles to disease management encountered in daily life by patients with T2DM and the factors affecting these obstacles. The following two research questions were addressed:

1. What are the obstacles encountered in daily life to coping with T2DM?
2. What are the factors that significantly affect these obstacles?

Sample and Participants

The sample for this study was composed of patients with T2DM who were hospitalized in the endocrinology departments of a university hospital and a state hospital in Turkey. Inclusion criteria were having a diagnosis of T2DM; being hospitalized in the internal medicine and endocrinology services department; being able to communicate verbally; and being free of neurological, cognitive, visual, and auditory problems. The desired sample size was calculated, using the formula of sample size determination for finite populations (over the incidence of diabetes as 13.7%; $p = .14$ for the occurrence of event, $q = .86$ for the nonoccurrence of the event; $t = 1.96$, $d = 0.05$), as 185 (Erdoğan, Nahcivan, & Esin, 2014). One hundred eighty-six qualified patients provided informed consent and were enrolled as participants in this study.

Data Collection

All patients with T2DM hospitalized in the endocrinology clinic of a university hospital and a state hospital between September 2016 and June 2017 were approached as potential participants. Study data were collected using face-to-face interviews that lasted for a mean duration of 20–25 minutes.

Data Collection Instruments

A demographics and clinical characteristics datasheet, DOQ, and Hospital Anxiety and Depression (HAD) scale were used for data collection.

Demographics and clinical characteristics datasheet

The 17 questions gathered information on participant demographics and clinical characteristics, including gender, age, marital status, educational level, smoking status, time since diagnosis, diabetes treatment status, diabetes follow-up status, blood glucose level, exercise, treatment compliance status, diabetes complications, and number of hospitalizations during the last year.

Diabetes obstacles questionnaire

The DOQ, published by Hearnshaw et al. in 2007, consists of eight subscales with 78 questions. The subscales include medication obstacles (10 items), self-monitoring (five items), knowledge and belief obstacles (10 items), obstacles in diagnosis (six items), obstacles in the relationship with healthcare professionals (18 items), lifestyle changes (13 items), obstacles in coping with diabetes (eight items), and obstacles in receiving suggestions and support (eight items). Each of the subscales is graded on a 5-point Likert scale ranging from "totally agree" to "totally disagree." The average score for each subscale is added together to obtain the total scale score. Scores ranged from 2 points for "totally agree" to –2 points for "totally disagree." Negative scores indicate that the respondent does not experience any difficulty with the item. The average score obtained for each subscale reflects the degree of difficulty experienced by the respondent (Hearnshaw et al., 2007). A validity and reliability study of the Turkish version of the DOQ was carried out by Kahraman et al. (2016). In the reliability study, 10 questions were removed from each subscale because they were not relevant to the Turkish population. The internal consistency reliability for DOQ subscales, as tested using Cronbach's alpha coefficient, ranged from .63 to .84, and the test–retest reliability of the subscales ranged from .87 to .97.

Hospital anxiety and depression scale

The HAD scale, originally developed by Zigmond and Snaith (1983), includes 14 questions, seven of which (odd numbers) are used to measure anxiety, with the other seven (even numbers) used to measure depression. Items are scored on a 4-point Likert-type scale (Zigmond & Snaith, 1983). A validity and reliability study of the Turkish version of the HAD scale was carried out by Aydemir, Guvenir, Küey, and Kültür (1997). In terms of reliability, the HAD scale earned a Cronbach's alpha of .85 for the anxiety subscale and .78 for the depression subscale. The test–retest reliability of the HAD scale was .72 for the anxiety subscale and .76 for the depression subscale. The cutoff point was 10/11 for the anxiety subscale and 7/8 for the depression subscale, with those scoring above these cutoff points considered at risk (Aydemir et al., 1997).

Ethical Considerations

Before data were collected, approval was received from the Pamukkale University Non-interventional Clinical Research Ethic Committee (Approval Number 60116787-020/29027, date of approval: May 5, 2016), a written permit was obtained from each of the participating hospitals, and all of the participants provided informed consent. Furthermore, permission to use their results was secured from the authors who conducted the validity and reliability study on the DOQ.

Data Analysis

IBM SPSS Statistics Version 22.0 (IBM, Inc., Armonk, NY, USA) was used for statistical analysis. To assess the sociodemographic and disease-associated characteristics of participants, distribution of numbers and percentages, mean scores, and standard deviations for the DOQ and HAD scale were calculated. Correlation analysis was used to evaluate the relationship between diabetes obstacles and hospital depression anxiety level. Before conducting regression analysis, univariate analysis (independent-samples t test, one-way analysis of variance, and correlation analysis) was used to determine the relationship between independent variables and the obstacles encountered in coping with T2DM in daily life.

These analyses were made to determine the independent variables to be used in the multiple linear regression model. In addition, multiple linear regression analysis was performed to identify the basic predictors concerning obstacles to coping with the disease that are encountered daily by patients with T2DM. In addition to the levels of anxiety and depression, demographic and disease-associated independent variables that were found to be significant in the univariate analysis (gender, educational level, smoking status, type of disease treatment, blood glucose level, exercise habits, and treatment compliance status) were included in the multiple linear regression. For the regression analysis, the results were considered as statistically significant at $p < .05$.

Results

Slightly more than half of the participants were male ($n = 101$, 54.3%). Most were less than 65 years old ($n = 120$, 64.5%), most (88.7%) were married, 88.2% had an educational level of primary school or less, most (80.6%) were nonsmokers, half (48.9%) had lived with diabetes for more than 10 years, and most ($n = 141$, 75.8%) were currently being treated with insulin (Table 1).

Most of the participants (78.5%) self-reported as performing blood glucose measurements regularly. Nearly two thirds (60.2%) did not exercise regularly, and nearly two thirds (60.8%) had a moderate level of treatment compliance. Neuropathy was the most frequently noted complication experienced (45.7%). In terms of the frequency of follow-ups, 39.2% had been admitted to a hospital at least once for diabetes within the most recent 1- to 6-month period, whereas 66.7% had been hospitalized at least once within the previous year (Table 1).

The mean scores for depression and anxiety were 8.62 ± 4.20 and 9.23 ± 4.68, respectively, which are above and below the respective cutoff points for these measures. The highest mean subscale score on the DOQ was obstacles to coping with diabetes (2.57 ± 3.78), followed by obstacles to self-monitoring (1.31 ± 3.62), obstacles to diagnosis (0.38 ± 2.81), and lifestyle changes (0.16 ± 6.55). Furthermore, the results indicate that the participants did not experience medication obstacles, knowledge and belief obstacles, obstacles to receiving suggestions and support, or obstacles to their relationship with healthcare professionals (Table 2).

A statistically significant correlation was found between the hospital depression anxiety level of the participants and the obstacles they encountered in coping with T2DM in daily life (Table 3).

The R^2 for this regression model was .285, indicating that approximately 28% of the variance in overall obstacles was explained by the independent variables (i.e., treatment compliance level, anxiety and depression level, and smoking, educational level; Table 4). The Durbin–Watson statistic was 1.854 (below 2.50), which did not reveal an autocorrelation among the residuals, confirming the suitability of using regression for analysis. On the basis of the results of the

TABLE 1.
Demographic and Clinical Characteristics of Participants (N = 186)

Characteristic	n	%
Gender		
Female	85	45.7
Male	101	54.3
Age (years)		
≤ 65	120	64.5
> 65	66	35.5
Married		
Yes	165	88.7
No	21	11.3
Education		
Primary school or less	164	88.2
High school or less	15	8.1
College or higher	7	3.7
Smoker		
Yes	36	19.4
No	150	80.6
Time since diagnosis, years		
≤ 5	43	23.1
6–10	52	28.0
> 10	91	48.9
Type of treatment of the disease		
Oral medication	18	9.7
Insulin	141	75.8
Oral medication + insulin	27	14.5
Diabetes follow-up		
None	15	88.1
1–6 months	73	39.2
7–12 months	46	24.7
Rarely	52	28.0
Measurement of blood glucose		
Yes	146	78.5
No	40	21.5
Exercise		
Yes	74	39.8
No	112	60.2
Treatment compliance		
Good	62	33.3
Moderate	113	60.8
Bad	11	5.9
Diabetes complications		
Retinopathy	21	11.3
Nephropathy	8	4.3
Neuropathy	85	45.7
Diabetic foot	47	25.3
≥ 2 complications	25	13.4
Hospitalization in the last year		
Once	124	66.7
≥ 2 times	62	33.3

TABLE 2.
Overall and Subscale Scores for the Diabetes Obstacles Questionnaire (N = 186)

Obstacle	Mean	SD
Medication obstacles	−4.27	4.58
Self-monitoring obstacles	1.31	3.62
Knowledge and belief obstacles	−4.04	5.04
Obstacles in diagnosis	0.38	2.81
Obstacles in the relationship with healthcare professionals	−8.52	7.22
Lifestyle changes obstacles	0.16	6.56
Obstacles in coping with diabetes	2.57	3.78
Obstacles in receiving suggestions and support	−0.99	4.14
Overall total	−13.63	21.72

TABLE 3.
Relationship Between the Diabetes Obstacles Questionnaire and Hospital Anxiety and Depression Scale (N = 186)

	DOQ	
Scale	r	p
Anxiety	.399	< .001
Depression	.350	< .001

Note. DOQ = Diabetes Obstacles Questionnaire.

TABLE 4.
Multiple Linear Regression Analysis of the Independent Variables of the Diabetes Obstacles Questionnaire

Independent Variable	β	t	p
Education	−.130	−1.950	.053
Treatment compliance	.289	4.309	< .001***
Smoking	−.138	−2.107	.036**
Anxiety	.208	2.587	.010**
Depression	.158	2.001	.047**

Note. R^2 = .285, Durbin–Watson = 1.854.
**p < .01. ***p < .001.

regression analysis, the level of treatment compliance was the most significant predictor of obstacles to coping with T2DM (β = .289, p < .001). Other significant predictors included, by order of importance, anxiety level (β = .208, p < .05) and depression level (β = .158, p < .05), smoking status (β = −.138, p < .05), and educational level (β = −.130, p = .053), respectively (Table 4).

Discussion

To successfully manage diabetes, obstacles to coping must be identified to encourage compliance with diabetes standards in self-management and clinical interventions (Nam et al., 2011). Therefore, the types of daily obstacles experienced by participants in coping with T2DM and factors affecting these obstacles were examined in this study. Participants experienced obstacles in four areas of the DOQ, including "coping with disease," "self-monitoring," "obstacles in the diagnosis of disease," and "making changes in lifestyle."

"Coping with disease" in daily life was the most significant obstacle identified in this study, showing that participants experienced serious deficiencies in accepting and coping with T2DM. Patients with T2DM are subject to many requirements, such as compliance with treatment, lifestyle adaptations, and behavioral changes (Geisel-Marbaise & Stummer, 2009). In a study of older adults with diabetes in the United States, medication use and complex treatment plans were found to constitute significant obstacles in coping with disease (Munshı et al., 2013). In another study performed in England, motivation and lack of self-efficacy were identified as significant obstacles to coping with disease (Harwood et al., 2013). The results of this study indicate that participants experienced serious obstacles in coping with diabetes and support the importance of interventions.

"Self-monitoring" was identified as the second most important obstacle in this study. The participants identified significant difficulties with subscale items, including perceiving difficulties, disappointment, apprehension, and annoyance about measuring blood glucose. For all chronic diseases, including diabetes, a primary element of self-care is individual ability to manage healthcare. Monitoring is the most important basic self-care behavior in diabetes management. Best practice includes regular blood glucose follow-up, use of medications, foot evaluation, follow-up of acute and chronic complications, and active participation in all health-related decisions (Wilkinson & Whitehead, 2009). Pilv et al. (2012) identified fear and disappointment as significant obstacles to self-monitoring. Larenjo et al. (2015) indicated that glycemic control promotes feelings of stress and discomfort in patients, which exacerbates obstacles. Moreover, fear of injections leads to problems in self-monitoring and compliance with treatment. Patient self-monitoring is very important to the optimal management of chronic diseases such as diabetes, and poor self-monitoring may result in acute and chronic complications and impaired health and quality of life (Munshı et al., 2013).

"Diagnosis of disease" was identified as another significant obstacle to coping in this study. Obstacles in diagnosis affect whether patients take disease seriously, which may result in low compliance (Nam et al., 2011). The attitudes of physicians toward a diagnosis affect their behaviors with regard to the disease and self-management (Nam et al., 2011). Interviews conducted with individuals with diabetes in Malaysia identified that negative feelings regarding diagnosis prevented diabetes mellitus management (Mohamed, Romli, Ismail, & Winkley, 2017). These results highlight the importance of diagnosis as a potential obstacle to disease management in patients.

"Making changes in lifestyle" was also identified as a significant obstacle to coping in this study. It is known that patients who are not able to make required lifestyle changes do not gain sufficient control over their disease condition (IQVIA Institute for Human Data Science, 2017). Studies have shown that patients with T2DM experience obstacles to changing dietary, exercise, and other behavioral habits.

Byers et al. (2016) identified the difficulty of making changes in lifestyle as a significant obstacle to self-management, indicating that it was difficult to adhere to healthy diets and that family members encouraged their making healthy dietary choices. Again, Booth et al. (2013) identified making lifestyle changes as one of six obstacles to disease coping. A similar result was found in this study.

One of the goals of this study was to identify factors that predict the presence of obstacles. On the basis of the results of multiple linear regression analysis, the presence of obstacles was found as the most significant predictor treatment compliance ($\beta = .289$, $p < .001$). This means that, as the compliance to treatment increases, patients' obstacles to diabetes decrease. This outcome highlights the importance of addressing treatment compliance to reduce obstacles to coping with diabetes. Noncompliance is frequent among patients with diabetes. The need for insulin and two or more medications have both been associated with low treatment compliance levels (Nam et al., 2011). Low compliance to T2DM treatment has been linked in previous studies to higher levels of blood glucose (Doggrell & Warot, 2014; Krapek et al., 2004) and increased short- and long-term risks of complications (Stolar, 2010), which in turn, increase disease burden (Keskek et al., 2014). On the basis of the findings of this study, obstacles to patient management of diabetes may be decreased by interventions that encourage compliance.

The anxiety levels among participants in this study were relatively low, whereas levels of depression were relatively high. Studies have reported that patients with diabetes face a higher risk of depression (Sayın et al., 2019; Siddiqui, 2014). Thus, the findings in this study are in line with those of earlier studies. Anxiety and depression levels were shown in this study to increase obstacles, including noncompliance with treatment and adherence to dietary restrictions. In the literature, depressive symptoms have been estimated to affect 24%–38% of patients with T2DM, and using insulin and differences in lifestyle have been identified as risk factors for depression.

Depression has been shown to have a negative effect on necessary lifestyle changes (e.g., medication, exercises, diet) and to decrease treatment compliance. Again, poor glycemic control and hypoglycemia were associated with depression and anxiety. Invasive practices such as continuous blood glucose monitoring, hypoglycemia, and fear of injection are sources of anxiety in patients with diabetes mellitus (Groot, Golden, & Wagner, 2016). The importance of addressing patient anxiety and depression levels to decrease obstacles to disease management was highlighted in this study. Smoking was identified in this study as another predictor of coping efficacy. Patients who smoke have lower levels of treatment compliance (Ahmed, Karter, Warton, Doan, & Weisner, 2008). The results of this study revealed the importance of changing lifestyle behaviors such as smoking to promote disease coping and self-management efficacy. Thus, lifestyle behaviors should be evaluated when planning nursing interventions to decrease obstacles in coping with diabetes.

Level of education was another variable identified in this study as a predictor of obstacles in coping. Lower educational level has been associated with lower health literacy and socioeconomic status. Therefore, these factors limit access to healthcare (Paduch et al., 2017). Health literacy helps individuals manage their health and diseases. As having a low educational level leads to low health literacy, these patients face a higher likelihood of experiencing more obstacles.

Limitations of the Study

Because of the descriptive and cross-sectional nature of this study, the results have limited generalizability. Another limitation is that, although treatment compliance was a factor associated with obstacles to the management of diabetes, the reasons for noncompliance were not investigated. Therefore, it is suggested that community-based longitudinal studies be conducted in the future.

Conclusions

The participants in this study experienced obstacles in "coping with disease," "self-monitoring," "diagnosis of the disease," and "changes regarding lifestyle." Factors predicting the presence of these obstacles were compliance to treatment, smoking, educational level, and anxiety and depression levels.

On the basis of these results, nurses should be aware of the factors predicting obstacles and of the obstacles encountered by patients in coping with illness in daily life to promote effective management of diabetes. In addition, the findings of this study support the necessity of nurses paying special attention to patients with diabetes and the importance of conducting studies that identify interventions to reduce obstacles. Nurses should implement interventions such as counseling, support groups, and training and assess the impact of these interventions on reducing the obstacles encountered by patients in coping with illness in daily life.

Furthermore, in this study, levels of anxiety and depression were shown to negatively affect lifestyle changes (e.g., medication, exercises, diet) that are important to patient management of diabetes. The anxiety and depression levels and lifestyle behaviors of the patients should also be addressed. Therefore, effective control of diabetes is helpful to the treatment of diabetes, and effective management of anxiety and depression may decrease the obstacles encountered by patients in coping with illness in daily life.

Author Contributions

Study conception and design: ÖF, ŞT
Data collection: AŞZ, ÖF, ŞT
Data analysis and interpretation: ÖF, AK, ŞT
Drafting of the article: ÖF, AŞZ, ŞT
Critical revision of the article: AK

References

Ahmed, A. T., Karter, A. J., Warton, E. M., Doan, J. U., & Weisner, C. M. (2008). The relationship between alcohol consumption and glycemic control among patients with diabetes: The Kaiser Permanente Northern California Diabetes Registry. *Journal of General Internal Medicine, 23*(3), 275–282. https://doi.org/10.1007/s11606-007-0502-z

Aydemir, O., Guvenir, T., Küey, L., & Kültür, S. (1997). Validity and reliability of Turkish version of Hospital Anxiety and Depression scale. *Türk Psikiyatri Dergisi, 8*(4), 280–287.

Booth, A. O., Lowis, C., Dean, M., Hunter, S. J., & McKinley, M. C. (2013). Diet and physical activity in the self-management of type 2 diabetes: Barriers and facilitators identified by patients and health professionals. *Primary Health Care Research & Development, 14*(3), 293–306.

Boussageon, R., Gueyffier, F., & Cornu, C. (2014). Effects of pharmacological treatments on micro and macro vascular complications of type 2 diabetes: What is the level of evidence? *Diabetes and Metabolism Journal, 40*(3), 169–175. https://doi.org/10.1016/j.diabet.2013.12.010

Byers, D., Garth, K., Manley, D., & Chlebowy, D. (2016). Facilitators and barriers to type 2 diabetes self-management among rural African American adults. *Journal of Health Disparities Research and Practice, 9*(1), 164–174. Retrieved from https://digitalscholarship.unlv.edu/jhdrp/vol9/iss1/9

Chen, H. Y., Ruppert, K., Charron-Prochownik, D., Noullet, W. V., & Zgibor, J. C. (2011). Effects of depression and antidepressant use on goal setting and barrier identification among patients with type 2 diabetes. *The Diabetes Educator, 37*(3), 370–380. https://doi.org/10.1177/0145721711400662

Cho, N. H., Shaw, J. E., Karuranga, S., Huang, Y., da Rocha Fernandes, J. D., Ohlrogge, A. W., & Malanda, B. (2018). IDF Diabetes Atlas: Global estimates of diabetes prevalence for 2017 and projections for 2045. *Diabetes Research and Clinical Practice., 138*, 271–281. https://doi.org/10.1016/j.diabres.2018.02.023

Demirağ, H. E. (2009). *Diabetes risk assessment of the first degree relatives of patients with type-2 diabetes mellitus* (Unpublished master's thesis). Adnan Menderes University, Turkey. (Original work published in Turkish)

Doggrell, S. A., & Warot, S. (2014). The association between the measurement of adherence to anti-diabetes medicine and the HbA1c.

International Journal of Clinical Pharmacy, 36(3), 488–497. https://doi.org/10.1007/s11096-014-9929-6

Erdoğan, S., Nahcivan, N., & Esin, M. N. (Eds.). (2014). *Nursing research: Process, practice and critical*. Istanbul, Turkey: Nobel Medical Bookstore. (Original work published in Turkish)

Geisel-Marbaise, S., & Stummer, H. (2009). Diabetes adherence—Does gender matter? *Journal of Public Health, 18*, 219–226. https://doi.org/10.1007/s10389-009-0305-2

Gemeay, E. M., Moawed, S. A., Mansour, E. A., Ebrahiem, N. E., Moussa, I. M., & Nadrah, W. O. (2015). The association between diabetes and depression. *Saudi Medical Journal, 36*(10),1210–1215. https://doi.org/10.15537/smj.2015.10.11944

Groot, M., Golden, S. H., & Wagner, J. (2016). Psychological conditions in adults with diabetes. *American Psychologist, 71*(7), 552–562. https://doi.org/10.1037/a0040408

Harwood, E., Bunn, C., Caton, S., & Simmons, D. (2013). Addressing barriers to diabetes care and self-care in general practice: A new framework for practice nurses. *Journal of Diabetes Nursing, 17*(5), 186–191.

Haskett, T. (2006). Chronic illness management: Changing the system. *Home Health Care Management & Practice, 18*(6), 492–494. https://doi.org/10.1177/1084822306289988

Hearnshaw, H., Wright, K., Dale, E., Sturt, J., Vermeire, E., & Van Royen, P. (2007). Development and validation of the Diabetes Obstacles Questionnaire (DOQ) to assess obstacles in living with type 2 diabetes. *Diabetic Medicine, 24*(8), 878–882. https://doi.org/10.1111/j.1464-5491.2007.02137.x

International Diabetes Federation. (2015). *IDF diabetes atlas-7th Edition—2015*. https://www.idf.org/e-library/epidemiology-research/diabetes-atlas/13-diabetes-atlas-seventh-edition.html

IQVIA Institute for Human Data Science. (2017). *The development of the Type 2 diabetes treatment compliance and continuity in Turkey*. https://www.iqvia.com/-/media/iqvia/pdfs/institute-reports/diabetes-reports/turkiye-de-tip-2-diyabet-tedavisinde-uyum-ve-surekliligin-gelitirilmesi.pdf (Original work published in Turkish)

Kahraman, G., Güngör Tavsanli, N., Baydur, H., Özmen, D., & Özmen, E. (2016). Validity and reliability of the diabetes obstacles questionnaire in type-2 diabetic patients. *Anatolian Journal of Psychiatry, 17*(1, Suppl.), 33–45. (Original work published in Turkish)

Keskek, S. O., Kirim, S., Yanmaz, N., Sahinoglu-Keskek, N., Ortoglu, G., & Canataroglu, A. (2014). Direct medical cost of type 1 and type 2 diabetes in Turkey. *International Journal of Diabetes in Developing Countries, 34*, 77–81. https://doi.org/10.1007/s13410-013-0159-6

Krapek, K., King, K., Warren, S. S., George, K. G., Caputo, D. A., Mihelich, K., ... Lubowski, T. J. (2004). Medication adherence and associated hemoglobin A1c in type 2 diabetes. *Annals of Pharmacotherapy, 38*(9), 1357–1362.

Laranjo, L., Neves, A. L., Costa, A., Ribeiro, R. T., Couto, L., & Sá, A. B. (2015). Facilitators, barriers and expectations in the self-management of type 2 diabetes—A qualitative study from Portugal. *European Journal of General Practice, 21*(2), 103–110. https://doi.org/10.3109/13814788.2014.1000855

Meurs, M., Roest, A. M., Wolffenbuttel, B. H., Stolk, R. P., de Jonge, P., & Rosmalen, J. G. (2016). Association of depressive and anxiety disorders with diagnosed versus undiagnosed diabetes: An epidemiological study of 90,686 participants. *Psychosomatic Medicine, 78*(2), 233–241. https://doi.org/10.1097/PSY.0000000000000255

Mohamed, A. M., Romli, J., Ismail, K., & Winkley, K. (2017). Barriers and facilitators of effective diabetes self-management

among people newly diagnosed with type 2 diabetes mellitus (T2DM): A qualitative study from Malaysia. *Journal of Epidemiology and Community Health, 71*(1, Suppl.), A68. https://doi.org/10.1136/jech-2017-SSMAbstracts.139

Munshı, M. N., Segal, A. R., Suhl, E., Ryan, C., Sterthal, A., Gıustı, J., & Weinger, K. (2013). Assessment of barriers to improve diabetes management in older adults. *Diabetes Care, 36*, 543–549. https://doi.org/10.2337/dc12-1303

Nam, S., Chesla, C., Stotts, N. A., Kroon, L., & Janson, S. L. (2011). Barriers to diabetes management: Patient and provider factors. *Diabetes Research and Clinical Practice, 93*(1), 1–9. https://doi.org/10.1016/j.diabres.2011.02.002

Paduch, A., Kuske, S., Schiereck, T., Droste, S., Loerbroks, A., Sørensen, M., ... Ick, A. (2017). Psychosocial barriers to health care use among individuals with diabetes mellitus: A systematic review. *Primary Care Diabetes, 11*(6), 495–514. https://doi.org/10.1016/j.pcd.2017.07.009

Pilv, L., Rätsep, A., Oona, M., & Kalda, R. (2012). Prevalent obstacles and predictors for people living with type 2 diabetes. *International Journal of Family Medicine, 2012*, Article ID 842912. https://doi.org/10.1155/2012/842912

Rätsep, A., Kalda, R., Oja, I., & Lember, M. (2006). Family doctors' knowledge and self-reported care of type 2 diabetes patients in comparison to the clinical practice guideline: Cross-sectional study. *BMC Family Practice, 7*, 36. https://doi.org/10.1186/1471-2296-7-36

Roy, T., & Lloyd, C. E. (2012). Epidemiology of depression and diabetes: A systematic review. *Journal of Affective Disorders, 142*(Suppl.), S8–S21. https://doi.org/10.1016/S0165-0327(12)70004-6

Satman, I., Omer, B., Tutuncu, Y., Kalaca, S., Gedik, S., Dinccag, N., ... TURDEP-II Study Group. (2013). Twelve-year trends in the prevalence and risk factors of diabetes and prediabetes in Turkish adults. *European Journal of Epidemiology, 28*, 169–180. https://doi.org/10.1007/s10654-013-9771-5

Sayın, S., Sayın, S., Bursalı, B., & İpek, H. B. (2019). Risk of anxiety and depression in patients with type 2 diabetes and related factors. *Cukurova Medical Journal, 44*(2), 479–485. https://doi.org/10.17826/cumj.463589 (Original work published in Turkish)

Siddiqui, S. (2014). Depression in type 2 diabetes mellitus—A brief review. *Diabetes & Metabolic Syndrome: Clinical Research & Reviews, 8*(1), 62–65. https://doi.org/10.1016/j.dsx.2013.06.010

Song, M. S., & Kim, H. S. (2009). Intensive management program to improve glycosylated hemoglobin level and adherence to diet in patients with type 2 diabetes. *Applied Nursing Research, 22*, 42–47. https://doi.org/10.1016/j.apnr.2007.05.004

Stolar, M. (2010). Glycemic control and complications in type 2 diabetes mellitus. *The American Journal of Medicine, 123*(3, Suppl.), S3–S11. https://doi.org/10.1016/j.amjmed.2009.12.004

Turkish Ministry of Health, Public Health Institution. (2014). *Turkey diabetes programme 2015–2020* (2nd ed.). Ankara, Turkey: Kuban.

Wilkinson, A., & Whitehead, L. (2009). Evolution of the concept of self-care and implications for nurses: A literature review. *International Journal of Nursing Studies, 46*(8), 1143–1147. https://doi.org/10.1016/j.ijnurstu.2008.12.011

Wilkinson, A., Whitehead, L., & Ritchie, L. (2014). Factors influencing the ability to self-manage diabetes for adults living with type 1 or 2 diabetes. *The International Journal of Nursing Studies, 51*(1), 111–122. https://doi.org/10.1016/j.ijnurstu.2013.01.006

Zigmond, A. S., & Snaith, R. P. (1983). The Hospital Anxiety and Depression scale. *Acta Psychiatrica Scandinavica, 67*(6), 361–370.

4

Effectiveness of a Nurse-Led Web-Based Health Management in Preventing Women With Gestational Diabetes From Developing Metabolic Syndrome

Mei-Chen SU[1] • An-Shine CHAO[2] • Min-Yu CHANG[3] • Yao-Lung CHANG[4] • Chien-Lan CHEN[5] • Jui-Chiung SUN[6*]

ABSTRACT

Background: Women with gestational diabetes mellitus (GDM) are more likely to develop metabolic syndrome (MS). However, the effectiveness of web-based health management in preventing women at high risk of GDM from developing MS has rarely been studied.

Purpose: The aim of this study was to evaluate the longitudinal effects of nurse-led web-based health management on maternal anthropometric, metabolic measures, and neonatal outcomes.

Methods: A randomized controlled trial was conducted from February 2017 to February 2018, in accordance with the Consolidated Standards of Reporting Trials guidelines. Data were collected from 112 pregnant women at high risk of GDM who had been screened from 984 potential participants in northern Taiwan. Participants were randomly assigned to the intervention group ($n = 56$) or the control group ($n = 56$). The intervention group received a 6-month nurse-led, web-based health management program as well as consultations conducted via the LINE mobile app. Anthropometric and metabolic measures were assessed at baseline (Time 0, prior to 28 weeks of gestation), Time 1 (36–40 weeks of gestation), and Time 2 (6–12 weeks of postpartum). Maternal and neonatal outcomes were assessed at delivery. Clinical trial was registered.

Results: Analysis using the general estimating equation models found that anthropometric and metabolic measures were significantly better in the intervention group than the control group and varied with time. At Time 1, the levels of diastolic pressure ($\beta = -4.981$, $p = .025$) and triglyceride (TG; $\beta = -33.69$, $p = .020$) were significantly lower in the intervention group than the control group, and at Time 2, the incidence of MS in the intervention group was lower than that in the control group ($\chi^2 = 6.022$, $p = .014$). The number of newborns with low birth weight in the intervention group was lower than that in the control group ($\chi^2 = 6.729$, $p = .012$).

Conclusion/Implications for Practice: This nurse-led, web-based health management was shown to be effective in improving MS outcomes and may play an important role and show feasible clinical value in changing the current pregnancy care model.

KEY WORDS:
gestational diabetes mellitus, health management, metabolic syndrome, nurse-led, web-based.

Introduction

Gestational diabetes mellitus (GDM) refers to varying degrees of glucose intolerance that occur during pregnancy or are first diagnosed during pregnancy (Puhkala et al., 2017). GDM is a growing concern and is accompanied by disease burden and healthcare issues (Gilbert et al., 2019; Rasekaba et al., 2018). The high-risk factors associated with GDM include high maternal prepregnancy body weight, a family history of Type 2 diabetes, and previous pregnancy with glucose intolerance (Puhkala et al., 2013; Shen et al., 2019). Good control of blood glucose in GDM is important to minimize the risk of pregnancy-related complications such as premature birth, preeclampsia, and cesarean section births (Allehdan et al., 2019; Gilbert et al., 2019). Moreover, GDM has been associated with perinatal complications such as shoulder dystocia, fetal macrosomia, and neonatal death (Allehdan et al., 2019; Gilbert et al., 2019). Associations between GDM and increased risk of developing Type 2 diabetes (Rao et al., 2019; Werbrouck et al., 2019) and metabolic syndrome (MS) after delivery (Huvinen et al., 2018; Nouhjah et al., 2018) have been previously reported. Women with a history of GDM suffer from Type 2 diabetes in later life and face a seven-times-higher

[1] PhD, RN, Assistant Professor, School of Nursing, National Taipei University of Nursing and Health Sciences, Taipei City, Taiwan, ROC • [2] MD, Associate Professor, Attending Physician, Department of Obstetrics and Gynecology, New Taipei Municipal TuCheng Hospital, New Taipei City, Taiwan, ROC • [3] MSN, RN, Supervisor, Department of Nursing, New Taipei Municipal TuCheng Hospital, and Adjunct Lecturer, Department of Nursing, Asia Eastern University of Science and Technology, New Taipei City, Taiwan, ROC • [4] MD, Associate Professor and Attending Physician, Department of Obstetrics and Gynecology, Linkou Chang Gung Memorial Hospital, Taoyuan City, Taiwan, ROC • [5] BSN, RN, Head Nurse, Department of Nursing, Linkou Chang Gung Memorial Hospital, Taoyuan City, Taiwan, ROC • [6] PhD, RN, Assistant Professor, Department of Nursing, Chang Gung University of Science and Technology, Taoyuan City, Taiwan, ROC.

risk of MS and cardiovascular disease than women with no history of GDM (Hakkarainen et al., 2016; McKenzie-Sampson et al., 2018; Puhkala et al., 2017). MS is a clustering of cardiovascular disease risk factors, including dyslipidemia, hypertension, hyperglycemia, and abdominal obesity (Puhkala et al., 2017). A review study revealed that women with a history of GDM had a higher risk of developing MS than those without a history of GDM (relative risk [RR] = 2.36, 95% CI [1.77, 3.14]). Offsprings exposed to GDM in utero have a higher risk of developing MS than those not exposed to GDM in utero (RR = 2.07, 95% CI [1.26, 3.42]). Women diagnosed with GDM have an increased risk of developing MS during pregnancy (RR = 20.51, 95% CI [5.04, 83.55]; Pathirana et al., 2021). MS diagnoses are typically made at the first postpartum evaluation in accordance with the International Diabetes Federation classification (Alberti et al., 2005), with modifications made for Asian populations. A diagnosis is made if any three of the following five criteria are met: waist circumference (WC) of $\geq$ 80 cm, elevated blood pressure (BP; $\geq$ 130 or 85 mmHg), elevated TG ($\geq$ 150 mg/dl), reduced high-density lipoprotein (HDL) cholesterol (<50 mg/dl), and elevated fasting blood glucose (FBG; $\geq$ 100 mg/dl).

Women at high risk of GDM are encouraged to alter certain lifestyle habits and attend regular follow-up examinations. As pregnancy progresses, the burden on pregnant women and health services increase (Hakkarainen et al., 2016; McKenzie-Sampson et al., 2018; Puhkala et al., 2017). The general prevalence of GDM is rising, with medical and insurance systems facing difficulties in coping effectively with this burden (Carolan-Olah & Sayakhot, 2019). Although interventions such as yoga, physical activity classes, lifestyle adjustments, and face-to-face nutrition counseling are currently provided to women with GDM, these interventions are often limited by time and place restrictions that make it difficult for some women to access these health resources (H. Chen et al., 2018). Thus, there is a need for a sustainable, innovative, and effective care system for GDM women that includes self-care behavior education and strengthening (Carolan-Olah & Sayakhot, 2019; Mackillop et al., 2018).

In previous studies, web-based interventions have been shown to be effective in improving lifestyle modifications; implementing blood glucose self-monitoring; achieving blood-sugar-control, maternal, and neonatal outcomes that are equivalent to the outcomes experienced by pregnant women receiving standard hospital care; and effectively reducing the rate of cesarean section (Homko et al., 2012; Rasekaba et al., 2018; von Storch et al., 2019). Web-based interventions employ a tracking system to improve self-monitoring that uses dietary logs, physical logs, reminders, and graphic progress indicators and, through peer support or real-time feedback interactivity, allow women to interact with one another and their health providers (Carolan-Olah & Sayakhot, 2019). Using this type of intervention in diabetes prevention may empower women to obtain appropriate resources and make positive decisions about lifestyle change and chronic disease control (Given et al., 2015; Homko et al., 2012; Rasekaba et al., 2018).

Over the past two decades, Taiwan's total fertility rate has declined to one of the lowest in the world, with an average fertility rate of 1.3 children per woman (National Statistics, ROC, 2020). Consequently, developing health policies that prevent high-risk pregnancies, ensure a safe birth process, and protect the health of newborns and mothers should be prioritized. Systematic and meta-analysis appraisals of web-based interventions have been conducted for women at high risk of GDM (Rasekaba et al., 2018; Xie et al., 2020). However, only a few studies of MS and its postpartum components have been conducted in women who were found during early pregnancy to be at higher risk of developing GDM (Puhkala et al., 2013, 2017). Furthermore, long-term follow-up studies are lacking on the use of web-based interventions in preventing the development of MS in women at high risk of GDM.

The aim of this study was to examine the longitudinal effects on pregnant women at high risk of GDM of a nurse-led web-based health management program intervention that was initiated prior to 28 weeks of gestation and lasted through 6–12 weeks postpartum. Maternal anthropometric and metabolic profiles, including weight, body mass index (BMI), BP, FBG, TG levels, HDL levels, cholesterol levels, and WC, were used as the primary outcome measures. Pregnancy-related complications and neonatal outcomes were also accessed.

Methods

Study Design and Setting

This randomized controlled study without blinding was conducted between February 2017 and February 2018 during regular maternity clinic visits at a medical center in northern Taiwan that delivers approximately 4,000 births per year and has nine obstetricians on staff. The trial was registered at ClinicalTrails.gov. The randomization and concealed allocation procedures were independently handled by a statistician who did not participate in this study using random allocation software (Random Allocation Software 1.0.0) block arrangement random allocation (permuted block randomization), with the number of groups set to 2, the number of samples set to 112, and the area block equal sample set to 4. The random serial numbers and groups generated by the computer were placed in consecutively coded, sealed opaque envelopes.

Participants

The inclusion criteria included (a) singleton pregnancy, (b) less than 28 weeks of gestation, and (c) having at least one of the GDM risk factors listed by the National Institute for Health and Care Excellence (2015) modified for Asian populations (i.e., > 34 years old, prepregnancy BMI $\geq$ 24 kg/m^2, a macrosomia baby [weight $\geq$ 4.5 kg], history of GDM in a previous pregnancy, and family history of diabetes). Pregnant women with preexisting diabetes (Type 1 or 2), with limited mobility or inability to perform physical exercise, or < 18 years old were excluded.

G*Power Version 3.1.1 (Heinrich Heine University, Düsseldorf, Germany) was used to estimate the minimum sample size (Faul et al., 2007). An *F* test with three repeated measurements for two independent groups was used. According to Cohen's (1988) rule for effect size, a sample of 70 is required to detect the differences in changes with an effect size of 0.25, a power of .80, and an alpha of .05 and, assuming a dropout rate of 20%–25%, a minimum sample size of 94 for the randomized controlled trial was needed in this study. A total of 112 participants were enrolled.

Measures

The participants in both groups filled out a questionnaire with demographic and health information at Time 0 (prior to 28 weeks of gestation). Anthropometric and metabolic measures were accessed at Time 0, Time 1 (36–40 weeks of gestation), and Time 2 (6–12 weeks postpartum). Maternal and neonatal outcome assessments were conducted at delivery.

Demographic characteristics

Demographic and personal health information with respect to height, prepregnancy bodyweight, parity, age, marital status, work status, educational level, family history of diabetes, previous history of premature birth or abortion, GDM, and preeclampsia was gathered using a self-report survey.

Maternal anthropometry and metabolic measures

To determine the effect of web-based health management on women's outcomes, the maternal anthropometric and metabolic profiles (weight, BMI, BP, FBG, cholesterol, HDL, and TG) for each participant were evaluated. The metabolic measures for analysis after a 12-hour fast were determined. The results were obtained in a hospital setting using laboratory instruments tested by the hospital quality control team. The data were collected from the medical records at the antenatal clinic by a researcher.

Women are typically screened for GDM at 24–28 weeks of gestation by clinical order if risk factors such as advanced maternal age, previous history of GDM, and previous history of fetal macrosomia were present. The International Association of Diabetes and Pregnancy Study Groups' 75-g oral glucose tolerance test was used to diagnose GDM. The participants drank 75 g of glucose in 330 ml of water, and the samples were taken after 60 and 120 minutes and assessed in accordance with the criteria for FBG, 1-hour, and 2-hour oral glucose tolerance test plasma glucose concentrations mean values (92, 180, and 153 mg/dl, respectively) proposed by the Hyperglycemia and Adverse Pregnancy Outcome Study (International Association of Diabetes and Pregnancy Study Groups Consensus Panel et al., 2010).

Maternal and neonatal outcomes

Maternal outcomes compared the diabetic control between the groups. Weight and BMI were recorded at each visit, as was pregnancy-induced hypertension or preeclampsia, gestational age at birth, birth weight, and the proportion of babies who were large for their gestational age (> 90th percentile for gestation and gender), mode of birth, and severe perineal trauma. Neonatal outcomes of interest included birth-related injuries and neonatal intensive care unit (NICU) admission. The data were collected from the medical records at the antenatal clinic by a researcher.

Nurse-Led Web-Based Health Management Intervention and Control

Development of a nurse-led web-based health management program

The development of the nurse-led web-based health management program was guided by discussion with an obstetrician, gynecologist, dietitian, sports coach (who provided pregnancy exercise guidance), nurse, and information technology engineer. The analysis, design, development, implementation, and evaluation model of system design (Reinbold, 2013) was applied to create the nurse-led web-based health management program (Figure 1). Twenty-two women with GDM were recruited using purposive sampling, and data were collected using in-depth, semistructured and open-ended interviews to explore the design needs of web-based health management. Themes were then mapped onto the web design (Table 1). The evaluation involved a two-stage process. In the first step, we invited nursing information experts and obstetrics and gynecology experts with clinical practice experience with GDM and MS (*n* = 5) to review the content relevance, wording clarity, and style design. The content validity index values were .97–.99. User evaluations were based on real case scenarios to simulate how women would use the system in a self-management process at home. We invited pregnant women with high risk of GDM of 30–40 years old (*n* = 10). They measured weight and BP, kept a diet and exercise log, recorded in paper logbooks, and input their personal health information into the website for 7 days. To confirm the consistency and stability of paper and electronic records, the intraclass correlation should be between .81 and .96. The researcher also interacted with the testers in 7 days to check network stability, operational convenience, and information content. The users evaluated the content relevance, wording clarity, and style design, finding the content validity index to be .91–.99. After evaluation, we made several modifications based on the experts' and users' suggestions. For example, the normal range of various metabolic indicators of the health plan were provided to help women set clear goals; embedded advertising was removed from videos and hyperlinks; and details for specific data upload, dietary, and exercise records were provided.

Intervention group

The participants in the intervention group received the standard clinic-based education class and were invited to use the web-based health management program. Each participant had a unique account and website log-in password, which

Figure 1

Diagram Depicting the Five Steps of Analysis, Design, Development, Implementation, and Evaluation Model

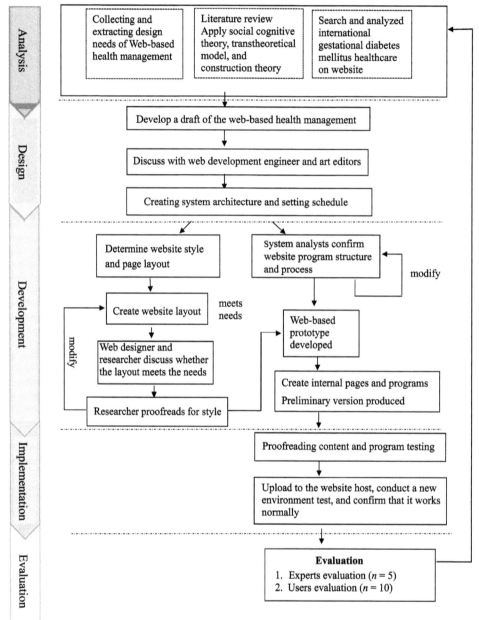

was encrypted using Secure Socket Layer. The website was enabled to count the number of log-ins by each participant and record user usage patterns. The system determined course participation, self-monitoring (records related to the diet diary and exercise log), and satisfaction with online health information. Each participant was required to log into the system at least once per week to fill in their weight measurements and complete the diet diary and exercise log. Reward points were given to participants every time they completed this task, and participants could redeem these points for gifts (e.g., maternity and baby products). This reward mechanism encouraged participants to record information frequently and develop

self-monitoring and management competencies. The intervention also included one-on-one, 20- to 30-minute LINE consultation sessions after each blood sample report that facilitated the provision of tailored health education, reinforced strategies, and elicited participant feedback.

Control group

Women in this group attended standard clinic-based care sessions. Women diagnosed with GDM were provided with a face-to-face health education program related to diabetes (same as the intervention group, conducted by the same

Table 1

Mapping of Themes Onto Website Constructs

Major Theme	Website Module
1. Membership and user-friendly website interface	1. Unique account and password to log in 2. Website manual

2. Access to reliable information and resources	Healthy lifestyle information
	    (1) What is gestational diabetes?
	    (2) How to avoid becoming diabetic?
	    (3) What to do if the oral glucose tolerance test check is abnormal?
	    (4) Healthy eating and exercise in GDM.
	    (5) Do I need to follow up after delivery?
	    (6) Life modification for GDM.

3. Provision of tailored and quick-link health information	1. Health plan in GDM: setting goals for blood sugar and metabolic indicator control levels 2. Weekly pregnancy and fetus changes: system automatically provides customized information on physical changes in the mother and fetus

4. Access to peer support	Social networking group
	    (1) Online discussions, browse previous discussions
	    (2) Interact with other participants or the researchers on Facebook and LINE groups to provide and receive emotional support

5. Self-monitoring and learning tools	1. Maternal health log
	    (a) diet diary
	    (b) exercise log
	    (c) recommendations for recipes and excise
	2. Maternal notepad
	    (a) my health data
	    (b) pregnant women's body changes
	    (c) baby growth
	    (d) pregnancy highlight for this week
	    (e) fetal movements
	3. Reminder service: motivated through e-mails, Facebook, and LINE messages

Note. GDM = gestational diabetes mellitus.

educator). This program comprised diet control and guidance related to exercise during pregnancy and maintaining a healthy lifestyle, with each session lasting approximately 1 hour. Because all of the participants were covered by Taiwan's national health insurance, participants followed the conventional schedule of examinations during pregnancy. Specifically, they received 10 examinations, with biweekly and weekly examinations conducted at 32–36 weeks and after 36 weeks, respectively.

Procedure

After institutional review board approval from the participating hospitals, three obstetrics and gynecological nurses with more than 5 years of respective experience assessed the eligibility of potential participants and obtained informed consent. These nurses were trained by the same researcher to ensure their understanding of the eligibility. To ensure the consistency and quality of the intervention, the intervention was carried out by one researcher. After the initial assessment, the qualified participants were transferred to the researcher to obtain consent. The researcher opened the envelopes in order and assigned the participants to the intervention group or control group according to the groups indicated on the envelope. The participants

were randomly assigned to the intervention group or control group, and all of the participants received standard maternity care. With the intervention group, the researcher took approximately 15–30 minutes instructing each participant on using the website and setting up a personal account. The participants were then provided with the URL link or QR code and log-in password for the website and instructed that they could use the website at any time during the 6-month study period. To avoid interaction between the two groups, only the intervention group was permitted to log in with their account and password on the web-based health management program and to view/use the information.

The participants in the intervention group were required to log into the website at least once per week to complete dietary, exercise, and self-management information. Their health status levels, weight, and postpartum WC were also measured. The recruitment procedure is shown in Figure 2.

Data Analysis

Data analysis was performed using SPSS/PC for Windows 20.0 (IBM, Inc., Armonk, NY, USA). A *t* test and a chi-square test were conducted to analyze the demographic variables of the participants and determine whether differences in essential

Figure 2

Consolidated Standards of Reporting Trials Flow Diagram

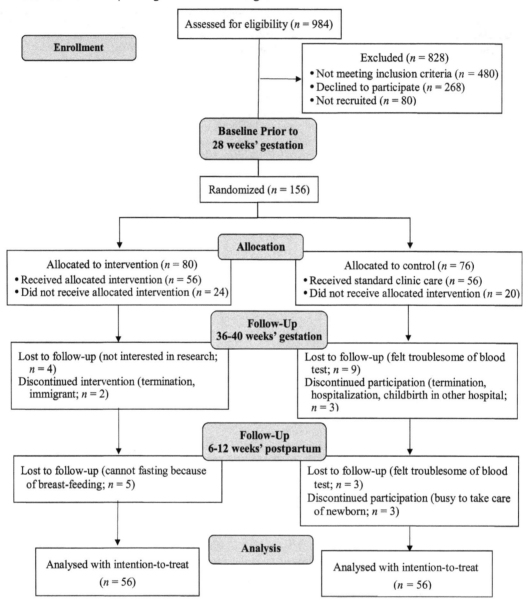

attributes were detected between the groups. The data related to MS indicators were processed using an independent-sample *t* test and a chi-square test to determine whether differences existed between the intervention and control groups. The significance level was set at a two-tailed *p* value of .05. Generalized estimating equations were applied to analyze intervention effectiveness. An intervention effectiveness evaluation was conducted after the covariates were controlled to assess the levels of MS indicators prior to and after the intervention. The aforementioned data were processed using intention-to-treat analysis.

Ethical Considerations

This study was approved by the regional ethics board in Taiwan (Chang Gung Memorial Hospital IRB No. 105-4129C). The researcher explained the purpose of the study, and all potential participants provided written consent prior to enrollment. The participants were informed they could withdraw during the study at any time for any reason without explanation.

Results

Demographic Characteristics

The mean ages of participants in the intervention and control groups were 35.71 (*SD* = 4.31) and 35.82 (*SD* = 4.28) years, respectively. Forty-five and 38 participants in the two groups, respectively, completed the follow-up test. The descriptive analysis results are shown in Table 2. No significant difference between the groups in terms of sociodemographic and clinical characteristics was identified.

Table 2

Baseline Characteristics and Components of Metabolic Syndrome, by Group (N = 112)

Variable	Intervention (*n* = 56)	Control (*n* = 56)	*p*
	n (%)	*n* (%)	
Age (years), *M* ± *SD*	35.71 ± 4.31	35.82 ± 4.28	.355
Education			.562
Less than high school	7 (12.5)	14 (25.0)	
College	12 (21.4)	11 (19.6)	
University	29 (51.8)	23 (41.1)	
Master's degree or more	8 (14.3)	8 (14.3)	
Work status			.510
Full time	32 (57.1)	37 (66.1)	
Part time	6 (14.3)	5 (8.9)	
None	16 (28.6)	14 (25.0)	
Marital status			.495 [a]
Married	56 (100)	54 (96.4)	
Divorced	0 (0.0)	2 (3.6)	
Gravidity			.313
Primipara	35 (62.5)	29 (51.8)	
Multipara	21 (37.5)	27 (48.2)	
Premature or abortion in any previous pregnancy	17 (30.4)	21 (37.5)	.162
GDM in any previous pregnancy	3 (5.4)	5 (8.9)	.118 [a]
Family history of DM	26 (46.4)	27 (48.2)	1.000
Preeclampsia in any previous pregnancy	3 (5.4)	2 (3.6)	1.000 [a]
Oral glucose tolerance test			
Fasting glucose (≥ 92 mg/dl)	3 (8.1)	2 (5.9)	1.000 [a]
1-hour glucose (≥ 180 mg/dl)	2 (5.4)	5 (14.7)	.248 [a]
2-hour glucose (≥ 153 mg/dl)	3 (8.1)	6 (17.6)	.672 [a]
BMI (kg/m^2) [b], *M* ± *SD*	24.39 ± 5.45	25.15 ± 5.05	.446
18.2–23.9	31 (55.3)	27 (48.2)	.385
24–26.9	9 (16.1)	15 (26.8)	
≥ 27	16 (28.6)	14 (25.0)	
Waist circumference (cm) [b], *M* ± *SD*	76.20 ± 7.81	76.84 ± 7.83	.664
Waist circumference (≥ 80 cm) [b]	19 (33.9)	24 (42.9)	.944
Fasting glucose (mg/dl), *M* ± *SD*	80.79 ± 15.5	79.80 ± 14.0	.823
Fasting glucose (≥ 100 mg/dl)	3 (5.4)	5 (8.9)	.716 [a]
Systolic blood pressure (mmHg), *M* ± *SD*	125.89 ± 20.7	126.50 ± 21.6	.880
Systolic blood pressure (≥ 130 mmHg)	21 (37.5)	21 (37.5)	1.000
Diastolic blood pressure (mmHg), *M* ± *SD*	75.61 ± 13.0	75.09 ± 12.3	.829
Diastolic blood pressure (≥ 85 mmHg)	9 (16.1)	12 (21.4)	.333
HDL cholesterol (mg/dl), *M* ± *SD*	71.52 ± 17.1	70.55 ± 13.8	.743
HDL cholesterol (< 50 mg/dl)	4 (7.1)	4 (7.1)	1.000
Triglycerides (mg/dl), *M* ± *SD*	183.89 ± 70.84	200.63 ± 109.4	.132
Triglycerides (≥ 150 mg/dl)	36 (64.2)	40 (71.4)	.544
Total cholesterol (mg/dl), *M* ± *SD*	216.32 ± 47.8	222.61 ± 46.9	.494
Total cholesterol (≥ 200 mg/dl)	37 (66.1)	37 (66.1)	1.000
Metabolic syndrome using IDF criteria	11 (19.6)	14 (25.0)	.463

Note. GDM = gestational diabetes mellitus; BMI = body mass index; HDL = high-density lipoprotein; IDF = International Diabetes Federation.
[a] Fisher's exact test; [b] Prepregnancy.

Effect of Intervention on Risk Factors of Metabolic Syndrome

After the intervention, at Time 1, the levels of diastolic BP (β = −4.98, p = .025) and TG (β = −33.69, p = .020) were significantly lower in the intervention group than the control group. Similarly, at Time 2, the intervention group had more favorable TG (β = −21.21, p = .036) and total cholesterol (β = −41.25, p = .006) levels than the control group (Table 3). As shown in Table 4, the weight gain differences between the groups were nonsignificant. However, BMI during pregnancy increased by 4.07 kg/m^2 (95% CI [3.7, 4.4]) in the intervention group and 4.75 kg/m^2 (95% CI [4.2, 5.3]) in the control group (p = .025). At Time 2, the BMI increase was 1.24 kg/m^2 (95% CI [0.9, 1.6]) in the intervention group and 1.93 kg/m^2 (95% CI [1.3, 2.5]) in the control group (p = .045). The intervention group had seven fewer participants with a WC of $\geq$ 80 cm than the control group (p = .042).

Generalized estimating equations were used to analyze the BMI levels at prior to pregnancy, Time 0, Time 1, and Time 2. The results indicate that BMI increased with the number of pregnancy weeks in both groups. Subsequently, a significant interaction effect between groups and measurement

times was observed. The results revealed that, on average, the average BMI level of the intervention group was 0.708 and 1.512 lower at Time 1 and Time 2, respectively, than that in the control group for the same time periods (p < .001). Thus, the web-based intervention was associated with a significant lowering in participant BMI levels. The follow-up results at Time 2 also showed that the number of individuals with MS decreased from 11 to 3 in the intervention group and from 14 to 10 in the control group, indicating that the intervention group achieved better performance in reversing MS (χ^2 = 6.022, p = .014).

Effect of the Intervention on Maternal and Neonatal Outcomes

As shown in Table 5, no differences were found between groups in terms of birth method and NICU admission. The numbers of low birth weight and large-sized newborns in the intervention group were lower than those in the control group (χ^2 = 6.729, p = .012). In terms of pregnancy complications, two participants in the intervention group were diagnosed with preeclampsia, whereas three participants in the control group separately developed

Table 3

Generalized Estimating Equation (GEE) of Baseline and Follow-Up Assessment of Changes in Metabolic Syndrome Markers in Two Groups (N = 112)

Characteristic	Intervention (*n* = 56)		Control (*n* = 56)		Group × Time Interaction Effect in the GEE Model		
	Mean	**SD**	**Mean**	**SD**	**ß**	**95% CI**	**p**
Systolic blood pressure							
Time 0	125.89	20.74	126.50	21.57			
Time 1	120.18	13.15	126.48	19.97	−5.69	[−12.47, 3.48]	.242
Time 2	120.60	16.78	125.92	21.04	−4.71	[−12.61, 4.03]	.101
Diastolic blood pressure							
Time 0	75.61	12.97	75.09	12.32			
Time 1	71.16	9.35	75.59	12.46	−4.98	[−9.33, 0.63]	.025*
Time 2	73.20	10.38	75.39	13.58	−2.73	[−7.98, 2.68]	.307
Fasting blood glucose							
Time 0	80.79	15.50	79.80	14.01			
Time 1	77.64	7.91	75.73	10.40	1.18	[−4.11, 6.48]	.662
Time 2	81.36	7.49	78.42	10.69	2.24	[−4.19, 8.67]	.495
Triglyceride							
Time 0	183.89	70.84	200.63	109.41			
Time 1	199.88	89.12	236.91	99.10	−33.69	[−77.38, 10.01]	.020*
Time 2	178.62	94.23	221.79	140.46	−41.25	[−89.04, −23.46]	.006**
Cholesterol							
Time 0	216.32	47.82	222.61	46.87			
Time 1	231.74	52.86	248.95	43.43	−10.36	[−28.34, 7.62]	.259
Time 2	213.62	52.06	241.45	46.29	−21.21	[−34.69, 2.26]	.036*
High-density lipoprotein							
Time 0	71.52	17.11	70.55	13.78			
Time 1	70.36	16.33	69.09	15.88	0.47	[−4.77, 5.70]	.861
Time 2	68.31	16.07	70.18	16.74	−4.73	[−11.16, 1.70]	.149

*p < .05. **p < .01. ***p < .001.

Table 4

Baseline Data and Changes From Baseline

Variable	Prepregnancy	Mean Weight Change From Baseline	
		36–40 Weeks of Gestation	6–12 Weeks of Postpartum
	M ± SD	Mean (95% CI/*p*)	Mean (95% CI/*p*)
Weight change (kg)			
Intervention	63.8 ± 15.4	10.6 [9.7, 11.5]	3.2 [2.2, 4.2]
Control	62.4 ± 13.6	11.7 [10.5, 12.9]	4.8 [3.3, 6.2]
Difference between groups		−1.1 (.144)	−1.6 (.071)
BMI change (kg/m²)			
Intervention	24.4 ± 5.4	4.07 [3.7, 4.4]	1.24 [0.9, 1.6]
Control	25.2 ± 5.1	4.75 [4.2, 5.3]	1.93 [1.3, 2.5]
Difference between groups		−0.68 (.025)	−0.69 (.045)
Waist circumference change (cm /no. of ≥ 80 cm)			
Intervention	76.2 ± 7.81 /19		3.55 [2.7, 4.0] /13
Control	76.8 ± 7.83 /24		4.39 [3.7, 5.1] /20
Difference between groups			−0.84 (.141) /−7 (.042)
Metabolic syndrome change [a]			
Intervention	11		3
Control	14		10
Difference between groups			−7 (.014)

Note. BMI = body mass index.
[a] Case numbers met the criteria of metabolic syndrome.

preeclampsia, postpartum hemorrhage, and a fourth-degree perineal tear.

Discussion

This study used an online self-management and learning system to improve conventional health management approaches, thereby helping participants improve MS risk factors. The prevalence of MS in the participants at Time 2 was 15.7%, which is slightly lower than the results obtained in other studies (Nouhjah et al., 2018; Puhkala et al., 2013). The dropout

rate was 19.6% and 32.1% in the intervention and control groups, respectively. The stated reasons for withdrawal in the control group included the trouble involved in scheduling and making additional visits for blood tests at nonoutpatient times, switching doctors or hospitals for pregnancy examinations, tocolytic treatments, and preeclampsia-related hospitalization. The main stated reason for withdrawal in the intervention group was the burden of maintaining the dietary log. After delivery, participants did not fast for 12 hours before taking a blood test because of the need to breastfeed. Moreover, both groups were busy caring for their newborns and viewed

Table 5

Maternal and Neonatal Outcomes in Participants (N = 94)

Variable	Intervention (*n* = 50)	Control (*n* = 44)	*p*
	n (%)	*n* (%)	
Cesarean delivery	19 (38.0)	17 (38.6)	.950
Admitted to NICU	6 (12.0)	5 (11.4)	.925
Preeclampsia/other complications	2 (4.0)	3 (6.8)	.549
Premature (< 37 weeks of gestation)	11 (22.0)	13 (29.5)	.408
Neonatal birth weight (g), *M ± SD*	3,094.0 ± 502.1	2,879.0 ± 609.9	.023*
< 2,500	4 (8.0)	10 (22.7)	.012*
2,500–4,000	46 (92.0)	32 (72.7)	
> 4,000	0 (0.0)	2 (4.5)	

Note. NICU = neonatal intensive care unit.
*p < .05.

themselves as healthy and not in need of follow-up examinations. Similar rates of failure and participant difficulties in similar studies of telemedicine in GDM have been reported (Bartholomew et al., 2015). The dropout rate in the control group exceeded expectations, and the overall statistical power of 80% in this group may have biased the findings.

Effectiveness of the Intervention in Reducing the Risk Factors of Metabolic Syndrome

The intervention group had significantly improved TG levels at Time 1, and the intervention group outperformed the control group in terms of both TG and total cholesterol level at Time 2. This finding is consistent with previous studies that offered lifestyle interventions to women with GDM (Grotenfelt et al., 2020). Although a significant difference was also noted in diastolic BP, the difference was in the normal range and was not deemed clinically significant. In addition, there were no significant differences in systolic BP, FBG, and HDL, because the average values of these indicators were normal at Time 0, Time 1, and Time 2. Prepregnancy obesity and excessive weight gain during pregnancy are essential predictors of MS development in women with GDM (Shen et al., 2019; Xu et al., 2014), indicating the importance of effective weight control in MS prevention efforts. By comparing BMI between gestation and postpartum periods, the findings of this study revealed a significantly smaller increase in BMI in the intervention group compared to the control group. Furthermore, fewer participants in the intervention group had abnormal WC, demonstrating that the intervention group controlled their weight more effectively. This finding indicates that an intervention using web-based health management may be widely accepted and highly feasible for young women to facilitate weight, blood lipid level, and WC management.

Eight of the 11 participants in the intervention group who had been diagnosed with MS at Time 0 had successfully reversed the syndrome at Time 2. By contrast, 10 participants in the control group still had MS. The change in MS risk between the two groups was significant, which corresponds with prior findings. Puhkala et al. (2013) offered a lifestyle intervention program to women with GDM. Their results indicated that MS incidence in the control group was 1.5 times higher than that in the intervention group at 1 year postpartum and that MS incidence among individuals with prepregnancy obesity was three times that of individuals with a normal weight at 1 year postpartum. Furthermore, the results of a prior literature review and meta-analysis support that lifestyle interventions may effectively prevent GDM and reduce the incidence/ delay the development of GDM-related MS (Allehdan et al., 2019; Grotenfelt et al., 2020).

Notably, the level of effectiveness in decreasing MS (particularly in terms of the reversion of blood lipids) was significant in this study. The researchers reviewed the log-in conditions of diet diaries, finding that the participants consumed mainly high-calorie foods and staple foods and consumed few vegetables at the beginning of the intervention. Their daily diet recordings were similar. Because most of the participants had full-time jobs, they frequently ate high-calorie bento boxes for lunch. Some claimed that they deserved rich meals during pregnancy, particularly after overcoming morning sickness. Others used their unborn children as an excuse for eating whatever they wanted. However, the participants gradually ate a healthier diet after acquiring the correct knowledge related to nutrient consumption during pregnancy on the website, engaged in group discussions, and accepted suggestions from dietitians.

A previous literature review and meta-analysis supports that regular exercise prior to pregnancy and during early pregnancy has the potential to significantly reduce gestational weight gain (Wang et al. 2019). However, because of the many pregnancy-related taboos in Taiwan (e.g., being discouraged to carry heavy objects and being required to get more rest), 57.1% of Taiwanese women cease to engage in strenuous exercise after becoming pregnant (Tung et al., 2014). Using website guidance, this study encouraged women to engage in an active lifestyle during pregnancy. For example, the web-based health management system allowed the participants to participate in online exercises with customized exercise guidance. By maintaining a diet diary and exercise log on the website, sharing their exercise routines, and supporting others' posts in the discussion group, participants gradually reduced their MS risk.

Effects of the Intervention on the Participants and Their Newborns

No significant difference was observed between the two groups in terms of cesarean section, admission to NICUs, pregnancy complications, or premature birth, which corresponds to the results of similar studies (Given et al., 2015; Homko et al., 2012). The similar incidences of cesarean section in the two groups may be attributed to the Taiwanese belief that birth time affects one's fortunes in life (*Shen Chen Ba Zi*). Consequently, the main reason that Taiwanese mothers choose to undergo cesarean section is to deliver their child at a time deemed to be fortuitous. Whether having a cesarean section, usually conducted 2–4 weeks prior to the estimated date of birth, is associated with premature birth and pregnancy complications in overweight mothers requires further investigation. In addition, because Taiwan's national health insurance covers 10–14 pregnancy examinations, maternal–fetal problems are usually detected at an early stage. Furthermore, the two groups received similar examinations, leading to no difference in intervention effects on maternal–fetal health. Most newborns had a normal weight. However, the number of newborns with low birth weight in the intervention group was significantly lower than in the control group. This finding was different to those of other studies (Homko et al., 2012; Mackillop et al., 2018). It may be that the participants in this study had abnormal metabolic indicators, especially in terms of cholesterol and TGs. Previous studies have reported lower birth weight as associated with higher concentrations of total cholesterol (L. H. Chen et al., 2017; Nghiem-Rao et al., 2016). The intervention group had better cholesterol control, which may have contributed to this group having a more normal neonatal birth weight.

Limitations

The results of this study support the clinical value of web-based health management interventions delivered during pregnancy. However, this study is affected by several limitations. This study was conducted at a single medical center. Thus, the results may not be generalizable to other populations. Also, blinding was not possible because of the nature of the intervention. There was a high dropout rate at 6–12 weeks of postpartum, which may reflect a general trend among women of deemphasizing their own health to focus on taking care of their babies. Future studies should explore how to best balance being a mother and maintaining appropriate self-care. In this study, the normal BMI (18.2–23.9) and normal WC ratios were higher in the intervention group than the control group. Moreover, the TG (≥ 150 mg/dl), total cholesterol, and MS levels were higher in the control group than the intervention group. Although no statistically significant difference was found between the two groups, the abovementioned differences may have had potential clinical significance. It is suggested that different sampling methods be used in future research to reduce potential biases.

Conclusions

The results of this study demonstrated that a nurse-led web-based health management program has the potential to effectively reduce BMI, WC, diastolic BP, cholesterol, and TG levels. This type of program may have a feasible clinical role to play in changing the current pregnancy care model. The findings may serve as a reference for health policy development in the future and provide meaningful suggestions for clinical practice.

The advantages of this study included the experimental design used, the random assignment of subjects, and the relatively long length of follow-up (early pregnancy through 6–12 weeks postpartum). Web-based health management represents an innovative use of current technologies for the prevention of MS in women with GDM, particularly in the Taiwan context. Pregnancy and childbirth are important health transition periods for women. Health providers should understand the factors affecting this transition and provide professional consultation and follow-up care using "anytime/anywhere" web-based programs to assist women with GDM at high risk. We suggest that web-based health management programs become a routine part of maternal and neonatal care because of the ability of this type of platform to provide information (e.g., health tracking, reminders and monitoring of metabolic risk factors after delivery) that is tailored to each user for the effective prevention of MS in women with GDM.

Acknowledgments

This study was supported by grants from the Ministry of Science and Technology in Taiwan (MOST 104-2511-S-255-004-MY2). We gratefully acknowledge all of the participants for their generous cooperation.

Author Contributions

Study conception and design: MCS, ASC, MYC, JCS
Data collection: MSC, ASC, MYC
Data analysis and interpretation: MCS, ASC, MYC, JCS
Drafting of the article: MCS, MYC, JCS
Critical revision of the article: MCS, ASC, JCS

References

Alberti, K. G., Zimmet, P., & Shaw, J., IDF Epidemiology Task Force Consensus Group. (2005). The metabolic syndrome—A new worldwide definition. *The Lancet, 366*(9491), 1059–1062. https://doi.org/10.1016/S0140-6736(05)67402-8

Allehdan, S. S., Basha, A. S., Asali, F. F., & Tayyem, R. F. (2019). Dietary and exercise interventions and glycemic control and maternal and newborn outcomes in women diagnosed with gestational diabetes: Systematic review. *Diabetes & Metabolic Syndrome: Clinical Research & Review, 13*(4), 2775–2784. https://doi.org/10.1016/j.dsx.2019.07.040

Bartholomew, M. L., Soules, K., Church, K., Shaha, S., Burlingame, J., Graham, G., Sauvage, L., & Zalud, I. (2015). Managing diabetes in pregnancy using cell phone/Internet technology. *Clinical Diabetes, 33*(4), 169–174. https://doi.org/10.2337/diaclin.33.4.169

Carolan-Olah, M., & Sayakhot, P. (2019). A randomized controlled trial of a web-based education intervention for women with gestational diabetes mellitus. *Midwifery, 68*, 39–47. https://doi.org/10.1016/j.midw.2018.08.019

Chen, H., Chai, Y., Dong, L., Niu, W., & Zhang, P. (2018). Effectiveness and appropriateness of mHealth interventions for maternal and child health: Systematic review. *JMIR Mhealth Uhealth, 6*(1), Article e7. https://doi.org/10.2196/mhealth.8998

Chen, L. H., Chen, S. S., Liang, L., Wang, C. L., Fall, C., Osmond, C., Veena, S. R., & Bretani, A. (2017). Relationship between birth weight and total cholesterol concentration in adulthood: A meta-analysis. *Journal of Chinese Medical Association, 80*(1), 44_49. https://doi.org/10.1016/j.jcma.2016.08.001

Cohen, J. (1988). *Statistical power analysis for the behavioral sciences* (2nd ed.). Erlbaum.

Faul, F., Erdfelder, E., Lang, A. G., & Buchner, A. (2007). G*Power 3: A flexible statistical power analysis program for the social, behavioral, and biomedical sciences. *Behavior Research Methods*, *39*, 175–191.

Gilbert, L., Gross, J., Lanzi, S., Quansah, D. Y., Puder, J., & Horsch, A. (2019). How diet, physical activity and psychosocial well-being interact in women with gestational diabetes mellitus: An integrative review. *BMC Pregnancy and Childbirth*, *19*, Article No. 60. https://doi.org/10.1186/s12884-019-2185-y

Given, J. E., Bunting, B. P., O'Kane, M. J., Dunne, F., & Coates, V. E. (2015). Tele-Mum: A feasibility study for a randomized controlled trial exploring the potential for telemedicine in the diabetes care of those with gestational diabetes. *Diabetes Technology & Therapeutics*, *17*(12), 880–888. https://doi.org/10.1089/dia.2015.0147

Grotenfelt, N. E., Wasenius, N., Eriksson, J. G., Huvinen, E., Stach-Lempinen, B., Koivusalo, S. B., & Rönö, K. (2020). Effect of maternal lifestyle intervention on metabolic health and adiposity of offspring: Findings from the Finnish Gestational Diabetes Prevention Study (RADIEL). *Diabetes & Metabolism*, *46*(1), 46–53. https://doi.org/10.1016/j.diabet.2019.05.007

Hakkarainen, H., Huopio, H., Cederberg, H., Pääkkonen, M., Voutilainen, R., & Heinonen, S. (2016). The risk of metabolic syndrome in women with previous GDM in a long-term follow-up. *Gynecological Endocrinology*, *32*(11), 920–925. https://doi.org/10.1080/09513590.2016.1198764

Homko, C. J., Deeb, L. C., Rohrbacher, K., Mulla, W., Mastrogiannis, D., Gaughan, J., Santamore, W. P., & Bove, A. A. (2012). Impact of a telemedicine system with automated reminders on outcomes in women with gestational diabetes mellitus. *Diabetes Technology & Therapeutics*, *14*(7), 624–629. https://doi.org/10.1089/dia.2012.0010

Huvinen, E., Eriksson, J. G., Koivusalo, S. B., Grotenfelt, N., Tiitinen, A., Stach-Lempinen, B., & Rönö, K. (2018). Heterogeneity of gestational diabetes (GDM) and long-term risk of diabetes and metabolic syndrome: Findings from the RADIEL study follow-up. *Acta Diabetologica*, *55*(5), 493–501. https://doi.org/10.1007/s00592-018-1118-y

International Association of Diabetes and Pregnancy Study Groups Consensus Panel. Metzger, B. E., Gabbe, S. G., Persson, B., Buchanan, T. A., Catalano, P. A., Damm, P., Dyer, A. R., de Leiva, A., Hod, M., Kitzmiler, J. L., Lowe, L. P., McIntyre, H. D., Oats, J. J., Omori, Y., & Schmidt, M. I. (2010). International Association of Diabetes and Pregnancy Study Groups recommendations on the diagnosis and classification of hyperglycemia in pregnancy. *Diabetes Care*, *33*(3), 676–682.

Mackillop, L., Hirst, J. E., Bartlett, K. J., Birks, J. S., Clifton, L., Farmer, A. J., Gibson, O., Kenworthy, Y., Levy, J. C., Loerup, L., Rivero-Arias, O., Ming, W. K., Velardo, C., & Tarassenko, L. (2018). Comparing the efficacy of a mobile phone-based blood glucose management system with standard clinic care in women with gestational diabetes: Randomized controlled trial. *JMIR Mhealth Uhealth*, *6*(3), Article e71. https://doi.org/10.2196/mhealth.9512

McKenzie-Sampson, S., Paradis, G., Healy-Profitós, J., St-Pierre, F., & Auger, N. (2018). Gestational diabetes and risk of cardiovascular disease up to 25 years after pregnancy: A retrospective cohort study. *Acta Diabetologica*, *55*, 315–322. https://doi.org/10.1007/s00592-017-1099-2

National Institute for Health and Care Excellence. (2015). *Diabetes in pregnancy: Management from preconception to the postnatal period*. https://www.nice.org.uk/guidance/ng3/chapter/1-Recommendations#gestational-diabetes-2

National Statistics, ROC. (2020). *Statistical yearbook of interior. Fertility rates of childbearing age women*. https://www.moi.gov.tw/files/site_stuff/321/2/year/year.html (Original work published in Chinese)

Nghiem-Rao, T. H., Dahlgren, A. F., Kalluri, D., Cao, Y., Simpson, P. M., & Patel, S. B. (2016). Influence of gestational age and birth weight in neonatal cholesterol response to total parenteral nutrition. *Journal of Clinical Lipidology*, *10*(4), 891–897.e1. https://doi.org/10.1016/j.jacl.2016.03.005

Nouhjah, S., Shahbazian, H., Shahbazian, N., Jahanfar, S., Jahanshahi, A., Cheraghian, B., Mohammadi, Z. D., Ghodrati, N., & Houshmandi, S. (2018). Early postpartum metabolic syndrome in women with or without gestational diabetes: Results from life after gestational diabetes Ahvaz cohort study. *Diabetes& Metabolic Syndrome: Clinical Research & Review*, *12*(3), 317–323. https://doi.org/10.1016/j.dsx.2017.12.027

Pathirana, M. M., Lassi, Z. S., Ali, A., Arstall, M. A., Roberts, C. T., & Andraweera, P. H. (2021). Association between metabolic syndrome and gestational diabetes mellitus in women and their children: A systematic review and meta-analysis. *Endocrine*, *71*, 310–320. https://doi.org/10.1007/s12020-020-02492-1

Puhkala, J., Kinnunen, T. I., Vasankari, T., Kukkonen-Harjula, K., Raitanen, J., & Luoto, R. (2013). Prevalence of metabolic syndrome one year after delivery in Finnish women at increased risk for gestational diabetes mellitus during pregnancy. *Journal of Pregnancy*, *2013*, Article 139049. https://doi.org/10.1155/2013/139049

Puhkala, J., Raitanen, J., Kolu, P., Tuominen, P., Husu, P., & Luoto, R. (2017). Metabolic syndrome in Finnish women 7 years after a gestational diabetes prevention trial. *BMJ Open*, *7*(3), Article e014565. https://doi.org/10.1136/bmjopen-2016-014565

Rao, U., de Vries, B., Ross, G. P., & Gordon, A., Cochrane Pregnancy and Childbirth Group. (2019). Fetal biometry for guiding the medical management of women with gestational diabetes mellitus for improving maternal and perinatal health. *Cochrane Database Systematic Review*, *9*, Article CD012544. https://doi.org/10.1002/14651858.CD012544.pub2

Rasekaba, T. M., Furler, J., Young, D., Liew, D., Gray, K., Blackberry, I., & Lim, W. K. (2018). Using technology to support care in gestational diabetes mellitus: Quantitative outcomes of an exploratory randomised control trial of adjunct telemedicine for gestational diabetes mellitus (TeleGDM). *Diabetes Research & Clinical Practice*, *142*, 276–285. https://doi.org/10.1016/j.diabres.2018.05.049

Reinbold, S. (2013). Using the ADDIE model in designing library instruction. *Medical Reference Services Quarterly*, *32*(3), 244–256. https://doi.org/10.1080/02763869.2013.806859

Shen, Y., Li, W., Leng, J., Zhang, S., Liu, H., Li, W., Wang, L., Tian, H., Chen, J., Qi, L., Yang, X., Yu, Z., Tuomilehto, J., & Hu, G. (2019). High risk of metabolic syndrome after delivery in pregnancies complicated by gestational diabetes. *Diabetes Research and Clinical Practice*, *150*, 219–226. https://doi.org/10.1016/j.diabres.2019.03.030

Tung, C. T., Lee, C. F., Lin, S. S., & Lin, H.-M. (2014). The exercise patterns of pregnant women in Taiwan. *The Journal of Nursing Research*, *22*(4), 242–249. https://doi.org/10.1097/jnr.0000000000000056

von Storch, K., Graaf, E., Wunderlich, M., Rietz, C., Polidori, M. C., & Woopen, C. (2019). Telemedicine-assisted self-management program for Type 2 diabetes patients. *Diabetes Technology & Therapeutics*, *21*(9), 514–521. https://doi.org/10.1089/dia.2019.0056

Wang, J., Wen, D., Liu, X., & Liu, Y. (2019). Impact of exercise on maternal gestational weight gain: An updated meta-analysis of randomized controlled trials. *Medicine (Baltimore)*, *98*(27), Article e16199. https://doi.org/10.1097/MD.0000000000016199

Werbrouck, A., Schmidt, M., Putman, K., Benhalima, K., Verhaeghe, N., Annemans, L., & Simoens, S. (2019). A systematic review on costs and cost-effectiveness of screening and prevention of Type 2 diabetes in women with prior gestational diabetes: Exploring uncharted territory. *Diabetes Research and Clinical Practice*, *147*, 138–148. https://doi.org/10.1016/j.diabres.2018.11.012

Xie, W., Dai, P., Qin, Y., Wu, M., Yang, B., & Yu, Y. (2020). Effectiveness of telemedicine for pregnant women with gestational diabetes mellitus: An updated meta-analysis of 32 randomized controlled trials with trial sequential analysis. *BMC Pregnancy and Childbirth*, *20*(1), Article No. 198. https://doi.org/10.1186/s12884-020-02892-1

Xu, Y., Shen, S., Sun, L., Yang, H., Jin, B., & Cao, X. (2014). Metabolic syndrome risk after gestational diabetes: A systematic review and meta-analysis. *PLOS ONE*, *9*(1), Article e87863. https://doi.org/10.1371/journal.pone.0087863

5

Facilitators of Self-Initiated HIV Testing Among Youths

Oluwamuyiwa Winifred ADEBAYO[1]* • Joseph P. DE SANTIS[2] • Karina A. GATTAMORTA[3] •
Natalia Andrea VILLEGAS[4]

ABSTRACT

Background: Youth experience disparities in HIV infection but have significantly low rates of HIV testing that lead to late diagnoses, increased transmission rates, and adverse health outcomes. There is limited knowledge regarding self-initiated HIV testing, which is a promising strategy for improving testing rates among youth.

Purpose: This study aimed to identify the facilitators of self-initiated HIV testing among youth.

Method: Thirty youths aged 18–24 years were recruited to participate in a qualitative descriptive study. Potential participants were recruited from a combination of HIV testing sites, including community testing events, a community-based organization, an adolescent health clinic, and a college campus. A demographic and sexual history questionnaire and audio-recorded interviews were used to collect data. Transcribed interviews were analyzed using qualitative content analysis.

Results: Salient themes and subthemes that explain the study findings are as follows: testing within the context of a sexual relationship (e.g., infidelity), support and influence from social relationships (e.g., family support), taking the initiative for health (e.g., signs and symptoms of infection), HIV testing preferences (e.g., free testing), and HIV testing experiences (e.g., provision of other health services).

Conclusions: The findings of this study advance scholarly understanding regarding the predictors of self-initiated testing and provide critical information necessary to further improve evidence-based nursing clinical practice and develop public health nursing interventions that target self-initiated HIV testing. Encouraging self-initiated HIV testing is an effective approach to increasing testing rates and, consequently, preventing new HIV transmissions in this vulnerable population.

KEY WORDS:
self-initiated HIV testing, youth, HIV testing, qualitative descriptive.

Introduction

In the United States, more than 1.1 million people currently live with HIV infection (Centers for Disease Control and Prevention [CDC], 2019a). Youth, defined by CDC (2019b) as individuals aged 13–24 years, account for more than one fifth of all new HIV diagnoses in the United States, and individuals aged 20–24 years account for 79% of new HIV infections among youth (CDC, 2019b). In comparison with other age groups, HIV-infected youth experience worse health outcomes in the United States and are the least likely to be linked to care (CDC, 2019b).

HIV testing is an essential point of care that facilitates the identification and counseling of people at risk for HIV infection and linkage of HIV-infected individuals to care, leading to the prevention of new HIV infections (CDC, 2020; U.S. Preventative Services and Task Force [USPSTF], 2013). However, youth have the lowest rates of HIV testing of all age groups in the general population (CDC, 2019b; Van Handel et al., 2016). In a nationally representative sample, only 33% of youth aged 18–24 years who had sexual intercourse reported having received HIV testing (Van Handel et al., 2016). An estimated 44% of HIV-infected youth are unaware of infection (CDC, 2019b). This is the highest percentage of undiagnosed HIV infection among any age group in the general population in the United States, which exacerbates HIV transmission in this population (CDC, 2019b).

An integrative literature review by Adebayo and Gonzalez-Guarda (2017) on the factors associated with HIV testing among youth in the United States synthesized 44 studies and identified several notable findings. Youth who were female, relatively older, and Black or African American and/or who identified as lesbian, gay, or bisexual were more likely to undergo testing for HIV infection (Adebayo & Gonzalez-Guarda, 2017). Some modifiable facilitators associated with HIV testing included sexual risk behaviors; higher perception of vulnerability to HIV infection; and having convenient, accessible, and

[1]PhD, RN, Assistant Professor, College of Nursing, Penn State University, USA • [2]PhD, ARNP, ACRN, FAAN, Associate Professor, School of Nursing and Health Studies, University of Miami, USA • [3]PhD, Research Associate Professor, School of Nursing and Health Studies, University of Miami, USA • [4]PhD, RN, IBCLC, Associate Professor, School of Nursing, University of North Carolina at Chapel Hill, USA.

private HIV testing locations (Adebayo & Gonzalez-Guarda, 2017). Barriers to HIV testing included misconceptions regarding HIV infection transmission, fear of HIV testing procedure and results, and not knowing the location of HIV testing sites (Adebayo & Gonzalez-Guarda, 2017). Even more significantly, this study showed that the absence of an offer of HIV testing by a clinician is a salient barrier to HIV testing among youth (Adebayo & Gonzalez-Guarda, 2017).

Persistently low rates of HIV testing suggest that clinician-initiated HIV testing (i.e., clinician assessment of sexual risk and recommendation of HIV testing) is insufficient to meet the testing needs of youth (Adebayo & Gonzalez-Guarda, 2017; Talib et al., 2013; Van Handel et al., 2016). Clinicians' assessment biases related to sexual orientation, sexual risk behaviors, and recommending or providing preventive HIV services to youth currently limit clinician-initiated HIV testing (Eisenberg et al., 2017; Leonard et al., 2010). In addition, youth experience barriers such as inability to afford clinician visits and fear of or shame at disclosing sexually risky behaviors that further limit clinician's recommendations of HIV testing (Murchison et al., 2017; Phillips et al., 2015; Wallace et al., 2011).

Self-initiated HIV testing, defined as testing completed after a self-appraisal of the need, process, and benefits of HIV testing without the immediate recommendation of a clinician, is an effective strategy for increasing HIV testing, especially among youth (Adebayo & Salerno, 2019; Ma et al., 2016; Talib et al., 2013). In the process of self-initiated testing, the individual is responsible for appraising their own risk behaviors, deciding that HIV testing is needed, seeking out HIV test sites, and initiating and completing HIV testing (Adebayo & Salerno, 2019; Joore et al., 2017; Ma et al., 2016). Previous studies involving adults have found self-initiated HIV testing to be associated with an increased likelihood of subsequent HIV testing, the adoption of risk reduction behaviors such as more frequent condom use, having fewer sexual partners, and achieving better sexual health outcomes (e.g., absence of other sexually transmitted infections [STIs]; Fonner et al., 2012; Ren et al., 2017; Udeagu et al., 2017). Resources that facilitate self-initiated HIV testing may mitigate the experienced barriers to HIV testing, including clinicians' biases that prevent offering HIV tests, stigma, fear of testing procedures or results, limited access to clinical institutions for testing, and the cost of clinician visits (Jürgensen et al., 2012; Pai, 2014; Salako et al., 2012).

Despite these remarkable benefits, limited knowledge is available about self-initiated HIV testing among youth or about the resources necessary to encourage testing. Self-initiated HIV testing shows promising advantages for improving testing rates among youth. The implications of self-initiated HIV testing among youth in addition to the benefits described above include individual sexual risk assessments and increased linkage to care and resources that will further prevent HIV transmission. Therefore, the purpose of this qualitative study was to explore the facilitators of self-initiated HIV testing among a sample of youth aged 18–24 years in South Florida.

Methods

Design

Owing to the knowledge gap in understanding regarding self-initiated HIV testing among youth, a qualitative descriptive design (Sandelowski, 2000) was adopted in this study. Most of the previous studies on HIV testing among youth were conducted using quantitative designs, which limits the findings by identifying factors associated with HIV testing without an understanding of how they influence testing behavior (Adebayo & Gonzalez-Guarda, 2017). A qualitative design approach was deemed particularly suited for this study, as we sought a thorough exploration and understanding of the experiences of youth who self-initiated testing for HIV infection (Sandelowski, 2000).

Ethical Considerations

The protocol, procedures, and study materials used in this study were approved by the institutional review board (Protocol #20170027) at the University of Miami. Before study participation, the principal investigator (PI; first author) reviewed the study purpose, data collection materials, and rights to refuse or stop the study at any time with youth who signified interest in the research study. Potential participants verbalized their understanding and did not state any questions or concerns before the study commenced. Study participants were assigned a random study identification number, which was unrelated to any identifiable participant information, to protect confidentiality. Study files were stored in a locked cabinet in a locked room that was secured at the school of nursing.

Procedure and Sample

The participants were recruited directly from HIV testing sites in South Florida through purposive sampling, targeting youth who had sought and completed HIV testing (Polit & Beck, 2012). Data collection was conducted from March to June 2017. The PI met with the staff at the HIV testing sites, explained the purpose of the study, and obtained letters of support. The staff performing HIV testing introduced the research study to the youth after the completion of testing. If a youth verbalized interest, the PI further explained the study, screened for eligibility, and ascertained that the participants self-initiated HIV testing (i.e., without an immediate recommendation from a clinician). Eligibility to participate in this study were as follows: (a) aged 18–24 years, (b) able to speak and understand English fluently, (c) able to provide informed consent, and (d) had self-initiated HIV testing.

The PI interviewed youth who met screening criteria and provided verbal informed consent in a private area at the HIV testing site. A demographic and sexual history questionnaire and audio-recorded interviews using a semistructured interview guide (see Table 1) were used to collect data from participants. The interview questions elicited information from participants about their knowledge of HIV testing, about facilitators of self-initiated HIV testing, and about experiences initiating and completing testing. The semistructured interview guide allowed participants' responses to determine the probes for subsequent questions, which prevented external influences on participants' perspectives. The interviews were approximately 30–60 minutes in length. Data collection ended when no new themes emerged, indicating that saturation had been achieved (Polit & Beck, 2012). Participants received US$20 after the completion of data collection.

Analytic Strategy

Data collection and analysis occurred concurrently, enabling the phenomenon under study to be understood holistically (Polit & Beck, 2012; Sandelowski, 2000). Qualitative content analysis is the method of choice for qualitative descriptive studies and was used to analyze the data from this study (Sandelowski, 2000). The first author and trained transcriptionists performed verbatim transcriptions. Upon verbatim transcription, the first author read the transcripts thoroughly to obtain an overall idea of what the participants were reporting. In the first level of coding, each participant's sentence was coded with as many keywords as possible, mainly using the participant's own words. In the second level of coding, keywords identified from Level 1 were categorized into clusters, which are larger groups that are mutually exclusive. The first and second authors reviewed and discussed the first and second levels of coding. In the third level of coding, broad themes were identified that formed an umbrella for more than one cluster identified in the second level of coding.

Rigor

Several steps were implemented to ensure rigor throughout the data collection and analysis process and to correctly represent the study participants, their experiences, and conclusions (Polit & Beck, 2012). We ensured credibility (i.e., confidence in the results of the study as a representation and interpretation of the data) by collecting data using open-ended questions (Cypress,

Table 1

Semistructured Interview Guide

Question
1. Do you consider yourself vulnerable to HIV infection? Why or why not?
2. Tell me about anything that happened that makes you think you could become HIV infected.
3. Tell me about your impression/perception/understanding of the meaning of HIV testing.
4. When did you decide to test for HIV infection?
5. Why did you choose to test today?
6. Tell me about your choice of this test location.
7. Tell me what you expected to gain from HIV testing.
8. Tell me what could improve your experience of HIV testing.

2017; Polit & Beck, 2012). These questions allowed the participants to interpret and lead responses. In addition, data were analyzed using codes derived from the data itself rather than external codes (Polit & Beck, 2012; Sandelowski, 2000). To ensure dependability (i.e., consistency in the methods of data collection and analysis) and transferability (i.e., the applicability of study methods and findings to similar contexts, environments, or populations), the first author kept audit trails and field notes, detailing the events that surrounded the study, participants, and reflections on the study process (Cypress, 2017). The second author reviewed audit trails carefully to verify that the conditions and process of data collection were similar and that resulting findings were consistent. The study team established confirmability (i.e., the corroboration of findings) by reviewing the themes, participant quotes, and interpretations to verify congruence and to validate findings (Cypress, 2017).

Results

Sixty youths were identified as potential participants across HIV testing sites. After discussing the study requirements, 13 individuals met the inclusion criteria but declined to participate either without reason ($n = 9$) or citing lack of time to participate ($n = 4$), and 17 individuals agreed to proceed with the study but did not meet inclusion criteria for age. The remaining 30 individuals met the inclusion criteria and were enrolled in the study. Most of the participants were female ($n = 21$, 70%) and Black or African American, non-Hispanic ($n = 17$, 56.7%). With regard to sexual risk behaviors, almost half of the participants reported having six or more lifetime sexual partners ($n = 14$, 46.7%). More than half did not use a condom during the most recent episode of sexual intercourse ($n = 17$, 56.7%). All of the participants reported a seronegative test result. A complete description of the participants' demographic and sexual history characteristics is summarized in Tables 2 and 3.

The findings from this study represent participants' acknowledgment of risks for HIV infection and the experiences that facilitate self-initiated HIV testing. The five themes and corresponding subthemes that further explain the experiences of the individual's self-initiation testing for HIV infection are described below (see Figure 1).

Theme 1: Testing Within the Context of a Sexual Relationship

This theme describes events in sexual relationships that heightened the risk of HIV infection and encouraged self-initiated HIV testing. The two subthemes below further illustrate this main theme.

Infidelity

Multiple participants ($n = 12$) in or just ending committed relationships reported that personal infidelity, partner infidelity, or suspicion of partner's infidelity facilitated HIV testing.

Table 2
Demographic Characteristics (N = 30)

Descriptive Variable	n	%
Gender		
Female	21	70.0
Male	8	26.7
Transgender	1	3.3
Age (years)		
18	2	6.7
19	4	13.3
20	4	13.3
21	7	23.4
22	6	20.0
23	4	13.3
24	3	10.0
Recruitment site		
Community testing events	17	56.7
Community-based organization for sexual minorities	2	6.7
Adolescent health clinic	6	20.0
College campus	5	16.7
Race		
Black/African American (not Hispanic)	17	56.7
Caucasian/White (not Hispanic)	3	10.0
Hispanic or Latino	8	26.7
Asian or Pacific Islander	1	3.3
More than one race	1	3.3
Educational level		
General educational development	1	3.3
Completed high school	22	73.4
Associate degree	3	10.0
Some college	3	10.0
Bachelor's degree	1	3.3
Employment status		
Not employed	6	20.0
Employed part-time (< 40hrs/week)	6	20.0
Employed full-time (≥ 40hrs/week)	18	60.0
Annual income		
Not applicable	5	16.7
Does not know	6	20.0
$1,000–$10,000	5	16.7
$11,000–$20,000	7	23.3
$21,000–$30,000	4	13.3
> $30,000	3	10.0

Infidelity heightened the perception of HIV vulnerability and encouraged self-initiated HIV testing.

> *Me and my boyfriend got in a big situation there. I just wanted to get tested because he had unprotected sex with another girl, and I was just afraid. I didn't want to get nothing if me and him will still have intercourse.* (Female, 22 years old)

A sense of security

Similar to the subtheme of infidelity, several participants (*n* = 7) indicated that self-initiated HIV testing provided a sense of

security in committed relationships. Participants described a sense of security as an assurance of a partner's fidelity, HIV infection-free status, and trust.

> *Yeah, in a way. I did it (HIV testing) a part for me, but part because I wanted him (boyfriend) to have a sense of, like security and, like clear ease of mind, too.* (Male, 20 years old)

Theme 2: Support and Influence From Social Relationships

This theme encompassed the relationships and interactions that provided "support" in the process of self-initiating HIV testing. These social relationships were sources of information and provided safe and comfortable environments to seek HIV testing while helping alleviate concerns related to testing. The subthemes emerging from this theme are discussed in the following paragraphs.

Family support

Most participants indicated that they would prefer or did not want family members to become aware of their HIV testing. However, the participants (*n* = 7) who received family support described it as an essential facilitator of self-initiated

Table 3
Sexual History Characteristics (N = 30)

Descriptive Variable	n	%
Types of sexual intercourse		
Oral	1	3.3
Vaginal	5	16.7
Oral and vaginal	14	46.7
Oral and anal	2	6.7
Oral, vaginal, and anal	8	26.6
Types of sexual relationships		
Same-sex	5	16.7
Opposite-sex	18	60.0
Bisexual	7	23.3
Number of sexual partners during lifetime		
1	3	10.0
2	1	3.3
3	4	13.3
4	6	20.0
5	2	6.7
6 or more	14	46.7
Number of sexual partners in the last 3 months		
0	3	10.0
1	18	60.0
2	4	13.4
3	1	3.3
4	1	3.3
5	0	0.0
6 or more	3	10.0
Condom used during the last sexual encounter		
No	17	56.7
Yes	13	43.3

Figure 1

Facilitators of Self-Initiated HIV Testing Among Youth

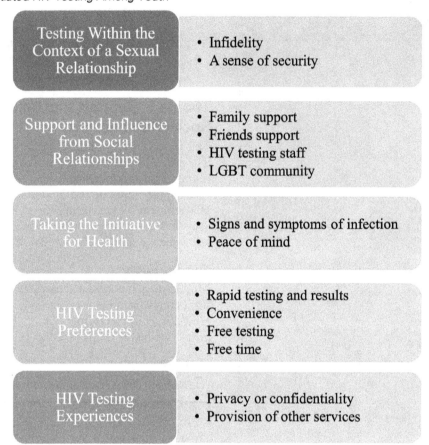

Note. LGBT = lesbian, gay, bisexual, or transgender.

HIV testing. Family support stemmed from being able to discuss sexual health with family members, family members being aware of the decision to seek testing, and advice from family members to seek testing. The quote below describes how the participant's siblings' testing experience and advice to get tested facilitated her own self-initiated HIV test.

> *I was scared because I didn't want to know...but after everyone (siblings) did it, I gained the confidence. Telling me all the possibilities of not knowing, and the damages it could do to you not knowing, made me more confident to just get it over with, and find out if anything's wrong.* (Female, 20 years old)

Family support also helped participants pay for HIV tests and deal with the fear of a possible seropositive result. Furthermore, in the presence of family support, participants described being able to seek testing freely without worry of family members finding out about tests or judging their sexual behaviors and actions.

> *Yeah, because like, say I did have it, I know I have the support system to like to be like, okay yeah you have it, now we have to take initiative to get like treatment for it, they'll be there, they're not gonna judge me or anything because they're gonna be there for me.* (Female, 18 years old)

Friends' support

The support of friends was an essential facilitator of self-initiated HIV testing described by multiple participants (*n* = 11). Friends' support was respectively identified as advice from friends to seek testing, experiences of friends' HIV testing or STI diagnoses, reminders from friends for ongoing testing events or free testing sites, and being accompanied by friends to seek testing. Having support from friends helped in the management of stigma associated with getting tested for HIV infection.

> *I feel like there's a stigma around STD testing like if you go, you just know you're dirty. So, the fact that she (friend) was willing to go with me, just like, it meant a lot. Cause a lot of people don't want to go by themselves or want that support system. So, she (friend) gave me that push to definitely go and want to do it.* (Female, 19 years old)

HIV testing staff

Another salient facilitator of self-initiated HIV testing described by most participants (*n* = 19) was the influence of the HIV testing staff. HIV testing staff facilitated self-initiated HIV testing by clearly explaining the process of HIV testing and obtaining results, engaging in friendly conversations beyond HIV infection risks and testing, and not making judgmental remarks or gestures. This interaction with HIV testing staff also helped with the management of stigma as well as the process and behavior of self-initiated HIV testing.

Initially, there's kinda like a stigma…. I think in general when someone is explaining to you the process more and explaining to you the term, you feel kind more engageful in that experience, and so I think it's kinda like positive, I think more comfortable, is the word to describe it, if anything. Yeah. I think. (Male, 23 years old)

Lesbian, gay, bisexual, and transgender community

The multiple participants ($n = 7$) who identified as sexual or gender minorities (i.e., lesbian, gay, bisexual, or transgender [LGBT]) described the influence of the LGBT community. Being a part of the LGBT community increased awareness of the high prevalence of HIV infection and instilled a desire to self-initiate testing.

In addition, LGBT events and organizations that encouraged HIV testing also helped participants deal with HIV-testing-related stigma and shame, develop the courage to seek HIV testing, and normalize the process of self-initiating HIV testing.

I started doing more LGBT-related events lately. And I would look and think more like the flyers that they had. Like before. I would be like let me not look at it. Because I can't. It's like embarrassing to even look at the flyers. But I would look at the flyer. I would take the flyers, and I would look at them. I would look at the places and the times, stuff like that. Um. That was. That was one of the biggest steps. Actually, looking at the information that they were giving me because I was ashamed to even look at the information. Then when I started looking at the information, I started thinking about going and doing testing or whatever. Um. And then, yeah. Finally, I went to testing. (Transgender female, 19 years old)

Theme 3: Taking the Initiative for Health

This theme describes the facilitation of self-initiated HIV testing by changes in physical health that indicated the presence of an STI and the desire and actions to assuage health concerns. Further detail about subthemes is provided in the following paragraphs.

Signs and symptoms of infection

A few of the participants ($n = 7$) discussed the desire to diagnose HIV infection early and how experiencing telltale signs and symptoms that might signify the presence of an STI facilitated self-initiated HIV testing. These participants explained that identifying HIV infection sooner rather than later would provide the option to engage in treatment early, take steps to stay healthy, and reduce the likelihood of premature death.

Basically, I look at myself like it's either you could find out now, or you could probably find it out at early time. You don't know the stuff you could

do to make it better. But if you keep waiting and waiting, you probably even not going to even know, make it—try to help you with treatments and stuff. You never know. Even if it doesn't go away, there is stuff that you could avoid if you find out early. (Female, 22 years old)

Peace of mind

The participants generally described feelings of fear and anxiety associated with concerns regarding HIV infection risk. Multiple participants ($n = 9$) described peace of mind as the sense of assurance stemming from the knowledge regarding their HIV status after testing. Being tested created a relaxed feeling, alleviated the stress of not knowing one's HIV status, and confirmed a state of good health.

Yeah, um. Peace of mind for sure. Just being much more relaxed. Even now that I don't even know my results yet, I just think that doing it alone kinda alleviates stress and kinda makes you feel like you're doing your thing in whatever direction. (Male, 23 years old)

Theme 4: HIV Testing Preferences

Under this theme, participants reported their preferences for HIV testing methods, the attributes of HIV testing sites, the costs associated with HIV testing, and the aspects of personal schedules that facilitated self-initiated HIV testing. These findings are discussed further as part of the following subthemes.

Rapid testing and results

Participants described rapid HIV testing as sites that allowed participants to complete HIV tests and receive results in "15 minutes" as opposed to spending "long hours." In managing class or work schedules, most participants ($n = 18$) spoke of sites that provided rapid HIV testing and said that the availability of rapid testing facilitated self-initiated HIV testing.

…It makes it easier and then we have our breaks so that we just get tested and then the situation of it, the way of it is fast. It's not like we're going to be sitting there for long hours, trying to wait on somebody to call us. You go in, get tested, and walk right out. It's a fast process; basically, the process is fast. (Female, 22 years old)

Convenience

Most participants ($n = 21$) discussed the convenience of testing sites as a significant facilitator of self-initiated HIV testing. Convenient HIV testing sites were locations visited regularly by participants such as nightclubs and community-based organizations; that either did not require transportation or a long commute or were within walking distance (e.g., testing vans) and that allowed walk-in visits or short-notice appointments.

…So you don't have to go out of your way to go to the clinic. The clinic I had to actually go there, wait

for my number to be called, and it takes hours. So, with stuff like that, you have to plan earlier throughout the day and prepare for that. Rather than the van, where it actually comes to where you are, and it doesn't come in the way of anything. It doesn't— What's the word I'm looking for...inconvenience you. It doesn't inconvenience you. (Male, 21 years old)

Free testing

Not having to pay for an HIV test was identified as a facilitator of self-initiated HIV testing by multiple participants (*n* = 11). Participants who reported being without health insurance sought free HIV testing. Similarly, not knowing places to get free HIV testing delayed self-initiated HIV testing.

Honestly. I don't.... I'm not aware where other test locations are. I really don't. I've been wanting. Like I Googled it to see where I can get it for free, and I couldn't find places online. And I think that also pushed me back also as whether to get tested for it or not because I remember 2 years ago I got it for free. So, I was like, there had to be places where they come and do locations for free. So, I was like...Oh my God, that's perfect. They did it right here. (Female, 21 years old)

Free time

Participants reported being busy with work or school, which led to difficulties in finding the time to be tested. Several participants (*n* = 8) reported that free time was necessary to self-initiate HIV testing.

Today is usually my really free day. I'm a really busy person, in general, so like. I've never been tested before, so like I didn't know how long it would take. So, I didn't want to go, have them tell me it's going to take an hour, and not have that hour. (Female, 19 years old)

Theme 5: HIV Testing Experiences

This theme summarized participant experiences at testing sites that facilitated self-initiated HIV testing. The relevant findings were the privacy of testing sites and test results and being able to access healthcare services in addition to HIV testing. The following paragraphs provide further detail on this theme.

Privacy or confidentiality

Several participants (*n* = 8) described privacy as a testing site without waiting rooms where people could identify them, sites without bold HIV testing signs, and sites that were located an appropriate distance away from residential areas to further decrease the risk of identification. Participants did not want their being tested for HIV infection or information about test results to be discovered by others without their consent.

I want to...I want to keep private. I'm not that comfortable for people knowing that I am (getting tested). (Female, 21 years old)

Provision of other services

Sites that provided services beyond testing facilitated self-initiated HIV testing among several participants (*n* = 5). Services discussed were testing sites that fostered a sense of community for LGBT youth, provided incentives like free condoms, provided testing for other STIs, and allowed consultation with healthcare professionals for other health needs.

...They tend to test everything all together. So, I was okay with that because I wanted to check everything at once. And the practitioner that I went with was very...she made me feel very comfortable about it. (Female, 21 years old)

Discussion

As one of the few initial studies exploring self-initiated HIV testing among youth, findings from this study provide unique, new insight into factors that facilitate self-initiated HIV testing.

Most of the participants were Black or African American (*n* = 17, 56.7%). Previous quantitative studies have noted that Black and African American youth are more likely to engage in HIV testing (Decker et al., 2015; Rakhmanina et al., 2014). This may be because of targeted messaging on HIV prevention and testing that provided education and intervention information for youth (Adebayo & Gonzalez-Guarda, 2017). Most participants in this study were female (*n* = 21, 70%). Several previous quantitative studies have shown that female youth are more likely to test for HIV infection (Decker et al., 2015; Rakhmanina et al., 2014; Talib et al., 2013). Moreover, two thirds of the participants in this study were aged 21 years or older (*n* = 20, 66.7%). Previous quantitative studies have also found relatively older youth to be significantly more likely to test for HIV infection (Decker et al., 2015; Rakhmanina et al., 2014; Talib et al., 2013). One reason for this finding may be that older youth tend to seek healthcare services independently of their parents or guardians. The presence of a parent or guardian and fear of their reactions are significant deterrents to HIV testing (Rakhmanina et al., 2014). Nurses and other healthcare professionals should assess youths' sexual health and sexual risk behaviors privately to provide the opportunity for responses free of parental/guardian influences.

For some participants, self-initiated HIV testing was embedded contextually in sexual relationships complicated by personal or partner infidelity and a desire to provide relational security. This suggests that youth may be more cognizant of the risks of HIV infection when in a committed sexual relationship. This finding is similar to those of previous quantitative studies, which show that youth in committed relationships are more likely to test for HIV infection than those who are not (Talib et al., 2013; Teitelman et al., 2015). An associated concern is that youth may depend mainly on changes in relationship commitment level rather than engagement in risky behaviors to increase their engagement in HIV testing. These findings indicate a need for further nursing assessment of knowledge related to HIV risks and education among youth.

Similar to previous studies, relationships with family members and friends facilitated self-initiated HIV testing (Leonard et al., 2014; Phillips et al., 2012). The influence of HIV testing staff was a unique element reported by most of the participants. Interactions with HIV testing staff who are nonjudgmental, friendly, open, and humorous are instrumental in helping youth with anxiety related to the process of completing self-initiated HIV testing. Educating nurses, HIV testing staff and counselors, and other healthcare professionals on the qualities of interactions that facilitate self-initiated HIV testing will help alleviate the stigma and fear that may delay or impede self-initiated HIV testing.

In addition, the participants reported taking the initiative for personal health when they discovered signs and symptoms of infection to achieve peace of mind regarding HIV serostatus. Although relatively fewer participants discussed this finding, it indicated that youth with these experiences possessed knowledge about HIV infection and the benefits of early diagnosis and treatment. This finding is important as it highlights that the inclusion of information on the availability of resources and treatment in the event of HIV diagnoses may help alleviate the fear of seropositive test results that often delays HIV testing in this population (Phillips et al., 2015; Schnall et al., 2015; Wallace et al., 2011).

Most of the participants had completed high school or a general educational development as their highest educational level (n = 23, 76.7%) and earned $20,000 or less per year (n = 23, 76.7%). Previous quantitative studies have noted that youth with lower levels of education and socioeconomic status are more likely to test for HIV infection (Decker et al., 2015; Inungu et al., 2011). Youth with lower educational levels and income may have jobs that pay less and require longer hours of work, which may make it more challenging to seek or afford HIV testing. Hence, there is a pressing need for rapid tests and results and free time to self-initiate HIV testing. The appeal of rapid testing and results is in the decreased wait time and the ability to test between other daily activities such as school and work. Sites that provide rapid HIV testing should advertise the estimated duration of HIV tests as an incentive to attract youth to self-initiate HIV testing. Similarly, HIV testing sites that offered free tests, were easily accessible with little to no transportation, or allowed appointments to be scheduled at short notice facilitated self-initiated HIV testing. This also indicates the need for publicizing information on free HIV-testing sites on directions to sites that are cost-effective for youth.

As reported in previous studies, privacy is a significant facilitator of HIV testing among youth (Phillips et al., 2015; Schnall et al., 2015). The participants in this study further described privacy as testing sites without bold HIV testing signs, with few people entering the room during testing, and with no waiting for testing or test results, which could lead to identification by others. These findings indicate the importance of ensuring and maintaining privacy during the testing process. Furthermore, youth should be reassured that their results will be kept confidential from those who perform the tests.

Testing sites that provided other services such as free condoms, testing for other STIs, and access to healthcare professionals encouraged self-initiated HIV testing among the participants. Youth who reported having limited time for HIV testing supported the decision to go to sites offering a "one-stop shop" (Hagell & Lamb, 2016) healthcare experience. Previous studies on access to care among youth confirm these findings and highlight the effectiveness of "one-stop shop" facilities, where youth are able to receive multiple healthcare services at the same time (Hagell & Lamb, 2016).

Limitations

This study was affected by several limitations. The study sample was largely female (n = 21, 70%) and African American (n = 17, 56.7%) and was recruited from community testing events with mobile testing vans (n = 17, 56.7%). Consequently, the current study should be interpreted within these contexts. However, this sample consisted of high-risk youth who were very vulnerable to HIV infection. Thus, findings may reflect the influences of self-initiated HIV testing in a similar population. In addition, the youth in this study all received seronegative HIV test results. Youth with seropositive HIV test results may have different experiences with sexual risk behaviors and experience unique facilitators or barriers to self-initiated HIV testing. Furthermore, this study aimed to examine only the facilitators to self-initiated HIV testing. Thus, the findings did not address barriers. To accurately capture barriers, future studies should include youth who have never self-initiated HIV testing.

Despite these limitations, this is one of the few initial qualitative studies to elicit the facilitators that are specifically related to the behavior of self-initiated HIV testing among youth. The findings of this research study may be used to support evidence-based practice and research to facilitate HIV testing among youth. Future nursing research will benefit from mixed methods approaches to understand the predictors of self-initiated HIV testing among youth and develop an intervention to improve self-initiated HIV testing.

Conclusions

In summary, HIV testing based on healthcare professional recommendations falls short in meeting the HIV testing needs of youth. Current clinical guidelines recommend one-time HIV testing for youth and adults aged 15–65 years and routine screening for individuals engaging in risky sexual behaviors or living in areas with high HIV prevalence (CDC, 2018; USPSTF, 2013). Most efforts to increase the rates of HIV testing have focused on encouraging healthcare professionals to offer HIV testing (CDC, 2018; USPSTF, 2013).

The findings from this study show that self-initiation of HIV testing by youth is facilitated by events in sexual relationships like infidelity; support from familial relationships, peers, the community, and HIV testing staff; the appearance of signs and symptoms of STIs; the desire to attain peace of mind; and HIV testing preferences and experiences. Nurses are at the front line of community and public healthcare and will benefit from knowledge on the facilitators of self-initiated HIV testing among youth. The practical implications of the findings of this study include educating nurses on the needs of youth for the self-initiation of HIV testing. Moreover, nurses should educate youth on sexual risks and the benefits of HIV testing, help youth identify social support systems (e.g., family, friends, community-based organizations), and link youth to appropriate and available resources (e.g., HIV testing sites, free testing). Furthermore, when structuring HIV testing services for youth, nurses and other healthcare professionals should advocate for HIV testing preferences and experiences such as rapid testing, privacy, convenience, and the provision of other health services that appeal to youth (e.g., additional STI testing).

Self-initiated HIV testing among youth provides an alternative way for youth to seek testing services independently. The findings from this study may inform current guidelines regarding different approaches to increasing HIV testing rates among youth. Furthermore, public health nursing is instrumental in addressing the HIV infection burden among youth. Initiatives that facilitate self-initiated HIV testing will increase rates of HIV testing among youth and consequently prevent HIV transmission in this population.

Acknowledgments

This study would not be possible without organizations and individuals that helped recruit participants. Special thanks to all the staff at Batchelor Children's Institute, Pridelines, and Community Health of South Florida. We also want to appreciate Drs. Jessica Williams (School of Nursing, The University of North Carolina at Chapel Hill), Ana Garcia (Miller School of Medicine, University of Miami), and Anthony Roberson (School of Nursing, Western Carolina University) for their mentorship and contributions to this research study.

Author Contributions

Study conception and design: OWA, JPDS
Data collection: OWA
Data analysis and interpretation: All authors
Drafting of the article: All authors
Critical revision of the article: JPDS

References

Adebayo, O. W., & Gonzalez-Guarda, R. M. (2017). Factors associated with HIV testing in youth in the United States: An integrative review. *Journal of the Association of Nurses in AIDS Care, 28*(3), 342–362. https://doi.org/10.1016/j.jana.2016.11.006

Adebayo, O. W., & Salerno, J. P. (2019). Facilitators, barriers, and outcomes of self-initiated HIV testing: An integrative literature review. *Research and Theory for Nursing Practice, 33*(3), 275–291. https://doi.org/10.1891/1541.6577.33.3.275

Centers for Disease Control and Prevention. (2018). *HIV testing.* https://www.cdc.gov/hiv/testing/index.html

Centers for Disease Control and Prevention. (2019a). *Statistics overview.* https://www.cdc.gov/hiv/statistics/overview/

Centers for Disease Control and Prevention. (2019b). *HIV among youth.* https://www.cdc.gov/hiv/group/age/youth/index.html

Centers for Disease Control and Prevention. (2020). *HIV testing.* https://www.cdc.gov/hiv/testing/index.html

Cypress, B. S. (2017). Rigor or reliability and validity in qualitative research: Perspectives, strategies, reconceptualization, and recommendations. *Dimensions of Critical Care Nursing, 36*(4), 253–263. https://doi.org/10.1097/dcc.0000000000000253

Decker, M. R., Rodney, R., Chung, S.-E., Jennings, J. M., Ellen, J. M., & Sherman, S. G. (2015). HIV testing among youth in a high-risk city: Prevalence, predictors, and gender differences. *AIDS Care, 27*(5), 555–560. https://doi.org/10.1080/09540121.2014.986048

Eisenberg, M. E., Lust, K., Mathiason, M. A., & Porta, C. M. (2017). Sexual assault, sexual orientation, and reporting among college students. *Journal of Interpersonal Violence,* 886260517726414. https://doi.org/10.1177/0886260517726414

Fonner, V. A., Denison, J., Kennedy, C. E., Oreilly, K., & Sweat, M. (2012). Voluntary counseling and testing (VCT) for changing HIV-related risk behavior in developing countries. *Cochrane Database of Systematic Reviews, 12*(9), CD001224. https://doi.org/10.1002/14651858.cd001224.pub4

Hagell, A., & Lamb, S. (2016). Developing an integrated primary health care and youth work service for young people in Lambeth: Learning from the Well Centre. *Journal of Children's Services, 11*(3), 233–243. https://doi.org/10.1108/JCS-10-2015-0029

Inungu, J., Lewis, A., Younis, M. Z., Wood, J., O'Brien, S., & Verdun, D. (2011). HIV testing among adolescents and youth in the United States: Update from 2009 behavioral risk factor surveillance system. *Open AIDS Journal, 5*, 80–85. https://doi.org/10.2174/1874613601105010080

Joore, I. K., Geerlings, S. E., Brinkman, K., Van Bergen, J. E. A. M., & Prins, J. M. (2017). The importance of registration of sexual orientation and recognition of indicator conditions for an adequate HIV risk-assessment. *BMC Infectious Diseases, 17*(1), 178. https://doi.org/10.1186/s12879-017-2279-y

Jürgensen, M., Tuba, M., Fylkesnes, K., & Blystad, A. (2012). The burden of knowing: Balancing benefits and barriers in HIV testing decisions. A qualitative study from Zambia. *BMC Health Services Research, 12*, 2. https://doi.org/10.1186/1472-6963-12-2

Leonard, L., Berndtson, K., Matson, P., Philbin, M., Arrington-Sanders, R., & Ellen, J. M. (2010). How physicians test: Clinical practice guidelines and HIV screening practices with adolescent patients. *AIDS Education and Prevention, 22*(6), 538–545. https://doi.org/10.1521/aeap.2010.22.6.538

Leonard, N. R., Rajan, S., Gwadz, M. V., & Aregbesola, T. (2014). HIV testing patterns among urban YMSM of color. *Health

Education & Behavior, 41(6), 673–681. https://doi.org/10.1177/1090198114537064

Ma, M., Malcolm, L., Diaz-Albertini, K., & Klinoff, V. A. (2016). HIV testing characteristics among Hispanic adolescents. *Journal of Community Health, 41*(1), 11–14. https://doi.org/10.1007/s10900-015-0056-7

Murchison, G. R., Boyd, M. A., & Pachankis, J. E. (2017). Minority stress and the risk of unwanted sexual experiences in LGBQ undergraduates. *Sex Roles, 77*, 221–238. https://doi.org/10.1007/s11199-016-0710-2

Pai, N. P. (2014). Perspective on HIV self-testing in North America: A tale of two countries—US and Canada. *Retrovirology: Research and Treatment, 6*, 7–15. https://doi.org/10.4137/RRT.S12953

Phillips, G., II, Hightow-Weidman, L. B., Arya, M., Fields, S. D., Halpern-Felsher, B., Outlaw, A. Y., Wohl, A. R., & Hidalgo, J. (2012). HIV testing behaviors of a cohort of HIV-positive racial/ethnic minority YMSM. *AIDS and Behavior, 16*(7), 1917–1925. https://doi.org/10.1007/s10461-012-0193-2

Phillips, G. II, Ybarra, M. L., Prescott, T. L., Parsons, J. T., & Mustanski, B. (2015). Low rates of human immunodeficiency virus testing among adolescent gay, bisexual, and queer men. *Journal of Adolescent Health, 57*(4), 407–412. https://doi.org/10.1016/j.jadohealth.2015.06.014

Polit, D., & Beck, C. (2012). *Nursing research: Generating and assessing evidence for nursing practice* (9th ed.). Wolters Kluwer Health/Lippincott Williams & Wilkins.

Rakhmanina, N., Messenger, N., Phillips, G. 2nd, Teach, S., Morrison, S., Hern, J., Payne, J., Ganesan, K., & Castel, A. D. (2014). Factors affecting acceptance of routine human immunodeficiency virus screening by adolescents in pediatric emergency departments. *Journal of Adolescent Health, 54*(2), 176–182. https://doi.org/10.1016/j.jadohealth.2013.07.027

Ren, X. L., Wu, Z. Y., Mi, G. D., McGoogan, J., Rou, K. M., & Zhao, Y. (2017). Uptake of HIV self-testing among men who have sex with men in Beijing, China: A cross-sectional study. *Biomedical and Environmental Sciences: BES, 30*(6), 407–417. https://doi.org/10.3967/bes2017.054

Salako, A. A., Jeminusi, O. A., Osinupebi, O. A., Sholeye, O. O., Abiodun, A. O., & Kuponiyi, O. T. (2012). Characteristics of clients accessing HIV counseling and testing services in a tertiary hospital in Sagamu, Southwestern Nigeria. *Nigerian Journal of Clinical Practice, 15*(4), 391–396. https://doi.org/10.4103/1119-3077.104509

Sandelowski, M. (2000). Whatever happened to qualitative description? *Research in Nursing & Health, 23*(4), 334–340. https://doi.org/10.1002/1098-240X(200008)23:4<334::AID-NUR9>3.0.CO;2-G

Schnall, R., Rojas, M., & Travers, J. (2015). Understanding HIV testing behaviors of minority adolescents: A health behavior model analysis. *Journal of the Association of Nurses in AIDS Care, 26*(3), 246–258. https://doi.org/10.1016/j.jana.2014.08.005

Talib, H. J., Silver, E. J., Coupey, S. M., & Bauman, L. J. (2013). The influence of individual, partner, and relationship factors on HIV testing in adolescents. *AIDS Patient Care and STDs, 27*(11), 637–645. https://doi.org/10.1089/apc.2013.0218

Teitelman, A. M., Calhoun, J., Duncan, R., Washio, Y., & McDougal, R. (2015). Young women's views on testing for sexually transmitted infections and HIV as a risk reduction strategy in mutual and choice-restricted relationships. *Applied Nursing Research, 28*(3), 215–221. https://doi.org/10.1016/j.apnr.2015.04.016

U.S. Preventative Services and Task Force. (2013). *Final update summary: Human immunodeficiency virus (HIV) infection: Screening.* https://www.uspreventiveservicestaskforce.org/Page/Document/UpdateSummaryFinal/human-immunodeficiency-virus-hiv-infection-screening

Udeagu, C. N., Shah, S., & Molochevski, M. (2017). Men who have sex with men seek timely human immunodeficiency virus confirmation and care after rapid human immunodeficiency virus self-test: Data from partner services program, New York City. *Sexually Transmitted Diseases, 44*(10), 608–612. https://doi.org/10.1097/OLQ.0000000000000648

Van Handel, M., Kann, L., Olsen, E. O., & Dietz, P. (2016). HIV testing among US high school students and young adults. *Pediatrics, 137*(2), e20152700. https://doi.org/10.1542/peds.2015-2700

Wallace, S. A., McLellan-Lemal, E., Harris, M. J., Townsend, T. G., & Miller, K. S. (2011). Why take an HIV test? Concerns, benefits, and strategies to promote HIV testing among low-income heterosexual African American young adults. *Health Education & Behavior, 38*(5), 462–470. https://doi.org/10.1177/1090198110382501

6

Health Literacy Levels of Women and Related Factors in Turkey

Sultan AYAZ-ALKAYA[1] • Fatma Ozlem OZTURK[2]*

ABSTRACT

Background: Health literacy is a complex issue affecting the health outcomes of women and their families.

Purpose: This study was conducted to determine the health literacy levels and related factors of women attending various courses in family centers of a municipality.

Methods: This cross-sectional research was conducted on a sample of women enrolled in various courses at eight family centers in a city center. The sample consisted of 837 women who agreed to participate. The participation rate was 76%. Two different health literacy scales were used to collect data for analysis.

Results: Of the women, 50.4% were over 40 years old, 35.2% were high school graduates, 89.6% were not working, 53.2% self-reported their monthly income as equal to their monthly expenses, 88.8% had social security, 28.4% had chronic diseases, 29.2% used medication regularly, 35.2% had visual problems, 7.8% had hearing problems, and 77.9% used the internet. According to the results of the Turkish Health Literacy Scale, 45.9% of the participants were in the inadequate category, 30.6% were in the inadequate and limited category, 16.0% were in the adequate category, and 7.4% were in the excellent category. Women aged 40 years and over, those who were elementary school graduates, those who had visual and hearing problems, those who used eyewear, those whose monthly income was less than expenses, and those who were non-internet users respectively had mean health literary scores that were significantly below the mean score for all participants ($p < .05$).

Conclusions/Implications for Practice: The largest number of participants was categorized has having a "low-insufficient" level of health literacy. Age, educational level, income, having visual and hearing problems, wearing glasses, and internet use were found to affect level of health literacy. For this reason, factors such as age, educational level, income, vision and hearing problems, use of eyeglasses, and internet use should be considered when planning initiatives to increase health literacy in women.

KEY WORDS:
women, women's health, health literacy, health promotion.

Introduction

Health literacy has become an important issue in recent years. Health literacy is defined as the cognitive and social skills that determine the motivation and ability of individuals to gain access to, understand, and use information in ways that promote and maintain good health (World Health Organization, n.d.). Individuals with high levels of health literacy are likely to use health services more effectively, make appropriate decisions, and protect their health (Ho et al., 2018; Tehrani et al., 2018). Low levels of health literacy result in more frequent use of emergency services, increased hospitalization and drug use, and lower utilization of preventive services. In addition, these factors lead to poorer health outcomes and increased healthcare costs (Maricic et al., 2020).

Health literacy levels vary from medium to low worldwide. In the United States, the percentage of adults with sufficient health literacy has been around 12% for at least the past decade (Goodman et al., 2013). In a 2015 study conducted in eight European countries (Austria, Bulgaria, Germany, Greece, Ireland, Netherlands, Poland, and Spain), 12% of respondents showed insufficient health literacy and 47% showed inadequate or limited health literacy (Sørensen et al., 2015). According to the findings of a study conducted in several Asian countries (Indonesia, Kazakhstan, Malaysia, Myanmar, Taiwan, and Vietnam), "problem-limited" was the most prevalent level of health literacy found, and the distribution of health literacy rates was similar across all of these countries (Duong et al., 2017). In Turkey, 64.6% of the general adult population was found to have inadequate or limited health literacy levels (Ozkan, 2018).

Although health literacy is an important issue affecting all of society, particular attention should be given to women. Women with higher levels of health literacy are better able to notice health problems, access healthcare in a timely

[1]PhD, RN, Professor, Faculty of Health Sciences, Department of Nursing, Gazi University, Ankara, Turkey • [2]PhD, RN, Lecturer, Faculty of Nursing, Department of Nursing, Ankara University, Ankara, Turkey.

manner, provide recommended treatments, and follow up on healthcare situations (Tehrani et al., 2018). In addition, women are one of the most sensitive and vulnerable groups in society because their maternal physiology threatens them with many risks and diseases. As women play an important role in maintaining and improving their own health as well as the health of their families, they are in a good position to positively influence the health of society at large. Therefore, the health literacy level of women affects not only themselves but also their children and families (Rakhshkhorshid & Sarasiyabi, 2017; Tehrani et al., 2018).

Health literacy is a complex issue that affects many women and may negatively affect their knowledge, ability to comply with healthcare plans and disease-prevention activities, and health outcomes for themselves and their children (Corrarino, 2013; Tehrani et al., 2018). Health literacy affects reproductive health services that target women. Information about contraception, safe sexual practices, healthy pregnancies, and postpartum preventive care is important to help women maintain their health and lead productive lives (Kilfoyle et al., 2016). Making informed decisions that lead to better health outcomes for themselves and their families is difficult for women in the absence of sufficient health-related knowledge. Therefore, health literacy is an important factor affecting a woman's ability to understand, process, and act on health-related information (Rakhshkhorshid & Sarasiyabi, 2017). Increasing the literacy rate of women may lead to improved health and reductions in the rates of illness and death (Tehrani et al., 2018). Therefore, more attention should be given to increasing health literacy in women. Nurses play a vital role in promoting health literacy, as they are the members of a profession that communicates and interacts actively with society and individuals (Loan et al., 2018).

Interventions designed to increase heath literacy typically include written educational materials prepared at an appropriate reading level that are designed to increase health knowledge, self-efficacy, and self-advocacy skills using clear communication, training, and counseling (Ayaz-Alkaya et al., 2020; Shieh et al., 2009). Determining a woman's health literacy is the first step toward improving this level (Corrarino, 2013). Studies in the literature that have investigated health literacy in women have measured health literacy using a single national or international instrument such as the Test of Functional Health Literacy in Adults (Maricic et al., 2020), Rapid Estimate of Adult Literacy in Medicine Revised (Jarahi et al., 2017), European Health Literacy Survey Questionnaire (Huang et al., 2020), and Iranian Health Literacy Questionnaire (Rakhshkhorshid & Sarasiyabi, 2017, Tehrani et al., 2018). In this study, health literacy level was evaluated using two scales. One of these scales was developed specifically for Turkish adults, and the other was adapted to Turkish culture from a different culture. This study differs from other studies in terms of its use of two different scales to assess health literacy in women, which enhances the sensitivity of the subsequent analysis and strengthens the validity of the findings.

This study was conducted to determine the health literacy and related factors of Turkish women attending courses at family centers in a municipality. The research questions were the following:

• What is the health literacy level of the participants?
• Do sociodemographic variables affect health literacy?
• Do visual and hearing problems affect health literacy?
• Does internet use affect health literacy?

Methods

Design and Participants

This was a cross-sectional research. The sample consisted of women enrolled in various courses at eight family centers in a metropolitan area ($N = 1,100$), who were presumed to be representative of adult women living in metropolitan areas in Turkey. The national employment rate of women in Turkey (29.1%; Turkish Statistical Institute, 2020) was similar to the rate in the city where this study was conducted. Unemployed women attend courses at family centers in preparation for seeking employment to contribute to family income and to make efficient use of their free time. Typical courses offered at family centers include knitting, dyeing, painting, jewelry design, computer, and skin care. Women may attend only one course at a time. The participants reside in the region where the family centers are located and share similar socioeconomic and cultural characteristics to others living in the same region. Any woman over the age of 18 years is eligible to register for family center courses. The sample consisted of the 837 women in these centers who agreed to participate. The participation rate was 76%.

Inclusion criteria were as follows: (a) aged 18–74 years, (b) currently registered for a course at a family center, and (c) agreed to participate in the research. Exclusion criteria were as follows: (a) over 74 years old and (b) having any neuropsychiatric disease.

Instruments

Data were collected using a personal information datasheet, the Turkish Health Literacy Scale-32 (THLS-32; developed for use in multiple cultural settings and later adapted for use in Turkey), and the Adult Health Literacy Scale (AHLS; developed specifically for use in Turkish populations). The use of more than one health literacy scale in this study was intended to increase the sensitivity of results.

The personal information datasheet was developed based on the literature (Ayaz-Alkaya & Terzi, 2019; Huang et al., 2020; Maricic et al., 2020) and consisted of closed-ended questions covering respondent age, educational level, working status, income level, social security, presence of chronic disease (diabetes, hypertension, heart failure, asthma, and hyperthyroidism), drug use, visual problems (myopia, hyperopia, blurred vision, dry eye, and wearing glasses), hearing problems (presbycusis and hearing impairment), and internet use.

The THLS-32 was developed by the European Health Literacy Research Consortium in 2012 (HLS-EU Consortium, 2012). The THLS-32 consists of 32 questions that evaluate the two dimensions of disease prevention and health promotion. The THLS-32 is scored using a 5-point Likert scale (1 = *very easy*, 2 = *easy*, 3 = *hard*, 4 = *very hard*, and 5 = *no idea*). The indexes were standardized with the help of the formula [index = (average − 1) × (50/3)] to generate a value range between 0 and 50. The obtained score is classified into four categories. Health literacy level scores of 0–25 points indicate inadequate health literacy, 26–33 points indicate limited health literacy, 34–42 points indicate adequate health literacy, and 43–50 points indicate excellent health literacy. The validity and reliability of this scale were tested by Okyay and Abacigil (2016), and its construct validity was examined using basic components (extraction method: principal components). Kaiser–Meyer–Olkin (KMO) value in evaluating the adequacy of sample size was found to be 0.90. The significance of the Bartlett's test results (χ^2 = 5206.808, SD = 496, $p < .001$) supports the factor analysis. To test the reliability of the scale, internal consistency (Cronbach's alpha) analysis was conducted, with a Cronbach's alpha coefficient of .93 found. In this study, the Cronbach's alpha of the scale was found to be .95.

The AHLS was developed by Sezer and Kadıoğlu (2014) to assess health-literacy competency in adults. This scale includes 22 items related to health information and drug use, and one figure used to assess knowledge of the location of organs in the body. Among the questions in the scale, 13 are yes/no, four are fill in the blanks, four are multiple-choice, and two are matching questions. The questions are scored separately according to question type. Total possible scores for this scale range from 0 to 23, with higher scores indicating a higher level of health literacy. The content and construct validities of this scale were examined, with the general content validity index found to be 90.71%. KMO criteria and Bartlett's test were used to test the construct validity of the scale using factor analysis. The KMO coefficient of .71 and Bartlett's test result of $p < .01$ indicate that the sample size used was sufficient for factor analysis. The Cronbach's alpha coefficient for the AHLS was .77. In this study, the Cronbach's alpha of the scale was found to be .73.

Data Collection

Research for this study was carried out between April 15, 2019, and May 15, 2019. Before data collection, the researcher informed the managers of the targeted family centers about the research. The researcher, with the managers, explained the research to the women who were attending courses at the family centers. Informed consent was obtained from each woman who agreed to participate. The women were informed that participation in this study was voluntary and that they could withdraw without prejudice at any time. Those who agreed to participate were given the study instruments in a sealed envelope. The researcher supervised the

completion and collection of these instruments. Data collection lasted approximately 20–25 minutes.

Ethical Considerations

Before data collection, ethical approval was obtained from Ankara University (Date: April 8, 2019, No. 09/157), and written permission was given by the Provincial Directorate of National Education. Written consent from each participant was obtained after reading the informed consent form.

Data Analysis

Data analysis was performed using SPSS Statistics Version 15.0 (SPSS Inc., Chicago, IL, USA). The distribution of data was evaluated using the Kolmogrov-Smirnov normality test. Descriptive variables were expressed as frequencies, percentages, mean, and standard deviation. Categorical data were compared using the chi-square test. Independent *t* tests were used in two groups, which had continuous variables, and one-way analysis of variance was used for more than two groups.

Results

Half (50.4%) of the participants were over 40 years old, 35.2% were high school graduates, 89.6% were not working, 53.2% stated that their monthly income was equal to expenses, 88.8% had social security, 28.4% had chronic diseases, 29.2% used medication regularly, 35.2% had visual problems, 7.8% had hearing problems, and 77.9% regularly used the internet (Table 1). The results from the THLS-32 showed that 45.9% of the participants were in the inadequate category, 30.6% were in the limited category, 16% were in the adequate category, and 7.4% were in the excellent category of health literacy.

In addition, on the basis of the THLS-32 results, being ≥ 40 years old, having an elementary school education, having visual and hearing problems, and using eyewear significantly increased the risk of being in the lower (inadequate and limited) categories of health literacy ($p < .05$). Furthermore, participants who were employed, had a monthly income in excess of expenses, had social security, had a chronic disease, or used the internet were significantly more likely to be in the higher (adequate and excellent) categories of health literacy ($p < .05$; Table 2).

On the basis of the AHLS results, being ≥ 40 years old, having an elementary school education, having visual and hearing problems, using eyewear, having a monthly income less than expenses, and not using the internet were each significantly associated with a lower health literacy score ($p < .05$; Table 3).

Discussion

Health literacy refers to the skills and competencies necessary to meet the complex requirements of health in modern society (Maricic et al., 2020). Health literacy is important because it affects not only women as the primary caregiver but also the family's health (Yuen et al., 2018). In this study, most of the participants scored in the inadequate or limited category of health literacy. Similarly, Huang et al. (2020) found most respondents to have inadequate (17.6%) or limited (49.3%) health literacy. The results of a meta-analysis study conducted by Charoghchian Khorasani et al. (2020) found that 31.7% of women had inadequate health literacy and 41.6% had marginal health literacy. Wang et al. (2015) reported that 51.0% of women had a low level of health literacy. Rakhshkhorshid and Sarasiyabi (2017) found that 100% of women of reproductive age had inadequate health literacy. The results of this study seem to be comparable with these and other findings reported in the literature. Women are

Table 1

Descriptive Characteristics of the Women (N = 837)

Descriptive Characteristic	n	%
Age (years)		
18–39	415	49.6
≥ 40	422	50.4
Educational level		
Primary school	250	29.9
Secondary school	171	20.4
High school	295	35.2
University	121	14.5
Working		
Yes	87	10.4
No	750	89.6
Income		
Less than expense	323	38.6
Equal to expense	445	53.2
More than expense	69	8.2
Social security		
Yes	738	88.2
No	99	11.8
Having any chronic disease		
Yes	238	28.4
No	599	71.6
Regular medication usage		
Yes	244	29.2
No	593	70.8
Visual problems		
Yes	295	35.2
No	542	64.8
Wearing glasses		
Yes	295	35.2
No	542	64.8
Hearing problems		
Yes	65	7.8
No	772	92.2
Internet use		
Yes	652	77.9
No	185	22.1

Table 2

Factors Related to Health Literacy Levels Based on Turkish Health Literacy Scale-32 Results (N = 837)

Factor	Inadequate and Limited		Adequate and Excellent		p
	n	%	n	%	
Age (years)					.001
18–39	297	71.6	118	28.4	
≥ 40	343	81.3	79	18.7	
Educational level					.001
Primary school	208	83.2	42	16.8	
Secondary school	135	78.9	36	21.1	
High school	217	73.6	78	26.4	
University	80	66.1	41	33.9	
Working					.011
Yes	57	65.5	30	34.5	
No	583	77.7	167	22.3	
Income					.009
Less than expense	260	80.5	63	19.5	
Equal to expense	336	75.5	109	24.5	
More than expense	44	63.8	25	36.2	
Social security					.036
Yes	556	75.3	182	24.7	
No	84	84.8	15	15.2	
Having any chronic disease					.019
Yes	169	71.0	69	29.0	
No	471	78.6	128	21.4	
Regular medication usage					.124
Yes	178	73.0	66	27.0	
No	462	77.9	131	22.1	
Visual problems					.002
Yes	244	82.7	51	17.3	
No	396	73.1	146	26.9	
Wearing glasses					.005
Yes	242	82.0	53	18.0	
No	398	73.4	144	26.6	
Hearing problems					.026
Yes	57	87.7	8	12.3	
No	583	75.5	189	24.5	
Internet use					< .001
Yes	477	73.2	175	26.8	
No	163	88.1	22	11.9	

key to maintaining and improving the health of both the community and the family. Therefore, increasing women's health literacy levels is vital.

Age, income, occupation, and education have all been reported to be associated with health literacy in previous studies (Huang et al., 2020; Rakhshkhorshid & Sarasiyabi, 2017; Tehrani et al., 2018). In this study, on the basis of both the results of the THLS-32 and AHLS, it was determined that

Table 3

Factors Related to Health Literacy Levels According to the Adult Health Literacy Scale (N = 837)

Factor	n	Mean	SD	p
Age (years)				< .001
18–39	415	12.47	3.69	
≥ 40	422	11.09	4.06	
Educational level				< .001
Primary school	250	9.87	3.95	
Secondary school	171	11.05	3.61	
High school	295	13.00	3.41	
University	121	13.73	3.58	
Working				.094
Yes	87	12.44	3.53	
No	750	11.70	3.98	
Income				< .001
Less than expense	323	10.82	4.21	
Equal to expense	445	12.51	3.55	
More than expense	69	11.46	4.06	
Social security				.623
Yes	738	11.80	3.96	
No	99	11.59	3.75	
Having any chronic disease				.433
Yes	238	11.60	4.40	
No	599	11.84	3.74	
Regular medication usage				.159
Yes	244	11.47	4.42	
No	593	11.90	3.72	
Visual problems				.009
Yes	295	11.29	4.20	
No	542	12.04	3.76	
Wearing glasses				.032
Yes	295	11.38	4.16	
No	542	11.99	3.80	
Hearing problems				.037
Yes	65	10.80	4.25	
No	772	11.86	3.90	
Internet use				< .001
Yes	652	12.48	3.54	
No	185	9.30	4.26	

the participants who were 40 years old and over, were elementary school graduates, and earned an income below their expenses were significantly more likely to be in the inadequate and limited categories of health literacy. In addition, the results of the THLS-32 indicate that the participants who were employed had a higher likelihood of being in the adequate category of health literacy. Consistent with this study, Huang et al. (2020) showed a relationship in the women's cohort between low health literacy and the variables low socioeconomic level, low educational level, and increasing age. Rakhshkhorshid and Sarasiyabi (2017) found a significant relationship between health literacy and age. In the same study, they also showed that

even educated people with more than 12 years of education lacked sufficient health literacy and that employed women had higher health literacy than housewives or unemployed women. Tehrani et al. (2018) found that the level of health literacy in almost half of their sample of women was not adequate and that those who were employed had better health literacy than housewives. This body of evidence supports that level of health literacy decreases as women get older and increases with educational and income levels. Increasing education is important to increasing the level of health literacy because better-educated individuals are better able to obtain the information necessary to address health problems. In addition, the higher level of health literacy found in working women may be explained by their generally higher level of education and better social support network than housewives. Therefore, the education and income levels of women should be increased. Employment increases income levels leading to higher health literacy. Women should be informed about health literacy from an early age to increase their health literacy.

Health literacy plays a crucial role in the management of chronic diseases. The ability to participate in self-management is compromised when a patient is unable to fully comprehend their diagnosis and treatment (Poureslami et al., 2017). In this study, the health literacy level of women with chronic diseases was adequate to excellent according to the THLS-32. This finding may be explained by the efforts of women with chronic diseases to obtain more information to manage their chronic diseases and to be healthier. Chronic diseases are complex conditions that require knowledge and skills to manage effectively. Similarly, Liu et al. (2020) highlighted the important role of health literacy in preventing chronic diseases. Improved health literacy has been associated with reductions in chronic-disease-related risk behaviors, higher self-reported health status, and decreased rates of hospitalization (Poureslami et al., 2017).

Health literacy level affects healthcare use and healthcare outcomes in people with visual and hearing impairments (T. Harrison et al., 2012; McKee et al., 2019). Individuals with hearing or visual difficulties or disabilities face important obstacles in accessing health services, which leads to inequalities. Although various causes of these inequalities, including poor health literacy and biological health differences (related to deafness etiologies), have been identified, communication barriers represent the main factor (Withers & Speight, 2017). Many users of American Sign Language learn language, health information, and even culture through their peers rather than family, causing them to struggle to detect and correct wrong information. Because of the environment in which communication is exchanged, insufficient health literacy may be an important cause of the low health information and worse health outcomes observed in deaf individuals (McKee et al., 2019). Visually impaired people with low levels of health literacy were found to be less likely to follow healthcare recommendations than their peers with higher health literacy levels (T. Harrison et al., 2012). In this study, the health literacy level of women with visual and hearing problems and of those who wear glasses was inadequate or limited based on the results of both the THLS-32 and AHLS. In T. C. Harrison et al. (2010), women with visual impairments stated that barriers to their ability to gain information in a format amenable to their processing skills undermined their ability to build health literacy capacity. McKee et al. (2015) found that 48% of deaf participants had inadequate health literacy and that deaf individuals were 6.9 times more likely than hearing participants to have inadequate health literacy. Thus, barriers to accessing health information should be identified, and best practices should be planned to increase the health literacy of women with visual and hearing problems.

Information and communication technologies are widely used to provide health services to communities. Internet usage helps promote health literacy (Jiang & Beaudoin, 2016; Kim & Xie, 2015). In this study, the participants who did not use the internet were found to have inadequate and limited levels of health literacy based on the results of both the THLS-32 and AHLS. Similarly, there is evidence that individuals with low health literacy experience difficulties in effectively using and interacting with technologies in healthcare settings (Kim & Xie, 2015). In Jiang and Beaudoin (2016), using the internet was identified as a factor that contributes positively to health literacy. Women who use the internet should be better able to access health information and assess services for health-related issues than their peers who do not. Health-related internet use helps people build health literacy. For this reason, women should be encouraged to use the internet to increase their health literacy level.

Strengths and Limitations

The strengths of this study included the use of a large, randomly selected sample and the application of locally and internationally developed scales with good reliability. However, the study has several limitations. The results may only be generalized to women enrolled and attending courses at the family centers where the study was conducted. Moreover, data collection was limited to women who were present in courses at the centers on the day of data collection and who agreed to participate. Therefore, the findings should not be generalized to the whole population. Finally, the cross-sectional design of this study did not allow causal inferences to be made.

Conclusions

In this study, the health literacy of most of the participants was at the low-insufficient level. Therefore, special efforts should be made to increase women's health literacy, which affects not only their personal health but also the health of their families. Strategies such as effective communication, development of health education materials, increasing educational opportunities, and promotion of internet use may be used to increase the level of health literacy in women. Factors such as age, educational level, income, visual and hearing problems, need to wear glasses, and internet use were found to affect the level of health literacy. Therefore, these factors should be considered when planning initiatives to increase health literacy in women. Interventional studies designed to increase the health literacy of women should be planned and implemented in future research.

Acknowledgments
We would like to thank the family center managers and all of the women who participated in this study.

Author Contributions
Study conception and design: SAA, FOO
Data collection: FOO
Data analysis and interpretation: SAA
Drafting of the article: SAA, FOO
Critical revision of the article: SAA, FOO

References

Ayaz-Alkaya, S., & Terzi, H. (2019). Investigation of health literacy and affecting factors of nursing students. *Nurse Education in Practice, 34,* 31–35. https://doi.org/10.1016/j.nepr.2018.10.009

Ayaz-Alkaya, S., Terzi, H., Işık, B., & Sönmez, E. (2020). A healthy lifestyle education programme for health literacy and health-promoting behaviours: A pre-implementation and post-implementation study. *International Journal of Nursing Practice, 26,* Article e12793. https://doi.org/10.1111/ijn.12793

Charoghchian Khorasani, E., Tavakoly Sany, S. B., Orooji, A., Ferns, G., & Peyman, N. (2020). Health literacy in Iranian women: A systematic review and meta-analysis. *Iranian Journal of Public Health, 49*(5), 860–874.

Corrarino, J. E. (2013). Health literacy and women's health: Challenges and opportunities. *Journal of Midwifery & Women's Health, 58*(3), 257–264. https://doi.org/10.1111/jmwh.12018

Duong, T. V., Aringazina, A., Baisunova, G., Nurjanah, G., Pham, T. V., Pham, K. M., Truong, T. Q., Nguyen, K. T., Oo, W. M., Mohamad, E., Su, T. T., Huang, H. L., Sørensen, K., Pelikan, J. M., Van den Broucke, S., & Chang, P. W. (2017). Measuring health literacy in Asia: Validation of the HLS-EU-Q47 survey tool in six Asian countries. *Journal of Epidemiology, 27*(2), 80–86. https://doi.org/10.1016/j.je.2016.09.005

Goodman, M., Finnegan, R., Mohadjer, L., Krenzke, T., & Hogan, J. (2013). *Literacy, numeracy, and problem solving in technology-rich environments among U.S. adults: Results from the program for the International Assessment of Adult Competencies 2012: First look* (NCES 2014-008, U.S. Department of Education). National Centre for Education Statistics. https://files.eric.ed.gov/fulltext/ED544452.pdf

Harrison, T., Guy, S., Mackert, M., Walker, J., & Pound, P. (2012). A study of the health literacy needs of people with visual impairments. *Research and Theory for Nursing Practice*, *26*(2), 142–160. https://doi.org/10.1891/1541-6577.26.2.142

Harrison, T. C., Mackert, M., & Watkins, C. (2010). Health literacy issues among women with visual impairments. *Research in Gerontological Nursing*, *3*(1), 49–60. https://doi.org/10.3928/19404921-20090731-01

HLS-EU Consortium. (2012). *Comparative report of health literacy in eight EU member states: The European health literacy survey (HLS-EU)*. Online Publication. http://www.health-literacy.eu

Ho, T. G., Hosseinzadeh, H., Rahman, B., & Sheikh, M. (2018). Health literacy and health-promoting behaviours among Australian–Singaporean communities living in Sydney metropolitan area. *Proceedings of Singapore Healthcare*, *27*(2), 125–131. https://doi.org/10.1177/2010105817741906

Huang, C. H., Talley, P. C., Lin, C. W., Huang, R. Y., Liu, I. T., Chiang, I. H., Lu, I. C., Lai, Y. C., & Kuo, K. M. (2020). Factors associated with low health literacy among community-dwelling women in Taiwan. *Women & Health*, *60*(5), 487–501. https://doi.org/10.1080/03630242.2019.1662872

Jarahi, L., Asadi, R., & Hakimi, H. R. (2017). General health literacy assessment of Iranian women in Mashhad. *Electronic Physician*, *9*(11), 5764–5769. https://doi.org/10.19082/5764

Jiang, S., & Beaudoin, C. E. (2016). Health literacy and the internet: An exploratory study on the 2013 HINTS survey. *Computers in Human Behavior*, *58*, 240–248. https://doi.org/10.1016/j.chb.2016.01.007

Kilfoyle, K. A., Vitko, M., O'Conor, R., & Bailey, S. C. (2016). Health literacy and women's reproductive health: A systematic review. *Journal of Women's Health*, *25*(12), 1237–1255. https://doi.org/10.1089/jwh.2016.5810

Kim, H., & Xie, B. (2015). Health literacy and internet- and mobile app-based health services: A systematic review of the literature. *Proceedings of the Association for Information Science and Technology*, *52*(1), 1–4. https://doi.org/10.1002/pra2.2015.145052010075

Liu, L., Qian, X., Chen, Z., & He, T. (2020). Health literacy and its effect on chronic disease prevention: Evidence from China's data. *BMC Public Health*, *20*, Article No. 690. https://doi.org/10.1186/s12889-020-08804-4

Loan, L. A., Parnell, T. A., Stichler, J. F., Boyle, D. K., Allen, P., VanFosson, C. A., & Barton, A. J. (2018). Call for action: Nurses must play a critical role to enhance health literacy. *Nursing Outlook*, *66*(1), 97–100. https://doi.org/10.1016/j.outlook.2017.11.003

Maricic, M., Curuvija, R. A., & Stepovic, M. (2020). Health literacy in female—Association with socioeconomic factors and effects on reproductive health. *Serbian Journal of Experimental and Clinical Research*, *21*(2), 127–132. https://doi.org/10.2478/sjecr-2018-0055

McKee, M. M., Paasche-Orlow, M. K., Winters, P. C., Fiscella, K., Zazove, P., Sen, A., & Pearson, T. (2015). Assessing health literacy in deaf American sign language users. *Journal of Health Communication*, *20*(2, Suppl.), 92–100. https://doi.org/10.1080/10810730.2015.1066468

McKee, M. M., Hauser, P. C., Champlin, S., Paasche-Orlow, M., Wyse, K., Cuculick, J., Buis, L. R., Plegue, M., Sen, A., & Fetters, M. D. (2019). Deaf adults' health literacy and access to health information: Protocol for a multicenter mixed methods study. *JMIR Research Protocols*, *8*(10), Article e14889. https://doi.org/10.2196/14889

Okyay, P., & Abacigil, F. (2016). *Turkey health literacy scale, reliability and validity* (1st ed., pp. 77–80). Ministry of Health. (Original work published in Turkish)

Ozkan, S. (2018). *Turkey health literacy levels and related factors research* (pp. 55–80). Turkish Ministry of Health General Directorate of Health Promotion. (Original work published in Turkish)

Poureslami, I., Nimmon, L., Rootman, I., & Fitzgerald, M. J. (2017). Health literacy and chronic disease management: Drawing from expert knowledge to set an agenda. *Health Promotion International*, *32*(4), 743–754. https://doi.org/10.1093/heapro/daw003

Rakhshkhorshid, M., & Sarasiyabi, A. S. (2017). Investigation of the health literacy level of women in reproductive age as a public health problem in Zahedan. *International Journal of Basic Science in Medicine*, *2*(2), 101–105. https://doi.org/10.15171/ijbms.2017.19

Sezer, A., & Kadıoğlu, H. (2014). Development of adult health literacy scale. *Journal of Anatolia Nursing and Health Sciences*, *17*(3), 165–170. (Original work published in Turkish)

Shieh, C., Mays, R., McDaniel, A., & Yu, J. (2009). Health literacy and its association with the use of information sources and with barriers to information seeking in clinic-based pregnant women. *Health Care for Women International*, *30*(11), 971–988. https://doi.org/10.1080/07399330903052152

Sørensen, K., Pelikan, J. M., Röthlin, F., Ganahl, K., Slonska, Z., Doyle, G., Fullam, J., Konilis, B., Agrafiotis, D., Uiters, E., Falcon, M., Mensing, M., Tchamov, K., Van Den Broucke, S., Brand, H., & HLS-EU Consortium. (2015). Health literacy in Europe: Comparative results of the European health literacy survey (HLS-EU). *European Journal of Public Health*, *25*(6), 1053–1058. https://doi.org/10.1093/eurpub/ckv043

Tehrani, H., Rahmani, M., & Jafari, A. (2018). Health literacy and its relationship with general health of women referring to health care centers. *Journal of Health Literacy*, *3*(3), 191–198. https://doi.org/10.22038/JHL.2018.36901.1021

Turkish Statistical Institute. (2020). *Labor statistics, July 2020*. https://data.tuik.gov.tr/tr/display-bulletin/?bulletin=isgucu-istatistikleri-temmuz-2020-33791 (Original work published in Turkish)

Wang, C., Kane, R. L., Xu, D., & Meng, Q. (2015). Health literacy as a moderator of health-related quality of life responses to chronic disease among Chinese rural women. *BMC Women's Health*, *15*, Article No. 34. https://doi.org/10.1186/s12905-015-0190-5

Withers, J., & Speight, C. (2017). Health care for individuals with hearing loss or vision loss a minefield of barriers to accessibility. *North Carolina Medical Journal*, *78*(2), 107–112. https://doi.org/10.18043/ncm.78.2.107

World Health Organization. (n.d.) *Health promotion—Track 2: Health literacy and health behaviour*. https://www.who.int/healthpromotion/conferences/7gchp/track2/en

Yuen, E. Y. N., Knight, T., Ricciardelli, L. A., & Burney, S. (2018). Health literacy of caregivers of adult care recipients: A systematic scoping review. *Health & Social Care in the Community*, *26*(2), e191–e206. https://doi.org/10.1111/hsc.12368

7

Machine-Based Hand Massage Ameliorates Preoperative Anxiety in Patients Awaiting Ambulatory Surgery

Cheng-Hua NI[1] • Li WEI[2] • Chia-Che WU[3] • Chueh-Ho LIN[4] • Pao-Yu CHOU[5] •
Yeu-Hui CHUANG[6,8] • Ching-Chiu KAO[7]*

ABSTRACT

Background: Hand massage therapies have been used to relieve anxiety and pain in various clinical situations. The effects of machine-based hand massage on preoperative anxiety in ambulatory surgery settings have not been evaluated.

Purpose: This prospective study was designed to investigate the effect of machine-based hand massage on preoperative anxiety and vital signs in ambulatory surgery patients.

Methods: One hundred ninety-nine patients aged 18 years and older who were scheduled to receive ambulatory surgery were recruited from the Taipei Municipal Wanfang Hospital in Taipei City, Taiwan. The patients were assigned randomly to the experimental group ($n = 101$), which received presurgical machine-based hand massage therapy, and the control group ($n = 98$), which received no intervention. The patients in both groups completed the Spielberger State-Trait Anxiety Inventory short form at preintervention (baseline) and postintervention.

Results: Within-group comparisons of Spielberger State-Trait Anxiety Inventory short form scores showed significant decreases between preintervention and postintervention scores in the experimental group (44.3 ± 11.2 to 37.9 ± 8.7) and no significant change in the control group. Within-group comparisons of vital signs revealed a significant increase in mean respiration rate between baseline and postintervention in both groups (both $ps < .05$). Blood pressure was found to have decreased significantly only in the control group at postintervention ($p < .05$). No significant preintervention to postintervention change in pulse was observed in either group.

Conclusions: The findings of this study indicate that machine-based hand massage reduces anxiety significantly in patients awaiting ambulatory surgery while not significantly affecting their vital signs.

KEY WORDS:
ambulatory surgery, anxiety, hand massage, preoperative, State-Trait Anxiety Inventory (STAI).

most common negative emotion in patients awaiting diagnostic procedures such as coronary angiography and may contribute to complications during these procedures (H. Li et al., 2016; Mei et al., 2017). Investigators have suggested that the preoperative waiting period in the hospital is an extended period during which patients tend to worry about their impending surgery/procedure (Gilmartin & Wright, 2008; Mitchell, 2003). Anxiety has been shown to affect the physiological and psychological status of patients adversely. In addition, preoperative anxiety has been identified as a predictor of postoperative pain (Brand et al., 2013; Kunikata et al., 2012) and has been associated with delayed recovery (Mavros et al., 2011). Furthermore, reducing anxiety in preoperative patients is important because undue anxiety may also interfere with patients' ability to learn and remember

[1]MS, RN, Supervisor, Department of Nursing, Center for Nursing and Healthcare Research in Clinical Practice Application, Wan Fang Hospital, Taipei Medical University, and Adjunct Assistant Professor, School of Nursing, College of Nursing, Taipei Medical University, Taiwan, ROC • [2]MD, PhD, Assistant Professor, Graduate Institute of Injury Prevention and Control, College of Public Health, Taipei Medical University, and Attending Physician, Division of Neurosurgery, Department of Surgery, Wan Fang Hospital, Taipei Medical University, Taiwan, ROC • [3]MD, PhD, Assistant Professor, School of Medicine, College of Medicine, Taipei Medical University, and Attending Physician, Department of Otolaryngology, Wan Fang Hospital, Taipei Medical University, Taiwan, ROC • [4]PhD, PT, Associate Professor, Master Program in Long-Term Care, College of Nursing, Taipei Medical University, Taiwan, ROC • [5]MS, RN, Head Nurse, Department of Nursing, and Center for Nursing and Healthcare Research in Clinical Practice Application, Wan Fang Hospital, Taipei Medical University, and Adjunct Instructor, School of Nursing, College of Nursing, Taipei Medical University, Taiwan, ROC • [6]PhD, RN, Professor, School of Nursing, College of Nursing, Taipei Medical University, and Center for Nursing and Healthcare Research in Clinical Practice Application, Wan Fang Hospital, Taipei Medical University, Taiwan, ROC • [7]MS, RN, Executive Director of Community Medicine, Center for Nursing and Healthcare Research in Clinical Practice Application, Wan Fang Hospital, Taipei Medical University, and Adjunct Assistant Professor, School of Nursing, College of Nursing, Taipei Medical University, Taiwan, ROC • [8]Contributed equally as corresponding author.

Introduction

Anxiety is recognized as a normal response of patients during the preoperative period. Anxiety has been identified as the

important postoperative home care instructions (Gilmartin & Wright, 2008).

The application of hand massage therapy in outpatients waiting for ambulatory surgery or diagnostic procedures has been evaluated in several previous studies (Brand et al., 2013; Kunikata et al., 2012; Nazari et al., 2012). Lower anxiety levels of anxiety have been reported in patients receiving hand massage therapy than in their peers who received routine nursing care only (Brand et al., 2013). Kunikata et al. (2012) measured autonomic activity and psychological indicators before and after a hand massage intervention, reporting a significant decrease in heart rate after the intervention, indicating a decrease in autonomic and sympathetic nerve activity and a promotion of relaxation. Furthermore, hand massage has been reported to reduce preoperative anxiety significantly in patients scheduled to receive ophthalmology surgery under local anesthesia (Kim et al., 2001; Nazari et al., 2012).

Various other applications of hand massage therapies have been used to relieve anxiety and pain in different clinical situations. For example, adding intraoperative hand reflexology during a minimally invasive conscious surgery for varicose veins was found to reduce patients' anxiety and the duration of postoperative pain (Hudson et al., 2015). Similarly, hand reflexology was shown to decrease anxiety in a clinical trial designed to study the effects of this intervention in patients waiting to receive a coronary angiography (Mobini-Bidgoli et al., 2017). Both hand massage and hand-holding methods delivered by nurses have been shown to reduce anxiety and to promote a sense of affinity in the patient toward the massage giver, with the one-on-one contact involved in massage associated with a positive anxiolytic effect (Kunikata et al., 2012).

Massage machines have been applied in clinical settings for years (Q. Li et al., 2019; Yoshida et al., 2014). Although the effects of manual hand massage on preoperative anxiety in ambulatory surgery patients have been studied previously (Kim et al., 2001; Nazari et al., 2012), to the best of our knowledge, the effect of machine-based hand massage on preoperative anxiety in ambulatory surgical settings has not yet been evaluated. Machine-based hand massage may be as effective as physical massage in ambulatory surgery patients awaiting ambulatory surgical procedures under local anesthesia. Therefore, the aim of this study was to evaluate the effects of machine-based hand massage on preoperative anxiety and vital signs in ambulatory surgery patients.

Methods

Study Design and Sample

This prospective study was conducted in the waiting area outside the surgical suites at Taipei Municipal Wanfang Hospital, Taipei, Taiwan. Patients awaiting ambulatory surgery aged 18 years and older were recruited using a random sampling approach from the Departments of Otolaryngology, Dermatology, Urology, and General Surgery from July 2016 to June 2017. Patients with catastrophic illness cards, a mental illness, or a malignant tumor and those who were scheduled for hand surgery were excluded. Screened patients waiting for surgery were asked to fill out a situational anxiety questionnaire and were instructed on how to complete it. Those who agreed to complete the questionnaire and were willing to participate in the study were enrolled as participants. All of the included patients ($n = 199$) were randomly assigned to either the experimental group ($n = 101$), which received presurgical hand massage therapy, or the control group ($n = 98$), which received no intervention.

Ethical Considerations

This study was approved by the Taipei Medical University Joint Institutional Review Board (approval number: N201512022). All of the participants provided signed informed consent to participate.

Intervention Procedure

The patient waiting area for ambulatory surgery was air-conditioned and had individually partitioned spaces and sofa-type seating with backs, allowing the patients to wait for surgery in comfort. The vital signs of patients in both groups were measured, and their basic demographic information was collected by the research assistants. The experimental equipment consisted of sphygmomanometers, ear thermometer, and hand massage machines. Participants in both groups received general, routine surgical nursing care. All of the participants were scheduled to undergo local surgery with local anesthesia and were discharged from the hospital on the same day.

To ensure the consistency of hand massage, the participants in the experimental group each received 15 minutes of hand massage administered using two identical commercial hand massagers (Breo iPalm 520 acupressure hand massager with heat compression; Chino, CA, USA) on each hand simultaneously. The hand massager temperature was set at 39°C. The machine was covered with plastic wrap for each use, which was replaced after each use to prevent cross-contamination. Patients in both groups completed the postintervention situational anxiety questionnaire after all of the experimental group participants had received hand massages.

Anxiety Evaluation

The short form of the Spielberger State-Trait Anxiety Inventory (STAI-S; Marteau & Bekker, 1992) was used to measure anxiety. The STAI-S is a self-administered scale suitable for use with adults and teenagers. This instrument comprises the situational anxiety and trait anxiety subscales, comprising 20 questions scored using a 4-point Likert scale. The STAI-S has been used in clinical settings to diagnose anxiety and to differentiate it from depression. A Chinese version of the STAI-S has been used widely in Taiwan to evaluate responses to various therapies (Lee et al., 2017; Wu et al., 2017). For the 10-item situational anxiety subscale, 1 represents *not at*

Table 1

Baseline Demographics and Clinical Characteristics of the Participants

Variable	Control (*n* = 98)		Hand Massage Therapy (*n* = 101)		*p* [a]
	Mean	**SD**	**Mean**	**SD**	
Age (years)	41.1	14.0	41.3	15.7	.93
Height (cm)	166.7	8.9	165.9	9.4	.32
Weight (kg)	67.3	14.6	65.3	14.5	.27
Pain score [b]	0.1	0.3	0.1	0.2	.12
Pulse rate (bpm)	79.1	13.6	77.9	13.2	.47
Respiration rate (bpm)	16.4	1.9	16.5	1.7	.88
Systolic pressure (mmHg)	132.9	22.7	133.2	21.9	.73
Diastolic pressure (mmHg)	78.9	13.2	77.4	13.4	.38
	n	**%**	***n***	**%**	
Gender					.35 [c]
Male	54	55.1	49	48.5	
Female	44	44.9	52	51.5	
Education					.44 [c]
Elementary	4	4.1	10	9.9	
Junior	7	7.1	7	6.9	
Senior	24	24.5	32	31.7	
Faculty	14	14.3	11	10.9	
Bachelor	35	35.7	30	29.7	
Master or above	14	14.3	11	10.9	
Religion					.63 [c]
Buddhist	35	35.7	36	35.6	
Catholic/Christian	48	49.0	54	53.5	
Muslim	15	15.3	11	10.9	
Marital status					.20 [d]
Unmarried	35	35.7	42	41.6	
Married	54	55.1	56	55.5	
Divorced	6	6.1	3	2.9	
Widowed	3	3.1	0	0	
Living status					.51 [d]
Alone	14	14.3	11	10.9	
With family	80	81.6	88	87.1	
With friends	4	4.1	2	2.0	
Working status					.04 [d,*]
No	21	21.4	33	32.7	
Yes	68	69.4	57	56.4	
Retired	6	6.1	11	10.9	
Cannot work with disease	3	3.1	0	0	
Smoking status					.29 [c]
No	65	66.3	77	76.2	
Yes	25	25.5	19	18.8	
Quit smoking	8	8.2	5	5.0	
Alcohol consumption [e]					.11 [d]
No	70	71.4	82	82.0	
Yes	21	21.4	16	16.0	
Quit drinking	7	7.2	2	2.0	

(continues)

Table 1

Baseline Demographics and Clinical Characteristics of the Participants, Continued

Variable	Control (*n* = 98)		Hand Massage Therapy (*n* = 101)		*p* [a]
	Mean	SD	Mean	SD	
Accompanied during surgery					.06 [c]
No	47	48.0	35	34.7	
Yes	51	52.0	66	65.3	
Know the expected duration of surgery [e]					.49 [c]
No	65	67.7	63	63.0	
Yes	31	32.3	37	37.0	
Surgery experience [e]					.28 [c]
No	31	31.6	39	39.0	
Yes	67	68.4	61	61.0	

[a] Mann–Whitney *U* test. [b] The scale of pain score: 1 to 10. [c] Chi-square test. [d] Fisher's exact test. [e] Numbers may not equal to total sample size due to missing value.
*p < .05.

all, 2 represents *somewhat*, 3 represents *moderately so*, and 4 represents *very much so*. For the 10-item trait anxiety subscale, reverse scoring is used, with scores ranging from 1 representing *very much so* to 4 representing *not at all*. Higher STAI-S scores indicate greater anxiety. The test–retest reliability is .89 for the Chinese version of the STAI-S.

Statistical Analysis

Continuous variables are presented as mean ± standard deviation (*SD*) by group and are compared using the two-sample *t* test or Mann–Whitney *U* test for nonnormally distributed variables. Categorical variables are presented as counts and percentages and compared using the chi-square test or Fisher's exact test. A two-sample *t* test was used to detect between-group differences at baseline and postintervention and to identify changes between baseline and postintervention. Paired *t* test was employed to compare within-group differences between baseline and postevaluation. A nonparametric Mann–Whitney *U* test was applied to compare the differences between the two groups for nonnormally distributed data. All of the assessments were two-sided, and *p* < .05 was used to determine statistical significance. All statistical analyses were

performed using SAS Version 9.4, Windows NT version (SAS Institute, Inc., Cary, NC, USA).

Results

The 101 experimental group participants received hand massage therapy before surgery, whereas the 98 participants in the control group received standard care only. The baseline characteristics of the participants are shown in Table 1. The distribution of baseline characteristics was similar between the two groups, with the exception of working status. Mean age was 41.1 ± 14.0 and 41.3 ± 15.7 years for the control group and experimental group, respectively. No significant differences were found between the two groups in terms of gender, education, religion, marital status, living status, smoking status, alcohol consumption, being accompanied during surgery, knowing the length of surgery, or surgery history. However, working status was significantly different between the two groups (Table 1).

Mean changes in STAI-S scores between baseline and postintervention are shown in Table 2. Mean STAI-S scores at baseline were 44.3 ± 11.2 in the experimental group and

Table 2

Mean Changes in STAI-S Scores, by Group

STAI-S Score	Control (*n* = 98)		Hand Massage Therapy (*n* = 101)		*p*
	Mean	SD	Mean	SD	
Baseline	42.6	9.7	44.3	11.2	.26 [a]
Postintervention	43.8	9.9	37.9	8.7	< .001 [a,*]
Change from baseline to postintervention	1.1	5.7	−6.4	7.5 [b,†]	< .001 [c,*]

Note. STAI-S = Spielberger State-Trait Anxiety Inventory short form.
[a] *T* test. [b] Paired *t* test. [c] Mann–Whitney *U* test.
*Significant difference between groups, *p* < .05.
†Significant difference between preintervention and postintervention, *p* < .05.

Table 3

Mean Changes in Vital Signs, by Group

Vital Sign	Control (n = 98)		Hand Massage Therapy (n = 101)		p^a
	Mean	SD	Mean	SD	
Pulse (bpm)					
Baseline	79.1	13.6	77.9	13.2	.47
Postintervention	78.9	13.7	78.9	11.5	.91
Change from baseline to postintervention	−0.2	9.2	1.0	7.8	.31
Respiration rate (bpm)					
Baseline	16.4	1.9	16.5	1.7	.88
Postintervention	17.5	4.5	17.3	1.7	.36
Change from baseline to postintervention	1.0	4.3 [b],*	0.8	1.7 [b],*	.59
Systolic pressure (mmHg)					
Baseline	132.9	22.7	133.2	21.9	.73
Postintervention	129.9	18.4	131.9	18.0	.28
Change from baseline to postintervention	−2.9	11.6 [b],*	−1.4	11.9	.58
Diastolic pressure (mmHg)					
Baseline	78.9	13.2	77.4	13.4	.38
Postintervention	76.9	10.6	77.8	11.6	.69
Change from baseline to postintervention	−2.1	7.5 [b],*	0.4	9.1	.08

[a] Mann–Whitney *U* test. [b] Paired *t* test.
*Significant difference between preintervention and postintervention, *p* < .05.

42.6 ± 9.7 in the control group. Statistically significant differences were found in mean STAI-S scores at postintervention, which were 37.9 ± 8.7 in the experimental group and 43.8 ± 9.9 in the control group (*p* < .05). Changes in STAI-S scores from baseline (preintervention) to postintervention were also significantly different between the two groups (1.1 ± 5.7 vs. −6.4 ± 7.5; *p* < .05). In addition, an analysis of the within-group comparison revealed that hand massage significantly decreased STAI-S scores (*p* < .05; Table 2).

Mean changes in vital signs between baseline and postintervention are shown in Table 3. No significant differences were found between the groups in terms of mean changes in preintervention and postintervention vital signs, including pulse, respiration rate, systolic pressure, and diastolic pressure. In addition, within-group comparison analysis revealed that postintervention respiration rates had significantly increased from baseline in both groups (*p* < .05), whereas blood pressure was found to have decreased significantly after the intervention only in the control group (*p* < .05; Table 3).

Discussion

The results of this study show a significant difference in preintervention/postintervention STAI-S scores between the two groups, indicating that the reduction in anxiety was significantly larger in the experimental group than in the control group. In addition, the within-group comparison revealed that the intervention significantly reduced STAI-S scores in the experimental group, whereas no significant preintervention/postintervention difference was found in STAI-S

scores in the control group. In terms of vital sign measurements, the within-group comparison revealed that the postintervention mean respiration rate was significantly higher in both groups and that postintervention blood pressure significantly decreased in the control group only. No significant postintervention change in pulse was found in either group.

Anxiety in the experimental group was significantly lower after the intervention. In addition, although the control group participants received routine preoperative care only, their vital signs were not significantly different from their peers in the experimental group. These results echo those of other studies on the effects of person-delivered hand massage therapy on preoperative and preprocedure anxiety. Although all of the patients in Brand et al. (2013) reported decreased anxiety before entering the operating suite, only those who had received the hand massage intervention exhibited significantly lower anxiety as measured using visual analog scores. The nurses who cared for those patients found that hand massage and reduced anxiety made it easier to set up intravenous lines in the preoperative area because of facilitated vasodilation and patients' overall level of comfort. In another study that used the STAI to measure anxiety in preoperative patients before and after a hand massage intervention (Kunikata et al., 2012), STAI scores decreased significantly after the hand massage. However, whereas patients' blood pressure and heart rates decreased after the intervention, their respiration rate did not. In contrast, in a clinical trial on pain and anxiety after cesarean section (Saatsaz et al., 2016), pain and anxiety as well as the physiological measures of blood pressure and respiration rate were reduced significantly after a hand massage intervention. As evidence remains unclear, the relationship between receiving a hand massage and changes in postoperative vital signs should be further investigated. Potential reasons for a direct relationship are that the improved blood flow and quality of sleep resulting from massage improves perceived anxiety and that massage therapy increases parasympathetic nervous system activity, releasing neurotransmitters and/or reducing cortisol levels.

Hand massage used as an alternative or complementary therapy may be implemented as a simple and effective nursing intervention in preoperative settings (Braithwaite & Ringdahl, 2017; Brand et al., 2013). In addition to the effects on patients' preoperative/preprocedure anxiety, providing hand massage therapy is of potential benefit to nurses as well. Nurses who have administered hand massage procedures to preoperative patients have reported gaining increased awareness of patients' psychological, emotional, and medical needs (Brand et al., 2013). Hand massage may be delivered by nurses or trained volunteers, with the results of studies on volunteer-administered intervention suggesting that family members and other caregivers may be easily trained to administer hand massage therapies both before a procedure and after hospital discharge (Gensic et al., 2017). Using a machine rather than a person to provide hand massages not only reduces the workload of caregivers but also provides consistent massages. Further side-by-side pretest and posttest studies related to the clinical application of machine-based hand massage in ambulatory settings are necessary to compare the effectiveness of machine-based hand massages with hand massages administered by nurses.

Strengths and Limitations

The strengths of this study include the random selection of ambulatory surgery patients and the administration of hand massage therapy consistently across patients, which enabled the effects of the intervention on anxiety and vital signs to be evaluated. One limitation was the lack of a side-by-side comparison of the results of machine-based hand massage with the results of nurse-administered hand massage, which would indicate the comparative efficacy of the two approaches. A second limitation was that the hospital personnel (mostly nurses) who provided routine care for the two groups of ambulatory surgery patients were not blinded to the group assignments, introducing the risk of performance bias. A third limitation was that, because nurse-administered hand massage is subject to variation among different nurses and different patients, an additional study is needed to compare the two methods and to evaluate the effectiveness of machine-based hand massage therapy in a larger, multicenter population.

Conclusions

Machine-based hand massage was shown to significantly reduce anxiety in ambulatory surgery patients. However, no dramatic effects of machine-based hand massage on vital signs were observed. Further studies are necessary to confirm the results of this study and to evaluate the effects of machine-based hand massage in comparison with the effects of nurse-delivered hand massage.

Acknowledgments

The authors would like to thank all participants in this study and Wan Fang Hospital, Taipei Medical University for financial support (Grant no. : 105-TMU-WFH-12).

Author Contributions

Study conception and design: CHN, LW, CCK
Data collection: CHN, YHC, CHL, PYC, CCK
Data analysis and interpretation: YHC, CCW, CHL, LW
Drafting of the article: CHN, LW, CCK
Critical revision of the article: CHN, PYC, LW, CCK

References

Braithwaite, C. M., & Ringdahl, D. (2017). Nurse-administered hand massage: Integration into an infusion suite's standard of care. *Clinical Journal of Oncology Nursing, 21*(4), E87–E92. https://doi.org/10.1188/17.CJON.E87-E92

Brand, L. R., Munroe, D. J., & Gavin, J. (2013). The effect of hand massage on preoperative anxiety in ambulatory surgery patients. *AORN Journal, 97*(6), 708–717. https://doi.org/10.1016/j.aorn.2013.04.003

Gensic, M. E., Smith, B. R., & LaBarbera, D. M. (2017). The effects of effleurage hand massage on anxiety and pain in patients undergoing chemotherapy. *JAAPA, 30*(2), 36–38. https://doi.org/10.1097/01.JAA.0000510988.21909.2e

Gilmartin, J., & Wright, K. (2008). Day surgery: Patients' felt abandoned during the preoperative wait. *Journal of Clinical Nursing, 17*(18), 2418–2425. https://doi.org/10.1111/j.1365- 2702.2008.02374.x

Hudson, B. F., Davidson, J., & Whiteley, M. S. (2015). The impact of hand reflexology on pain, anxiety and satisfaction during minimally invasive surgery under local anaesthetic: A randomised controlled trial. *International Journal of Nursing Studies, 52*(12), 1789–1797. https://doi.org/10.1016/j.ijnurstu.2015.07.009

Kim, M. S., Cho, K. S., Woo, H., & Kim, J. H. (2001). Effects of hand massage on anxiety in cataract surgery using local anesthesia. *Journal of Cataract and Refractive Surgery, 27*(6), 884–890. https://doi.org/10.1016/S0886-3350(00)00730-6

Kunikata, H., Watanabe, K., Miyoshi, M., & Tanioka, T. (2012). The effects measurement of hand massage by the autonomic activity and psychological indicators. *Journal of Medical Investigation, 59*(1–2), 206–212. https://doi.org/10.2152/jmi.59.206

Lee, W.-L., Sung, H.-C., Liu, S.-H., & Chang, S.-M. (2017). Meditative music listening to reduce state anxiety in patients during the uptake phase before positron emission tomography (PET) scans. *British Journal of Radiology, 90*(1070), Article 20160466. https://doi.org/10.1259/bjr.20160466

Li, H., Jin, D., Qiao, F., Chen, J., & Gong, J. (2016). Relationship between the Self-Rating Anxiety Scale score and the success rate of 64-slice computed tomography coronary angiography. *International Journal of Psychiatry in Medicine, 51*(1), 47–55. https://doi.org/10.1177/0091217415621265

Li, Q., Becker, B., Wernicke, J., Chen, Y., Zhang, Y., Li, R., Le, J., Kou, J., Zhao, W., & Kendrick, K. M. (2019). Foot massage evokes oxytocin release and activation of orbitofrontal cortex and superior temporal sulcus. *Psychoneuroendocrinology, 101*, 193–203. https://doi.org/10.1016/j.psyneuen.2018.11.016

Marteau, T. M., & Bekker, H. (1992). The development of a six-item short-form of the state scale of the Spielberger State-Trait Anxiety Inventory (STAI). *British Journal of Psychology, 31*(3), 301–306. https://doi.org/10.1111/j.2044-8260.1992.tb00997.x

Mavros, M. N., Athanasiou, S., Gkegkes, I. D., Polyzos, K. A., Peppas, G., & Falagas, M. E. (2011). Do psychological variables affect early surgical recovery? *PLOS ONE, 6*(5), Article e20306. https://doi.org/10.1371/journal.pone.0020306

Mei, L., Miao, X., Chen, H., Huang, X., & Zheng, G. (2017). Effectiveness of Chinese hand massage on anxiety among patients awaiting coronary angiography: A randomized controlled trial. *Journal of Cardiovascular Nursing, 32*(2), 196–203. https://doi.org/10.1097/JCN.0000000000000309

Mitchell, M. (2003). Patient anxiety and modern elective surgery: A literature review. *Journal of Clinical Nursing, 12*(6), 806–815. https://doi.org/10.1046/j.1365-2702.2003.00812.x

Mobini-Bidgoli, M., Taghadosi, M., Gilasi, H., & Farokhian, A. (2017). The effect of hand reflexology on anxiety in patients undergoing coronary angiography: A single-blind randomized controlled trial. *Complementary Therapies in Clinical Practice, 27*, 31–36. https://doi.org/10.1016/j.ctcp.2017.01.002

Nazari, R., Ahmadzadeh, R., Mohammadi, S., & Rafiei Kiasari, J. (2012). Effects of hand massage on anxiety in patients undergoing ophthalmology surgery using local anesthesia. *Journal of Caring Sciences, 1*(3), 129–134. https://doi.org/10.5681/jcs.2012.019

Saatsaz, S., Rezaei, R., Alipour, A., & Beheshti, Z. (2016). Massage as adjuvant therapy in the management of post-cesarean pain and anxiety: A randomized clinical trial. *Complementary Therapies in Clinical Practice, 24*, 92–98. https://doi.org/10.1016/j.ctcp.2016.05.014

Wu, P. Y., Huang, M. L., Lee, W. P., Wang, C., & Shih, W. M. (2017). Effects of music listening on anxiety and physiological responses in patients undergoing awake craniotomy. *Complementary Therapies in Medicine, 32*, 56–60. https://doi.org/10.1016/j.ctim.2017.03.007

Yoshida, S., Fujiwara, K., Kohira, S., & Hirose, M. (2014). Electromagnetic interference of implantable cardiac devices from a shoulder massage machine. *Journal of Artificial Organs, 17*(3), 243–249. https://doi.org/10.1007/s10047-014-0765-1

8

Preventing Alveolar Osteitis After Molar Extraction Using Chlorhexidine Rinse and Gel

Chia-Hui WANG[1,7] • Shu-Hui YANG[2,7] • Hsiu-Ju JEN[3] • Jui-Chen TSAI[4] • Hsi-Kuei LIN[5] • El-Wui LOH[6]*

ABSTRACT

Background: Alveolar osteitis (AO) may occur after molar extraction. Chlorhexidine (CHX) rinse and CHX gel are widely used to prevent AO. Although previous meta-analyses support the effectiveness of both CHX rinse and CHX gel in preventing AO, important issues regarding these two formulations have not been addressed adequately in the literature.

Purpose: A systematic review and meta-analysis of randomized controlled trials was conducted to determine the effectiveness of CHX rinse and CHX gel in preventing AO.

Methods: PubMed, EMBASE, SCOPUS, and Cochrane databases were searched for randomized controlled trials published before June 2018. The risk ratio (RR) was used to estimate the pooled effect of AO incidence using a random-effect model.

Results: The RRs of AO in patients treated with 0.12% CHX rinse (RR = 0.54, 95% CI [0.41, 0.72]) and 0.2% CHX rinse (RR = 0.84, 95% CI [0.52, 1.35]) were significantly lower than in those treated with the control. Moreover, a significantly lower RR was identified in patients treated with 0.2% CHX gel (RR = 0.47, 95% CI [0.34, 0.64]) than in those treated with the control. When CHX products of different concentrations were grouped together, patients treated with CHX rinse showed an RR of AO of 0.61 (95% CI [0.48, 0.78]) and those treated with CHX gel showed an RR of AO of 0.44 (95% CI [0.43, 0.65]). On the other hand, a meta-analysis of three trials that compared CHX rinse and CHX gel directly showed a significantly lower RR of AO in patients treated with CHX rinse than in those treated with CHX gel (RR = 0.56, 95% CI [0.34, 0.96]).

Conclusions/Implications for Practice: The results support the effectiveness of both CHX rinse and gel in reducing the risk of AO after molar extraction. Each formulation provides unique benefits in terms of ease of application and cost. On the basis of the results of this study, the authors recommend that CHX gel be used immediately after molar extraction because of the convenience and cost-effectiveness of this treatment and that CHX rinse be used by the patient after discharge at home in combination with appropriate health education and case management.

KEY WORDS:
chlorhexidine, rinse, gel, alveolar osteitis.

Introduction

Alveolar osteitis (AO), the inflammation of the alveolar bone when an intra-alveolar blood clot disintegrates or fails to form, is one of the most common complications occurring after third molar (wisdom-tooth) extraction (Cardoso et al., 2010). AO usually manifests 2–5 days after surgery and is one of the main reasons for seeking postsurgical emergency appointments (Lee et al., 2015). Patients may experience fetid breath and persistent and radiating pain, which is not easily relieved by analgesics. The AO incidence after tooth extraction ranged from 3.2% to 6.14% in studies with large sample sizes (Abu Younis & Abu Hantash, 2011; Congiusta & Veitz-Keenan, 2013; Sigron et al., 2014) and even up to 35% in early studies (Erickson et al., 1960). Moreover, the risk of AO has been reported to be associated with the degree of difficulty involved in molar tooth extraction (Ogunlewe

[1]PhD, RN, Supervisor, Department of Nursing, Taipei Medical University Shuang Ho Hospital, and Assistant Professor, School of Nursing, College of Nursing, Taipei Medical University, Taiwan, ROC • [2]BSN, RN, Department of Nursing, Taipei Medical University Shuang Ho Hospital, Taiwan, ROC • [3]BSN, RN, Head Nurse, Department of Nursing, Taipei Medical University Shuang Ho Hospital, and Adjunct Assistant Professor, School of Nursing, College of Nursing, Taipei Medical University, Taiwan, ROC • [4]MSN, RN, Consultant, Department of Nursing, Taipei Medical University Shuang Ho Hospital, and Adjunct Assistant Professor, School of Nursing, College of Nursing, Taipei Medical University, Taiwan, ROC • [5]DDS, Department of Dentistry, Taipei Medical University Shuang Ho Hospital, and Lecturer, School of Dentistry, College of Oral Medicine, Taipei Medical University, Taiwan, ROC • [6]PhD, Joint Appointment Medical Researcher, Center for Evidence-Based Health Care and Shared Decision Making Resource Center, Department of Medical Research, and Department of Dentistry, Taipei Medical University Shuang Ho Hospital; Researcher, Cochrane Taiwan, Taipei Medical University; and Assistant Professor, Graduate Institute of Clinical Medicine, College of Medicine, Taipei Medical University, Taiwan, ROC • [7]contributed equally.

et al., 2007) and is often higher after surgical extractions than after nonsurgical extractions (Nusair & Younis, 2007).

A series of pharmacological agents, including antibacterial agents, antifibrinolytic agents, antiseptic agents, obtundent dressings, steroidal anti-inflammatory agents, clot-support agents, and growth-factor-rich plasma (Blum, 2002; Haraji et al., 2012), have each been examined for their potential in preventing AO. Chlorhexidine (CHX), an antiseptic agent developed in the 1940s, inhibits the growth of bacteria by increasing their cytoplasmic permeability and causing cell lysis. This agent is widely used for antibacterial purposes in hygiene control and surgery (Balagopal & Arjunkumar, 2013). CHX is available in the market in the form of different hygiene and treatment products such as chewing gum, toothpaste, spray, rinse, gel, and varnishes. Previous meta-analyses on both the gel and rinse formulations (Caso et al., 2005; Yengopal & Mickenautsch, 2012; Zhou et al., 2017) have suggested a prophylactic effect of CHX in terms of reducing the risk of AO after molar extraction. Although a recent systematic review and meta-analysis provided additional information on this issue, the focus of the review was on specific types of formulation (Dobson et al., 2018; Teshome, 2017) and more-recent publications were not covered (Rodriguez Sanchez et al., 2017).

A new meta-analysis of randomized controlled trials (RCTs) was performed in this study to evaluate the effectiveness of CHX rinse and CHX gel, the two most common types of CHX prophylactics, in preventing AO after molar extraction.

Methods

Literature Search
A search of the PubMed, EMBASE, SCOPUS, and Cochrane databases up to June 2018 was conducted to identify relevant trials. The following MeSH search headings were used: "alveolar osteitis," "dry socket," "alveolitis sicca dolorosa," "fibrinolytic alveolitis," "chlorhexidine," "CHX," "molar extraction," "extraction," "molar removal," "molar surgery," and "surgery." These terms and their combinations were searched as text words. The "related articles" function in PubMed was used to broaden the scope of search. All of the abstracts, studies, and citations retrieved in this search were reviewed. In addition, other trials identified by manually searching the reference sections of the accessed articles and by contacting known experts in the field were reviewed. Furthermore, relevant unpublished trials registered on the ClinicalTrials.gov registry (http://clinicaltrials.gov/) and otherwise-unlisted articles searchable in Google Scholar were searched and reviewed as well. No language restrictions were applied.

Trial Selection
Trials that met the following criteria were included in the analysis: evaluating the efficacy of CHX rinse or gel in preventing AO in dental patients undergoing molar extraction or surgery, clearly stating the inclusion and exclusion criteria used to select

patients for participation, and adequately describing the molar extraction or surgical procedures. Trials or data were excluded from analysis that examined additional components such as active gel-containing CHX and metronidazole versus placebo gel that would confound the contribution of CHX or that compared the efficacy of different CHX implication protocols of dosage, administration time, and treatment period. When duplicated articles with overlapping data sets were identified, the trial with the larger population was included.

Data Extraction and Quality Assessment

Two reviewers independently extracted the following information from each trial: first author, year of publication, trial population characteristics, trial design, inclusion and exclusion criteria, matching criteria, definition of molar tooth extraction, and incidence of AO. The retrieved studies were assessed for eligibility by the two reviewers according to the specified inclusion criteria. The individually recorded decisions of the two reviewers were compared, and any disagreements were resolved by a third reviewer.

The quality of the retrieved trials was assessed using the revised Cochrane risk-of-bias tool for randomized trials Version 2 recommended by the Cochrane Collaboration (Higgins et al., 2019). Two reviewers conducted the assessment, and any disagreement was resolved by a third reviewer. Five domains were assessed, including bias arising from the randomization process, bias due to deviations from intended interventions (effect adhering to intervention), bias due to missing outcome data, bias in measuring outcomes, and bias in selecting the reported results.

Data Synthesis and Analysis

The statistical package Review Manager, Version 5.3 (Cochrane Collaboration, Oxford, England) was used to analyze the data. The meta-analysis was performed according to the recommendations in the Preferred Reporting Items for Systematic Reviews and Meta-Analyses guidelines (Moher et al., 2009). When necessary, standard deviations were estimated using the provided confidence interval (CI) limits, standard error, or range values.

Data were pooled only for trials that reported sufficiently similar clinical and methodological variables. A pooled estimate of risk ratio (RR) was computed using the DerSimonian and Laird random-effect model (DerSimonian & Laird, 1986). Heterogeneity among the trials was assessed using the I^2 test and a null hypothesis test, in which $p < .1$ was considered to represent significant outcome heterogeneity. Because the included trials used CHX in rinse or gel formulations at different CHX concentrations, subgroup analyses were conducted according to their packing materials (rinse or gel) and CHX concentrations to examine differences attributable to differences in composition.

Results

Trial Characteristics

The procedures used in sampling are summarized in Figure 1. The initial search yielded 202 records, of which 145 records were excluded because of duplication. After a brief reading of the title and abstract, a further 99 records, including 14 short publications, 45 reviews (narrative review and systematic review and meta-analysis), three non-RCTs, one cohort study, and 36 dentistry articles, were excluded because of lack of relevance to the scope of this review. The full contents of the remaining 46 records were retrieved for evaluation. Subsequently, 23 records were excluded, including four RCTs that tested CHX mixed with other materials; one RCT that was not restricted to molar extraction; 16 RCTs that tested CHX dosage,

administration time, or treatment period; and one RCT that used a duplicate sample. Of the remaining 23 trials, 20 were identified from the academic databases and three (Ahmedi et al., 2014; Shaban et al., 2014; Younus et al., 2014) were identified through Google Scholar. The data from these 23 trials were used in analysis, and their characteristics are presented in Table 1. The included studies were published between 1991 and 2017 and had sample sizes of 30–271 patients. Seven of the trials examined the effectiveness of CHX rinse, 13 examined the effectiveness of CHX gel, and three examined the comparative effectiveness of CHX rinse and CHX gel. In terms of controls, a subject–subject case–control design was used in 18 of the trials, and a split-mouth case–control design was used in five of the trials. All of the included trials restricted their subjects to single third molar or bilateral third molar extractions with the

Figure 1

Sampling Procedures

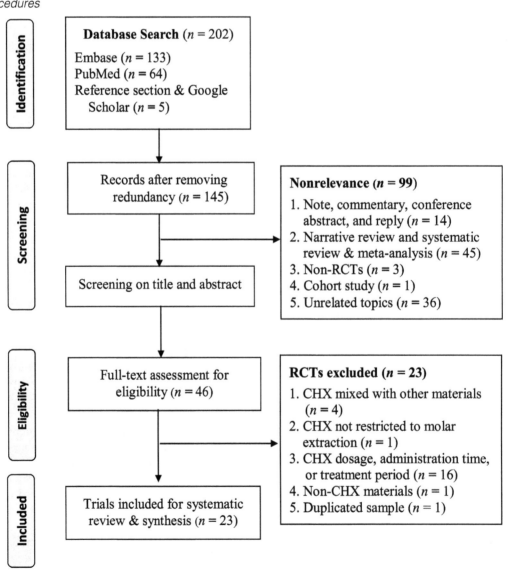

Note. RCT = randomized controlled trial; CHX = chlorhexidine.

Table 1

Characteristics of the Selected Randomized Controlled Trials

Trial/Author (Year)	Inclusion Criteria	No. of Patients (% Male)	Mean Age or Mean Age ± SD	Treatment
Rinse vs. control				
1. Berwick & Lessin (1990)	Bilateral max. third molars	I: 20 (NA) C: 20 (NA)	21.4	I: 0.12% CHX rinse for 1 min before surgery C: NSR after surgery
2. Channar et al. (2013)	Mand. third molar	I: 73 (NA) C: 72 (NA)	30.4 ± 5.2	I: 0.2% CHX rinse (15 ml for 30 s), twice daily for 7 days after surgery C: NSR
3. Delilbasi et al. (2002)	Mand. third molar	I: 62 (48.0) C: 59 (42.4)	I: 24.1 C: 24.2	I: 0.2% CHX rinse (15 ml for 30 s) before surgery and twice daily for 7 days after surgery C: NSR before surgery and twice daily for 7 days after surgery
4. Hermesch et al. (1998)	≥ 1 Mand. third molar	I: 136 (37.5) C: 135 (37.0)	I: 22.2 C: 22.4	I: 0.12% CHX rinse (15 ml for 30 s), twice daily for 7 days before and 7 days after surgery C: 11.6% alcohol (15 ml for 30 s), twice daily for 7 days before and 7 days after surgery
5. Larsen (1991)	Bilateral mand. third molars	I: 73 (43.8) C: 67 (44.8)	NA	I: 0.12% CHX rinse (15 ml for 30 s), twice daily for 7 days before and 7 days after surgery C: Identical solution without CHX (15 m; for 30 s), twice daily for 7 days before and 7 days after surgery
6. Osunde et al. (2017)	Mand. third molars	I: 50 (48) C: 50 (44)	I: 26.4 ± 5.1 C: 27.1 ± 5.9	I: Gargle with 0.12% CHX gluconate rinse twice daily C: Gargle with warm NSR twice daily
7. Ragno & Szkutnik (1991)	Mand. third molars	I: 80 C: 80	NA	I: 0.12% CHX rinse. Rinse with 15 ml before suture and then the day after surgery (15 ml for 30 s), twice daily for 7 days C: Placebo. Rinse with 15-ml placebo solution before suture and then the day after surgery (15 ml for 30 s), twice daily for 7 days
Gel vs. control				
8. Ahmedi et al. (2014)	Bilateral mand. third molars	I: 25 C: 25	NA	I: 2-ml 1% CHX digluconate gel into alveolus before suture C: NSR of alveolus before suture
9. Babar et al. (2012)	Mand. third molar	I: 50 (78) C: 50 (54)	29 ± 6	I: 0.2% CHX gel into alveolus C: No treatment
10. Freudenthal et al. (2015)	Mand. third molars	I: 48 (51) C: 47 (44)	I: 33 C: 34	I: 10-ml Cervitec gel (0.2% CHX and 0.2 sodium fluoride) into alveolus before suture C: 10-ml placebo gel (0.2% sodium fluoride) into alveolus before suture
11. Haraji et al. (2013)	Bilateral mand. third molars	I: 80 (48.8) C: 80 (48.8)	21.6 ± 2.5	I: 0.2% CHX gel into alveolus before suture C: Dry dressing into alveolus before suture
12. Haraji & Rakhshan (2014)	Bilateral mand. third molars	I: 45 (53.3) C: 45 (53.3)	22.1 ± 2.7	I: 0.2% CHX gel into alveolus before suture C: Dry dressing into alveolus before suture
13. Jesudasan et al. (2015)	Mand. third molars	I: 90 C: 90	I: 28 ± 6 C: 28 ± 7	I: 0.2% CHX gel into alveolus before suture C: No treatment before suture

(continues)

Table 1

Characteristics of the Selected Randomized Controlled Trials, Continued

Trial/Author (Year)	Inclusion Criteria	No. of Patients (% Male)	Mean Age or Mean Age ± SD	Treatment
14. Khan et al. (2015)	Max. or mand. first, second, or third molar	I: 128 C: 125	36.7 ± 11.0	I: Bite on gauze with 10-ml 0.2% CHX gluconate gel for 15 min C: Bite on gauze with placebo gel for 15 min
15. Requena-Calla & Funes-Rumiche (2016)	Mand. third molar	I: 20 (50) C: 20 (65)	I: 23.1 C: 22.9	I: 1-ml 0.12% CHX gel into alveolus before suture C: 1-ml placebo gel into alveolus before suture
16. Rubio-Palau et al. (2015)	Mand. third molars	I: 80 (48.7) C: 80 (51.7)	25.04	I: 10-ml 0.2% CHX bioadhesive gel in alveolus C: 10-ml placebo gel in alveolus
17. Shaban et al. (2014)	Bilateral mand. third molars	I: 41 (34.1) C: 42 (31.1)	24.2 ± 5.0	I: 0.2% CHX gel into alveolus C: No treatment
18. Torres-Lagares, Infante-Cossio, et al. (2006)	Mand. third molar	I: 17 (29.4) C: 13 (30.8)	I: 29 ± 10.2 C: 26.3 ± 6.0	I: 0.2% CHX adhesive gel into alveolus C: No treatment
19. Torres-Lagares, Gutierrez-Perez, et al. (2006)	Mand. third molar	I: 53 (37.7) C: 50 (28.0)	I: 27.8 ± 8.4 C: 25.7 ± 8.6	I: 0.2% CHX digluconate bioadhesive gel into alveolus C: Placebo gel into alveolus
20. Torres-Lagares et al. (2010)	Mand. third molar	I: 24 (78.6) C: 14 (91.7)	I: 32.5 ± 16.7 C: 32.0 ± 11.9	I: 10-ml 0.2% CHX bioadhesive gel in alveolus C: 10-ml placebo gel into alveolus
Rinse vs. gel				
21. Abu-Mostafa et al. (2015)	Max. or mand. molar	G: 160 R: 141	G: NA R: NA	G: 0.2% CHX bioadhesive gel into alveolus on the first and third day after surgery R: 0.12% CHX rinse from the second day, twice daily for 7 days
22. Hita-Iglesias et al. (2008)	Mand. third molar	G: 41 (34.2) R: 32 (15.6)	G: 28 R: 26	I: 0.2% CHX bioadhesive gel on wound, twice daily for 7 days C: 0.12% CHX rinse, twice daily for 7 days
23. Younus et al. (2014)	Mand. third molar	G: 50 (58) R: 50 (62)	G: 23.5 ± 5.1 R: 22.9 ± 5.2	G: 0.2% CHX gel in alveolus, 4 times daily for 7 days R: 10-ml 0.2% CHX rinse, 4 times daily for 7 days

Note. I = intervention group; C = control group; NA = not available; CHX = chlorhexidine; NSR = normal saline rinse; Mand. = mandibular; Max. = maxillary; min = minute; NaF = sodium fluoride; G = gel group; R = rinse group; s = seconds.

exceptions of Khan et al. (2015) and Abu-Mostafa et al. (2015), which allowed the extraction of any molar tooth.

The methodological quality of the eligible trials is presented in Table 2. All of the included trials reflected low risk of bias because of either deviations from intended interventions or missing outcome data. The low risk is likely attributable to the high level of motivation that the participants had in reducing postoperative pain and in returning for follow-up examinations. However, all of the included trials reflected some level of concern with regard to bias in reporting results, as none mentioned the registration of their protocols. Most of the included trials had either a low risk or some concerns for bias related to the randomization process, although one trial that compared CHX gel and the control and three trials that compared CHX rinse and CHX gel were found to reflect

a high risk of bias in the domain. The participants in those trials that compared CHX rinse and CHX gel would know their allocation sequences even if the allocation was random. Furthermore, the one trial that compared CHX gel and the control had a high risk of bias in randomization process because no treatment was provided to the controlled subjects. Finally, there was a mixture of classes of bias in terms of outcome measurement, with 13 deemed at a low risk, six deemed as having some concerns, and four deemed at a high risk.

Incidence of Alveolar Osteitis

Chlorhexidine rinse versus control

Five of the included trials compared the incidence of AO between a 0.12% CHX rinse group and a control group

(Berwick & Lessin, 1990; Hermesch et al., 1998; Larsen, 1991; Osunde et al., 2017; Ragno & Szkutnik, 1991), and two trials compared the incidence of AO between a 0.2% CHX rinse group and a control group (Channar et al., 2013, Delilbasi et al., 2002). These trials were analyzed in two subgroups, with the results presented in Figure 2. The RR of AO in patients treated with 0.12% CHX rinse was significantly lower than that in patients treated with the control (RR = 0.54, 95% CI [0.41, 0.72]), with no heterogeneity across trials ($I^2 = 0\%$, $p = .73$). Furthermore, the RR of AO in patients treated with 0.2% CHX rinse was significantly lower than that in patients treated with the control (RR = 0.84, 95% CI [0.52, 1.35]), with no significant heterogeneity across trials ($I^2 = 0\%$, $p = .82$). The overall RR of both CHX types was 0.61 (95% CI [0.48, 0.78]), with no subgroup difference ($I^2 = 56.4\%$, $p = .13$) and significant heterogeneity across trials ($I^2 = 0\%$, $p = .62$).

Chlorhexidine gel versus control

Thirteen of the included trials compared the incidence of AO between CHX gel and a control. Of these, 11 used 0.2% CHX gel, one used 0.12% CHX gel (Requena-Calla & Funes-Rumiche, 2016), and one used 1% CHX gel (Ahmedi et al., 2014). These trials were analyzed in three subgroups, with the results summarized in Figure 3. Patients treated with 0.12% CHX gel in the single trial did not show a difference compared with the control (RR = 0.33, 95% CI [0.01, 7.72]). However, patients treated with 0.2% CHX gel exhibited a significantly lower RR of AO compared with those treated with the control (RR = 0.47, 95% CI [0.34, 0.64]), with insignificant heterogeneity across trials ($I^2 = 21\%$, $p = .24$). Furthermore, patients treated with 1% CHX gel in the other single trial exhibited a lower risk of AO than those treated with the control, with borderline significance (RR = 0.14, 95% CI [0.02, 1.08]). The total effect for all of the trials included in the analysis

Table 2

Assessment of the Methodological Quality of Selected Trials Using the Revised Cochrane Risk-of-Bias Tool for Randomized Trials (Version 2)

Trial	Randomisation	Deviation From Intended Interventions	Missing Outcome	Measurement of Outcome	Reporting	Overall
CHX Rinse vs. control						
1. Berwick & Lessin (1990)	LR	LR	LR	LR	SC	SC
2. Channar et al. (2013)	SC	LR	LR	LR	SC	SC
3. Delilbasi et al. (2002)	LR	LR	LR	LR	SC	SC
4. Hermesch et al. (1998)	LR	LR	LR	SC	SC	SC
5. Larsen (1991)	LR	LR	LR	SC	SC	SC
6. Osunde et al. (2017)	LR	LR	LR	LR	SC	SC
7. Ragno & Szkutnik (1991)	LR	LR	LR	LR	SC	SC
CHX Gel vs. control						
8. Ahmedi et al. (2014)	LR	LR	LR	HR	SC	HR
9. Babar et al. (2012)	SC	LR	LR	HR	SC	HR
10. Freudenthal et al. (2015)	LR	LR	LR	LR	SC	SC
11. Haraji et al. (2013)	SC	LR	LR	LR	SC	SC
12. Haraji & Rakhshan (2014)	SC	LR	LR	LR	SC	SC
13. Jesudasan et al. (2015)	SC	LR	LR	LR	SC	SC
14. Khan et al. (2015)	SC	LR	LR	SC	SC	SC
15. Requena-Calla & Funes-Rumiche (2016)	SC	LR	LR	HR	SC	HR
16. Rubio-Palau et al. (2015)	SC	LR	LR	SC	SC	SC
17. Shaban et al. (2014)	HR	LR	LR	LR	SC	HR
18. Torres-Lagares, Infante-Cossio, et al. (2006)	SC	LR	LR	SC	SC	SC
19. Torres-Lagares, Gutierrez-Perez, et al. (2006)	LR	LR	LR	LR	SC	SC
20. Torres-Lagares et al. (2010)	SC	LR	LR	LR	SC	SC
CHX Rinse vs. gel						
21. Abu-Mostafa et al. (2015)	HR	LR	LR	SC	SC	HR
22. Hita-Iglesias et al. (2008)	HR	LR	LR	HR	SC	HR
23. Younus et al. (2014)	HR	LR	LR	LR	SC	HR

Note. LR = low risk; SC = some concerns; HR = high risk.

Figure 2

Forest Plot of Chlorhexidine Rinse (0.12% and 0.2%, Separately) Versus Control for Risk Ratio of Alveolar Osteitis

Study or Subgroup	CHX rinse Events	CHX rinse Total	Control Events	Control Total	Weight	Risk Ratio M-H, Random, 95% CI
1.1.1 0.12% CHX rinse vs Control						
Berwick 1990	7	39	9	38	7.6%	0.76 [0.31, 1.83]
Hermesch 1998	25	136	40	135	30.7%	0.62 [0.40, 0.96]
Larsen 1991	12	144	28	134	14.7%	0.40 [0.21, 0.75]
Osunde 2017	2	50	3	50	1.9%	0.67 [0.12, 3.82]
Ragno 1991	14	80	29	80	19.1%	0.48 [0.28, 0.84]
Subtotal (95% CI)		**449**		**437**	**74.0%**	**0.54 [0.41, 0.72]**
Total events	60		109			
Heterogeneity: Tau² = 0.00; Chi² = 2.04, *df* = 4 (*p* = .73); *I*² = 0%						
Test for overall effect: *Z* = 4.21 (*p* < .0001)						
1.1.2 0.2% CHX rinse vs Control						
Channar 2013	12	73	15	72	12.6%	0.79 [0.40, 1.57]
Delilbasi 2002	13	62	14	59	13.4%	0.88 [0.45, 1.72]
Subtotal (95% CI)		**135**		**131**	**26.0%**	**0.84 [0.52, 1.35]**
Total events	25		29			
Heterogeneity: Tau² = 0.00; Chi² = 0.05, *df* = 1 (*p* = .82); *I*² = 0%						
Test for overall effect: *Z* = 0.73 (*p* = .46)						
Total (95% CI)		**584**		**568**	**100.0%**	**0.61 [0.48, 0.78]**
Total events	85		138			
Heterogeneity: Tau² = 0.00; Chi² = 4.39, *df* = 6 (*p* = .62); *I*² = 0%						
Test for overall effect: *Z* = 4.00 (*p* < .0001)						
Test for subgroup differences: Chi² = 2.29, *df* = 1 (*p* = .13), *I*² = 56.4%						

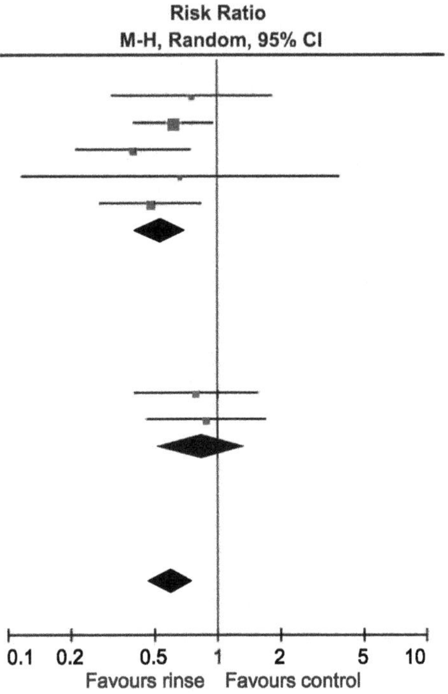

was significant (RR = 0.45, 95% CI [0.33, 0.62]), with insignificant heterogeneity (I^2 = 15%, p = .29) and differences between subgroups (I^2 = 0%, p = .52) across all trials.

Subgroup difference

To examine whether effectiveness in reducing the risk of AO differed between CHX rinse and CHX gel, all of the CHX rinse trials were analyzed in one group, whereas all of the CHX gel trials were analyzed in a separate group. The results are summarized in Figure 4. No significant subgroup difference was observed (I^2 = 53.7%, p = .14).

Chlorhexidine rinse versus chlorhexidine gel

Three trials compared the incidence of AO in the CHX rinse and CHX gel groups (Abu-Mostafa et al., 2015; Hita-Iglesias et al., 2008; Younus et al., 2014). The results of the meta-analysis showed a significantly lower incidence of AO in patients treated with CHX rinse than those treated with CHX gel (RR = 0.61, 95% CI [0.39, 0.95]; table not shown because of space limitations and may be obtained by contacting the corresponding author). No heterogeneity was observed across trials (I^2 = 41%, p = .18).

Discussion

In this study, using either CHX rinse or CHX gel after molar extraction was found to reduce the risk of AO. The subgroup analysis showed no difference between the CHX rinse trials and CHX gel trials in terms of AO risk. On the other hand, a meta-analysis of the three trials that compared CHX rinse and CHX gel suggested that CHX rinse is better than CHX gel in preventing AO.

It seems confusing at the first glance when looking at the insignificant difference between subgroups of all CHX rinse trials and all CHX gel trials and the significant effects resulting from the comparison of CHX rinse and CHX gel. This strongly suggests the presence of a methodology problem. The RR of a trial is affected by many factors, one of which is the treatment received by the control group. For example, saline control likely affords a certain level of AO prevention, whereas the option of no treatment probably has no AO prevention effect. Phenomena such as this affect the results to some extent and, unfortunately, are unable to be statistically adjusted for in the current study design. On the other hand, the number of trials used in the meta-analysis comparing CHX rinse and CHX gel was relatively small. Nevertheless, CHX gel appears to offer a few practical advantages over CHX rinse. First, only one application of CHX gel is required after molar extraction, whereas several days of CHX rinse are required. This implies that no further prescription is required for patients treated with CHX gel. However, an at-home CHX rinse must be prescribed for patients following the CHX rinse protocol along with additional health education to ensure compliance. In terms of cost, the market price of a 200-ml bottle of CHX rinse is approximately US$3. CHX rinse may be used by a single patient only because of hygienic concerns. By comparison, the market price of a 50-ml tube of CHX gel is approximately US$23.3.

Figure 3

Forest Plot of Chlorhexidine Gel (0.12%, 0.2%, and 1%, Separately) Versus Control for Risk Ratio of Alveolar Osteitis

Study or Subgroup	CHX gel Events	Total	Control Events	Total	Weight	Risk Ratio M-H, Random, 95% CI
1.2.1 0.12% CHX gel vs control						
Requena-Calla 2016	0	20	1	20	0.9%	0.33 [0.01, 7.72]
Subtotal (95% CI)		20		20	0.9%	0.33 [0.01, 7.72]
Total events	0		1			
Heterogeneity: Not applicable						
Test for overall effect: Z = 0.69 (P = 0.49)						
1.2.2 0.2% CHX gel vs control						
Babar 2012	4	50	18	100	7.5%	0.44 [0.16, 1.24]
Freudenthal 2015	11	48	9	47	11.8%	1.20 [0.55, 2.62]
Haraji 2013	9	80	26	80	14.2%	0.35 [0.17, 0.69]
Haraji 2014	6	45	16	45	10.5%	0.38 [0.16, 0.87]
Jesudasan 2015	2	90	9	90	3.8%	0.22 [0.05, 1.00]
Khan 2016	7	128	23	125	11.2%	0.30 [0.13, 0.67]
Rubio-Palau 2015	14	80	18	80	16.4%	0.78 [0.42, 1.45]
Shaban 2014	2	41	9	41	4.0%	0.22 [0.05, 0.97]
Torres-Lagares 2006a	3	17	4	13	4.9%	0.57 [0.15, 2.13]
Torres-Lagares 2006b	6	45	16	45	10.5%	0.38 [0.16, 0.87]
Torres-Lagares 2010	1	14	4	24	2.0%	0.43 [0.05, 3.46]
Subtotal (95% CI)		638		690	96.9%	0.47 [0.34, 0.64]
Total events	65		152			
Heterogeneity: Tau² = 0.06; Chi² = 12.67, df = 10 (p = .24); I² = 21						
% Test for overall effect: Z = 4.69 (p < .00001)						
1.2.3 1% CHX gel vs control						
Ahmedi 2014	1	25	7	25	2.2%	0.14 [0.02, 1.08]
Subtotal (95% CI)		25		25	2.2%	0.14 [0.02, 1.08]
Total events	1		7			
Heterogeneity: Not applicable						
Test for overall effect: Z = 1.89 (p = 0.06)						
Total (95% CI)		683		735	100.0%	0.45 [0.33, 0.62]
Total events	66		160			
Heterogeneity: Tau² = 0.05; Chi² = 14.12, df = 12 (p = .29); I² = 15%						
Test for overall effect: Z = 5.07 (p < .00001)						
Test for subgroup differences: Chi² = 1.32, df = 2 (p = .52); I² = 0%						

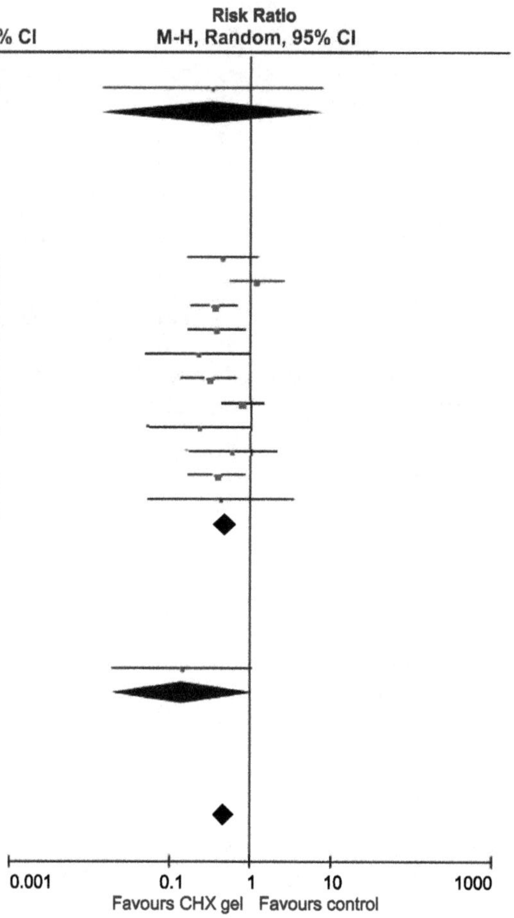

However, the gel can be used by 25 patients in a clinic (presuming 2 ml/patient) at a cost of less than US$1 per patient (price information obtained from the National Health Insurance, Taiwan). Certainly, the way that CHX products are applied affects their actual efficacies. For example, a recent RCT showed that irrigation of the molar surgical site with CHX had a better AO prevention effect than simply rinsing the mouth with CHX (Cho et al., 2018). Moreover, reducing the risk of AO reduces the need for return clinic visits because of extraction complications. In addition to benefits of treatment, side effects should be considered when evaluating treatment efficacy. Staining and bitter taste are two common side effects of CHX (Flötra et al., 1971; Tilliss, 1999) that have been at least partially addressed in newer CHX products (Raszewski et al., 2019). Practitioners may provide or recommend choices of CHX products to maximize their usage while minimizing their side effects and maintaining the targeted prophylactic effects. Another issue that should be noted is the potential that patients may exhibit an allergic reaction to CHX. A patch test involving 7,610 general dermatology patients using CHX digluconate (0.5% aqueous) revealed a 0.47% positive reaction in the sample (Liippo et al., 2011). Although the actual situation of CHX allergy in dentistry remains to be investigated (Pemberton & Gibson, 2012), precautions should be taken, especially among patients with a history of CHX contact allergy.

The trials included in our analysis showed considerable heterogeneity because of various backgrounds and clinical factors. Although most of the trials reported information on age and gender, which are known factors attributable to AO, some trials did not provide clear information on these basic variables. Whether all of the included trials examined young adults as revealed by most of the reported information could not be confirmed. Moreover, although we restricted the trials to molar extractions, we did not restrict the diagnostic criteria and molar extraction methods or narrow the target to a specific tooth (e.g., the third molar), nor did the standard used to diagnose AO. In addition, the experimental (i.e., methods of CHX rinse or CHX gel use) and control methods differed in the included trials. Other factors such as working experience and analgesics use that may affect the outcomes of surgery varied across the trials.

Figure 4

Subgroup Difference Between All Types of Chlorhexidine Rinse (0.12% and 0.2%) and All Types of Chlorhexidine Gel (0.12%, 0.2%, and 1%) for Risk Ratio of Alveolar Osteitis

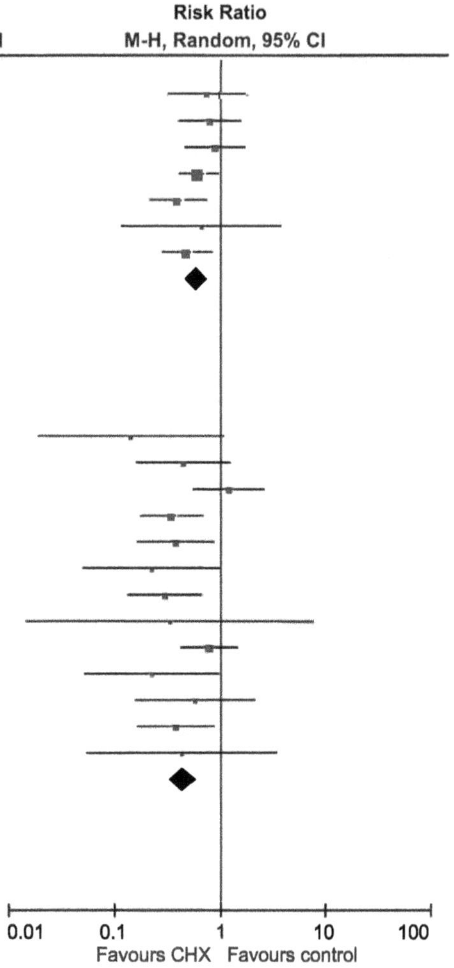

Our meta-analysis had some limitations. First, although molar extraction is a routine dental procedure worldwide, the number of RCTs related to AO and CHX rinse or gel is relatively low. Second, the included trials were conducted in a limited number of countries. Because overall oral health may vary across populations, the AO risk revealed in our results may differ slightly from the real-world situation in clinics.

Implication for Practice

Both CHX rinse and gel treatments may be used after molar extraction to reduce the risk of AO. Although this measure improves health outcomes and dental health service quality, it only increases the treatment costs slightly. The findings of this review support the use of CHX rinse or gel in molar extraction surgery, whether covered by national insurance or self-pay. For convenience and affordability, CHX gel applied immediately after molar extraction by the dentist is recommended.

The at-home CHX rinse is recommended as long as the dental clinic is able to provide appropriate health education and case management support.

Acknowledgments

This study was funded by the Taipei Medical University (grant number: TMU107-AE1-B05) and Taipei Medical University Shuang Ho Hospital (grant number: 106HCP-17).

Author Contributions

Study conception and design: CHW, SHY, EWL
Data collection: HJJ, JCT, HKL
Data analysis and interpretation: All authors
Drafting of the article: CHW, SHY
Critical revision of the article: EWL

References

*References marked with an asterisk indicate studies included in the meta-analysis.

Abu Younis, M. H., & Abu Hantash, R. O. (2011). Dry socket: Frequency, clinical picture, and risk factors in a Palestinian dental teaching center. *Open Dentistry Journal, 5*, 7–12. https://doi.org/10.2174/1874210601105010007

*Abu-Mostafa, N. A., Alqahtani, A., Abu-Hasna, M., Alhokail, A., & Aladsani, A. (2015). A randomized clinical trial compared the effect of intra-alveolar 0.2% chlorohexidine bio-adhesive gel versus 0.12% chlorohexidine rinse in reducing alveolar osteitis following molar teeth extractions. *Medicina Oral Patología Oral y Cirugía Bucal, 20*(1), e82–e87. https://doi.org/10.4317/medoral.19932

*Ahmedi, J., Ahmedi, E., Agani, Z., Hamiti, V., Reçica, B., & Tmava-Dragusha, A. (2014). The efficacy of 1% chlorhexidine gel on the reduction of dry socket occurrence following surgical third molar extraction-pilot study. *Open Journal of Stomatology, 4*(3), 152–160. https://doi.org/10.4236/ojst.2014.43023

*Babar, A., Ibrahim, M. W., Baig, N. J., Shah, I., & Amin, E. (2012). Efficacy of intra-alveolar chlorhexidine gel in reducing frequency of alveolar osteitis in mandibular third molar surgery. *Journal of the College of Physicians and Surgeons-Pakistan 22*(2), 91_94.

Balagopal, S., & Arjunkumar, R. (2013). Chlorhexidine: The gold standard antiplaque agent. *Journal of Pharmaceutical Sciences and Research, 5*(12), 270–274.

*Berwick, J. E., & Lessin, M. E. (1990). Effects of a chlorhexidine gluconate oral rinse on the incidence of alveolar osteitis in mandibular third molar surgery. *Journal of Oral and Maxillofacial Surgery, 48*(5), 444–448. https://doi.org/10.1016/0278-2391(90)90227-S

Blum, I. R. (2002). Contemporary views on dry socket (alveolar osteitis): A clinical appraisal of standardization, aetiopathogenesis and management: A critical review. *International Journal of Oral and Maxillofacial Surgery, 31*(3), 309–317. https://doi.org/10.1054/ijom.2002.0263

Cardoso, C. L., Rodrigues, M. T. V., Ferreira, O. Jr., Garlet, G. P., & de Carvalho, P. S. (2010). Clinical concepts of dry socket. *Journal of Oral and Maxillofacial Surgery, 68*(8), 1922–1932. https://doi.org/10.1016/j.joms.2009.09.085

Caso, A., Hung, L. K., & Beirne, O. R. (2005). Prevention of alveolar osteitis with chlorhexidine: A meta-analytic review. *Oral Surgery, Oral Medicine, Oral Pathology, Oral Radiology, and Endodontics, 99*(2), 155–159. https://doi.org/10.1016/j.tripleo.2004.05.009

*Channar, K. A., Dall, A. Q., Memon, A. B., & Lal, B. (2013). Prevention of alveolar osteitis in surgical removal of lower third molar. *Pakistan Oral & Dental Journal, 33*(2), 244–248.

Cho, H., David, M. C., Lynham, A. J., & Hsu, E. (2018). Effectiveness of irrigation with chlorhexidine after removal of mandibular third molars: A randomised controlled trial. *British Journal of Oral and Maxillofacial Surgery, 56*(1), 54–59. https://doi.org/10.1016/j.bjoms.2017.11.010

Congiusta, M. A., & Veitz-Keenan, A. (2013). Study confirms certain risk factors for development of alveolar osteitis. *Evidence-Based Dentistry, 14*(3), Article 86. https://doi.org/10.1038/sj.ebd.6400954

*Delilbasi, C., Saracoglu, U., & Keskin, A. (2002). Effects of 0.2% chlorhexidine gluconate and amoxicillin plus clavulanic acid on the prevention of alveolar osteitis following mandibular third molar extractions. *Oral Surgery, Oral Medicine, Oral Pathology, Oral Radiology, and Endodontics, 94*(3), 301–304.

DerSimonian, R., & Laird, N. (1986). Meta-analysis in clinical trials. *Controlled Clinical Trials, 7*(3), 177–188. https://doi.org/10.1016/0197-2456(86)90046-2

Dobson, M., Pillon, L., Kwon, O., & Innes, N. (2018). Chlorhexidine gel to prevent alveolar osteitis following mandibular third molar extractions. *Evidence-Based Dentistry, 19*(1), 16–17. https://doi.org/10.1038/sj.ebd.6401288

Erickson, R. I., Waite, D. E., & Wilkison, R. H. (1960). A study of dry sockets. *Oral Surgery, Oral Medicine, and Oral Pathology, 13*(9), 1046–1050. https://doi.org/10.1016/0030-4220(60)90316-9

Flötra, L., Gjermo, P., Rölla, G., & Waerhaug, J. (1971). Side effects of chlorhexidine mouth washes. *Scandinavian Journal of Dental Research, 79*(2), 119–125. https://doi.org/10.1111/j.1600-0722.1971.tb02001.x

*Freudenthal, N., Sternudd, M., Jansson, L., & Wannfors, K. (2015). A double-blind randomized study evaluating the effect of intra-alveolar chlorhexidine gel on alveolar osteitis after removal of mandibular third molars. *Journal of Oral and Maxillofacial Surgery, 73*(4), 600–605. https://doi.org/10.1016/j.joms.2014.08.035

Haraji, A., Lassemi, E., Motamedi, M. H. K., Alavi, M., & Adibnejad, S. (2012). Effect of plasma rich in growth factors on alveolar osteitis. *National Journal of Maxillofacial Surgery, 3*(1), 38–41. https://doi.org/10.4103/0975-5950.102150

*Haraji, A., & Rakhshan, V. (2014). Single-dose intra-alveolar chlorhexidine gel application, easier surgeries, and younger ages are associated with reduced dry socket risk. *Journal of Oral and Maxillofacial Surgery, 72*(2), 259–265. https://doi.org/10.1016/j.joms.2013.09.023

*Haraji, A., Rakhshan, V., Khamverdi, N., & Alishahi, H. K. (2013). Effects of intra-alveolar placement of 0.2% chlorhexidine bioadhesive gel on dry socket incidence and postsurgical pain: A double-blind split-mouth randomized controlled clinical trial. *Journal of Oral and Facial Pain and Headache, 27*(3), 256–262. https://doi.org/10.11607/jop.1142

*Hermesch, C. B., Hilton, T. J., Biesbrock, A. R., Baker, R. A., Cain-Hamlin, J., McClanahan, S. F., & Gerlach, R. W. (1998). Perioperative use of 0.12% chlorhexidine gluconate for the prevention of alveolar osteitis: Efficacy and risk factor analysis. *Oral Surgery, Oral Medicine, Oral Pathology, Oral Radiology, and Endodontics, 85*(4), 381–387. https://doi.org/10.1016/S1079-2104(98)90061-0

Higgins, J. P. T., Savović, J., Page, M. J., & Sterne, J. A. C.; on behalf of the ROB2 Development Group. (2019). *Revised Cochrane risk-of-bias tool for randomized trials (RoB 2).* https://www.riskofbias.info/welcome/rob-2-0-tool/current-version-of-rob-2

*Hita-Iglesias, P., Torres-Lagares, D., Flores-Ruiz, R., Magallanes-Abad, N., Basallote-Gonzalez, M., & Gutierrez-Perez, J. L. (2008). Effectiveness of chlorhexidine gel versus chlorhexidine rinse in reducing alveolar osteitis in mandibular third molar surgery. *Journal of Oral and Maxillofacial Surgery, 66*(3), 441–445. https://doi.org/10.1016/j.joms.2007.06.641

*Jesudasan, J. S., Wahab, P. U., & Sekhar, M. R. (2015). Effectiveness of 0.2% chlorhexidine gel and a eugenol-based paste on postoperative alveolar osteitis in patients having third molars extracted: A randomised controlled clinical trial. *British Journal of Oral and Maxillofacial Surgery, 53*(9), 826–830. https://doi.org/10.1016/j.bjoms.2015.06.022

*Khan, M. A., Bashir, S., Khan, F. R., Umer, F., Haider, S. M., & Hasan, T. (2015). Clinical efficacy of single dose chlorhexidine gel application in molar extractions—A randomized clinical trial. *Journal of the Pakinstan Dental Association, 24*(4), 175–181.

*Larsen, P. E. (1991). The effect of a chlorhexidine rinse on the incidence of alveolar osteitis following the surgical removal of impacted mandibular third molars. *Journal of Oral and Maxillofacial Surgery, 49*(9), 932–937. https://doi.org/10.1016/0278-2391(91)90055-Q

Lee, C. T., Zhang, S., Leung, Y. Y., Li, S. K., Tsang, C. C., & Chu, C. H. (2015). Patients' satisfaction and prevalence of complications on surgical extraction of third molar. *Patient Preference and Adherence, 9*, 257–263. https://doi.org/10.2147/PPA.S76236

Liippo, J., Kousa, P., & Lammintausta, K. (2011). The relevance of chlorhexidine contact allergy. *Contact Dermatitis, 64*(4), 229–234. https://doi.org/10.1111/j.1600-0536.2010.01851.x

Moher, D., Liberati, A., Tetzlaff, J., & Altman, D. G., for the PRISMA Group. (2009). Preferred reporting items for systematic reviews and meta-analyses: The PRISMA statement. *BMJ, 339*, Article b2535. https://doi.org/10.1136/bmj.b2535

Nusair, Y. M., & Younis, M. H. A. (2007). Prevalence, clinical picture, and risk factors of dry socket in a Jordanian dental teaching center. *The Journal of Contemporary Dental Practice, 8*(3), 53–63.

Ogunlewe, M. O., Adeyemo, W. L., Ladeinde, A. L., & Taiwo, O. A. (2007). Incidence and pattern of presentation of dry socket following non-surgical tooth extraction. *Nigerian Quarterly Journal of Hospital Medicine, 17*(4), 126–130.

*Osunde, O. D., Anyanechi, C. E., & Bassey, G. O. (2017). Prevention of alveolar osteitis after third molar surgery: Comparative study of the effect of warm saline and chlorhexidine mouth rinses. *Nigerian Journal of Clinical Practice, 20*(4), 470–473. https://doi.org/10.4103/1119-3077.180064

Pemberton, M. N., & Gibson, J. (2012). Chlorhexidine and hypersensitivity reactions in dentistry. *British Dental Journal, 213*(11), 547–550. https://doi.org/0.1038/sj.bdj.2012.1086

*Ragno, J. R. Jr., & Szkutnik, A. J. (1991). Evaluation of 0.12% chlorhexidine rinse on the prevention of alveolar osteitis. *Oral Surgery, Oral Medicine, and Oral Pathology, 72*(5), 524–526. https://doi.org/10.1016/0030-4220(91)90487-W

Raszewski, Z., Nowakowska-Toporowska, A., Weżgowiec, J., & Nowakowska, D. (2019). Design and characteristics of new experimental chlorhexidine dental gels with anti-staining properties. *Advances in Clinical and Experimental Medicine, 28*(7), 885–890. https://doi.org/10.17219/acem/94152

*Requena-Calla, S., & Funes-Rumiche, I. (2016). Effectiveness of intra-alveolar chlorhexidine gel in reducing dry socket following surgical extraction of lower third molars. A pilot study. *Journal of Clinical and Experimental Dentistry, 8*(2), e160–e163. https://doi.org/10.4317/jced.52444

Rodriguez Sanchez, F., Rodriguez Andres, C., & Arteagoitia Calvo, I. (2017). Does chlorhexidine prevent alveolar osteitis after third molar extractions? Systematic review and meta-analysis. *Journal of Oral and Maxillofacial Surgery, 75*(5), 901–914. https://doi.org/10.1016/j.joms.2017.01.002

*Rubio-Palau, J., Garcia-Linares, J., Hueto-Madrid, J. A., Gonzalez-Lagunas, J., Raspall-Martin, G., & Mareque-Bueno, J. (2015). Effect of intra-alveolar placement of 0.2% chlorhexidine bioadhesive gel on the incidence of alveolar osteitis following the extraction of mandibular third molars. A double-blind randomized clinical trial. *Medicina Oral Patología Oral y Cirugía Bucal, 20*(1), e117–e122. https://doi.org/10.4317/medoral.20009

*Shaban, B., Azimi, H. R., Naderi, H., Janani, A., Zarrabi, M. J., & Nejat, A. (2014). Effect of 0.2% chlorhexidine gel on frequency of dry socket following mandibular third molar surgery: A double-blind clinical trial. *Journal of Dental Materials and Techniques, 3*(4), 175–179. https://doi.org/10.22038/jdmt.2014.3348

Sigron, G. R., Pourmand, P. P., Mache, B., Stadlinger, B., & Locher, M. C. (2014). The most common complications after wisdom-tooth removal: Part 1: A retrospective study of 1,199 cases in the mandible. *Swiss Dental Journal, 124*(10), 1052–1056.

Teshome, A. (2017). The efficacy of chlorhexidine gel in the prevention of alveolar osteitis after mandibular third molar extraction: A systematic review and meta-analysis. *BMC Oral Health, 17*(1), Article 82. https://doi.org/10.1186/s12903-017-0376-3

Tilliss, T. S. (1999). Use of a whitening dentifrice for control of chlorhexidine stain. *The Journal of Contemporary Dental Practice, 1*(1), 9–15.

*Torres-Lagares, D., Gutierrez-Perez, J. L., Hita-Iglesias, P., Magallanes-Abad, N., Flores-Ruiz, R., Basallote-Garcia, M., & Gonzalez-Martin, M. (2010). Randomized, double-blind study of effectiveness of intra-alveolar application of chlorhexidine gel in reducing incidence of alveolar osteitis and bleeding complications in mandibular third molar surgery in patients with bleeding disorders. *Journal of Oral and Maxillofacial Surgery, 68*(6), 1322–1326. https://doi.org/10.1016/j.joms.2009.08.022

*Torres-Lagares, D., Gutierrez-Perez, J. L., Infante-Cossio, P., Garcia-Calderon, M., Romero-Ruiz, M. M., & Serrera-Figallo, M. A. (2006). Randomized, double-blind study on effectiveness of intra-alveolar chlorhexidine gel in reducing the incidence of alveolar osteitis in mandibular third molar surgery. *International Journal of Oral and Maxillofacial Surgery, 35*(4), 348–351. https://doi.org/10.1016/j.ijom.2005.08.002

*Torres-Lagares, D., Infante-Cossio, P., Gutierrez-Perez, J. L., Romero-Ruiz, M. M., Garcia-Calderon, M., & Serrera-Figallo, M. A. (2006). Intra-alveolar chlorhexidine gel for the prevention of dry socket in mandibular third molar surgery. A pilot study. *Medicina Oral, Patología Oral y Cirugía Bucal, 11*(2), E179–E184.

Yengopal, V., & Mickenautsch, S. (2012). Chlorhexidine for the prevention of alveolar osteitis. *International Journal of Oral and Maxillofacial Surgery, 41*(10), 1253–1264. https://doi.org/10.1016/j.ijom.2012.04.017

*Younus, S., Ghumman, N. U., Latif, K., & Chishty, M. S. (2014). Efficacy of chlorhexidine gel vs chlorhexidine rinses in reducing incidence of dry socket in mandibular third molar surgery. *Pakistan Oral & Dental Journal, 34*(2), 249–252.

Zhou, J., Hu, B., Liu, Y., Yang, Z., & Song, J. (2017). The efficacy of intra-alveolar 0.2% chlorhexidine gel on alveolar osteitis: A meta-analysis. *Oral Diseases, 23*(5), 598–608. https://doi.org/10.1111/odi.12553

9

The Effect of Semirecumbent and Right Lateral Positions on the Gastric Residual Volume of Mechanically Ventilated, Critically Ill Patients

Zahra FARSI[1]* • Maa'soumeh KAMALI[2] • Samantha BUTLER[3] • Armin ZAREIYAN[4]

ABSTRACT

Background: Delay in stomach discharge is a challenge for patients who are tube fed and may result in serious side effects such as pneumonia and malnutrition.

Purpose: This study was designed to determine the respective effects of the semirecumbent (SR) supine and right lateral (RL) with a flatbed positions on the gastric residual volume (GRV) of mechanically ventilated, critically ill adult patients.

Methods: A randomized, crossover clinical trial design was used to investigate GRV in 36 critically ill, ventilated adult patients who were hospitalized in the intensive care unit. GRV was measured at 3 hours after three consecutive feedings. GRV was first measured in all of the participants in the supine position; after which, participants were randomly assigned into one of two therapeutic positioning groups (Group A: assessment in the SR position and then the RL position; Group B: assessment in the RL position and then the SR position).

Results: GRV was significantly lower in both the SR and RL positions than in the supine position. GRV in the SR and RL positions did not vary significantly. The in-group measurements for GRV did not significantly differ for any of the three positions. In Group A, GRV was significantly lower at each subsequent measurement point.

Conclusion/Implications for Practice: Positioning patients in the RL and SR positions rather than in the supine position is an effective strategy to reduce GRV. Furthermore, placing patients in either the RL or SR position is an effective intervention to promote faster digestion and feedings.

KEY WORDS:
gastric residual, positioning, right lateral, semirecumbent, supine, tube feeding.

Introduction

Enteral tubes are placed in patients who have a functional and accessible gastrointestinal (GI) tract but are not able to consume or absorb sufficient nutrients to sustain adequate nutrition and hydration. A wide variety of enteral tubes may be placed through the nares, mouth, stomach, or small intestine to provide liquid nutrition, fluids, and medications directly into the GI tract of patients in intensive care units (ICUs; Lord, 2018). Tubes may be wide or narrow and gastric or intestinal. They may be inserted nasally or through oropharyngeal placement. Although the use of enteral feeding tubes is beneficial, as with most healthcare interventions, there are risks. Critically ill patients with enteral tubes are at a greater risk of delayed gastric emptying (DGE) because of an increase of gastric residual volume (GRV), regurgitation or vomiting, gastroesophageal reflux, aspiration, and ventilator-associated pneumonia (Chen, Tzeng, Gau, Kuo, & Chen, 2013; Nasiri, Farsi, Ahangari, & Dadgari, 2017; Reignier et al., 2013) as well as of GI changes such as abdominal distension, constipation, vomiting, diarrhea, increased abdominal circumference, and subjective discomfort (Poveda, Castilho, Nogueira, Ferretti-Rebustini, & Silva, 2018). DGE increases with medical severity and is often seen in patients with trauma, shock, respiratory failure, gastroparesis, electrolyte disorders, poorly controlled diabetes mellitus, gastric outlet obstruction, ileus, recent surgery, cytokines, trauma, sepsis, and feeding intolerance and those requiring narcotic pain medications (Chen et al., 2013; Guo, 2015; Montejo et al., 2010). Approximately 50% of adults requiring mechanical ventilation (MV) experience DGE (Nguyen et al., 2008). DGE may cause a constant feeling of fullness, nausea, and vomiting, which negatively impacts nutritional status and increases aspiration risk, gastroesophageal reflux, pneumonia, and hospital length of stay (LOS; Dutch Dieticians Oncology Group, 2017; Guo, 2015; Stewart, 2014).

Controlling GRV is important for patient well-being and medical stability (Stewart, 2014). Several methods are currently used to control GRV, including changing the method

[1]PhD, Associate Professor, Faculty of Nursing, Research Department and Community Health Department, Aja University of Medical Sciences, Tehran, Iran • [2]MSc, Researcher, Student Research Committee, Faculty of Nursing, Aja University of Medical Sciences, Tehran, Iran • [3]PhD, Assistant Professor, Harvard Medical School and Boston Children's Hospital, Boston, Massachusetts, USA • [4]PhD, Associate Professor, Faculty of Nursing, Community Health Department, Aja University of Medical Sciences, Tehran, Iran.

of feeding (such as feeding after the pyloric outlet), prescribing medications to increase GI motility (such as metoclopramide, cisapride, herbal medicine, and pressure medicine), using acupuncture, and changing body position (DeLegge, 2011; Heydari & Emami Zeydi, 2014). Often, patients are moved and their positions are changed every 3 hours to prevent pressure sores. The right lateral (RL) position on a bed flat has been shown to reduce regurgitation and aspiration in adults (Hussein, 2012). The semirecumbent (SR) position, the upright positioning of the head and torso, while lying on the back has been found to decrease the aspiration of gastric contents in comparison with the supine position (Gocze et al., 2013). An angle of 45° has been identified as the most effective position for accelerating gastric emptying, as the gastric contents gravitate toward the duodenum in the SR position more easily than in other positions (Gocze et al., 2013). The prone position has been used for some patients but is often not well tolerated. Therefore, technical considerations preclude its routine use, and it has been associated with an increased rate of serious complications in ventilated adults (Gattinoni et al., 2001; Guerin et al., 2004). Furthermore, GRV does not differ significantly between the prone and supine positions (van der Voort & Zandstra, 2001). Findings across research studies on gastric emptying are inconsistent in adult patients (Chen et al., 2013; Gocze et al., 2013; Sanaka et al., 2013). One study reported that the gastric emptying of saline solutions was faster when lying in the RL position compared with the left lateral (LL) position, whereas no difference was found between lying in the RL and sitting positions. On the contrary, another study showed that gastric emptying of water occurred more quickly when a patient is in the RL position compared with the sitting position (Sanaka et al., 2013). In one investigation of the rate of gastric emptying of glucose solution, no significant difference was found between lying on the RL, lying on the LL, or the sitting position (Burn-Murdoch, Fisher, & Hunt, 1980).

Understanding the most appropriate position for critically ill and ventilated adult patients may facilitate reductions in the incidence of pneumonia, reflux, hospital LOS, mortality, and morbidity. This study aimed to assess the effects of the SR and RL positions on the GRV of mechanically ventilated, critically ill adults hospitalized in the ICU. It was hypothesized that patients in the SR position should exhibit rates of gastric emptying that are higher than those in other positions, as the gastric content should gravitate toward the duodenum in the SR position more easily than in other positions.

Methods

Design

A randomized, crossover clinical trial was implemented. A repeated-measures design was used in which each participant was assigned randomly to a sequence of different interventions.

This crossover trial was "balanced," whereby all participants received two interventions (RL and SR positions) and participated for the same number of periods (3-hour interval between interventions), with all receiving three GRV measurements.

Participants and Setting

The study participants included 36 mechanically ventilated, critically ill patients in two medical ICUs in Bea'sat Hospital, Tehran, Iran, who were recruited between April and June 2017. Both ICUs were similar in terms of equipment, facilities, and patients and were considered as a single setting for the purposes of this study. Criteria for inclusion included between 18 and 65 years old, nasogastric tube (NGT) feeding only, requiring noninvasive MV 48 hours before and throughout the duration of the intervention, and no limitations to altering body position. The exclusion criteria included experiencing acute GI disorders, concern for GI motility, pregnancy, medications to increase GI motility taken within the last 2 weeks or during the study, change to nutrition regimen, transfer or discharge of the patient from the ICU, and discontinuing/weaning from MV. Patients were recruited using a convenient sampling method and were randomly assigned into one of two study groups using a random-numbers table and sealed envelope technique. We used a random-numbers table to generate the random sequence. Numbers were placed in the envelopes and were opened sequentially only after each participant's name was written on the appropriate envelope. To minimize the potential for bias, the researcher assistant who enrolled patients into this study was blinded to the random allocation sequence. All direct patient care was completed by an experienced ICU nurse with a master's degree.

Sample Size

A standard, two-sequence, two-period crossover design ($m = 1$) was used for trials with the objective of establishing therapeutic equivalence between the two different interventions. An 80% ($1 - \beta = 0.8$) power with a confidence level of 99% was adopted to establish therapeutic equivalence. On the basis of the results of a previous study, the variance was estimated as 8.03^2 ($\sigma_m^2 = 8.03)^2$. The true mean difference was 5.36 (Aslani, Hanifi, Ahmadi, & Fallah, 2014). Furthermore, we assumed that the equivalence limit was 25% ($\delta = 0.25$). A minimum of 50% difference was assumed for the equivalence limit based on the standard of the sample size in the crossover studies (Chow, Shao, & Wang, 2008). Thus, a minimum of 18 participants were required in each group for this study.

$$n = \frac{(Z_\alpha + Z_{1-\beta})^2 \sigma_m^2}{2(-\delta)^2} = \frac{(2.58 + 1.28)^2 (8.03)^2}{2(5.36 - 0.25)^2} = 18.38$$

Ethical Approval

This study followed the principles of the Declaration of Helsinki, was approved by the Ethics Committee of the

AJA University of Medical Sciences under Code No. IR. AJAUMC.REC.1394.48, and was registered with the Iranian Registry of Clinical Trials (http://www.irct.ir/) under No. IRCT2015110623446N6. The legal guardians of the participants were fully informed regarding which aspects of care were related to this study, the purpose of the study, the potential benefits of the interventions to the participants, the intended health-promotion benefits of the research, and the minimal risk and minimal burden involved in participation. Then, if they agreed, the patients' legal guardians provided written informed consent on behalf of the participants. All information regarding individual participants was kept confidential, and during all phases of the study, the legal guardians of the participants could withdraw their consent to participate without affecting the quality of care provided.

Procedure and Data Collection

The medical status of participants was collected using physical examinations conducted by the resident physician, reviews of medical records, and assessments of illness severity using the Acute Physiology and Chronic Health Evaluation (APACHE) III. The APACHE III scale measures illness severity using multiple variables including age, heart rate, mean blood pressure, temperature, respiratory rate, partial pressure of oxygen in arterial blood (PaO_2), arterial pH, alveolar–arterial O_2 difference ($AaDO_2$), hematocrit, white blood cell count, serum creatinine, 24-hour urine output, serum blood urea nitrogen, serum sodium, serum albumin, serum bilirubin, serum glucose, comorbidities, and the Glasgow Coma Scale (Knaus et al., 1991). Blood samples were collected for the APACHE III measurement. The total APACHE III scale score was classified into three levels (0–40: mild, 41–80: moderate, and > 80: severe), with a total possible score ranging from 0 to 299. In previous research, higher APACHE scale scores have been associated with higher rates of mortality and morbidity (Knaus et al., 1991). The NGT was replaced every 7 days per hospital protocol. All of the participants received a premade complete diet through NGT. The nutritional recipe provided 100 cc of nutrition and included seven cups of a meal powder mixed with 90-cc water (1 kcal/cc). The total number of calories and the required volume per individual patient were calculated by a nutritionist and a critical care medicine fellow using the Harris–Benedict equation, which takes into account the gender, body weight, height, age, and activity level of the patient, to determine the most appropriate volume. The metric basal metabolic rate (BMR) formula was used to determine the total daily energy expenditure (calories) for each participant:

Women: BMR = 655 + (9.6 × weight in kg) + (1.8 × height in cm) – (4.7 × age in years)

Men: BMR = 66 + (13.7 × weight in kg) + (5 × height in cm) – (6.8 × age in years)

As the participants were sedentary (little or no exercise), the patients' BMR was multiplied by 1.2 to calculate the total

calories (Douglas et al., 2007). All feedings were bolus feedings, with 3 hours between each NGT feeding. In both groups, the intervention began after confirmation of NGT placement just before feeding, using aspiration of gastric fluid by syringe, and testing of content acidity along with auscultation of bowel sounds. Laryngoscopy was used if the position of NGT was uncertain. The gastric fluid was returned to the stomach. The next feeding was adjusted according to the intake during the previous meal (Dietitians Association, Australia, 2015). GRV was measured at three different points in time (Stage 1: 3 hours after the first feeding, Stage 2: 3 hours after the second feeding, and Stage 3: 3 hours after the third feeding of the study). Each GRV measurement was taken in a different interventional position. Stage 1 was always in the supine position on a bed flat. Positioning during Stages 2 and 3 varied by study group. For Group A, Stage 2 was in the SR position with the head of bed at an incline of 45° and Stage 3 was in the RL position. For Group B, Stage 2 was in the RL position and Stage 3 was in the SR position. Each positional change occurred immediately before an NGT feeding.

In this study, the presence of GI symptoms (abdominal distention, vomiting, and regurgitation) was evaluated and recorded. If any negative symptoms occurred, appropriate interventions were provided. Moreover, the feedings were postponed if medically indicated. If during the intervention, patients required a diagnostic or therapeutic procedure (e.g., x-ray, endotracheal suctioning) that required a change in the patient's body position, the study was stopped and postponed until the next day.

Data Analysis

The statistical analyst was blinded to the study goals and descriptions of each study group. The data were analyzed using SPSS Software Version 18. The Kolmogorov–Smirnov test was used to examine the normal distribution of the variables. The Fisher's exact test was used to examine differences in gender between the two groups. The Mann–Whitney U test was used to examine the differences in age between the two groups. The independent sample t test was used to examine the difference in the APACHE III scale score in both groups and the difference in GRV between the SR and RL positions at the three data collection points. The repeated-measures analysis of variance was used to assess the differences between the GRV in different positions over the three data collection points. A level of $p < .05$ was considered significant.

Results

Participant Characteristics

Of the 52 patients admitted to the hospital during the study recruitment period, 36 met the inclusion criteria, provided informed consent, and were included in the final analysis (Figure 1). The participants in the two intervention groups (Groups A and B) were similar in terms of gender ($p = .72$);

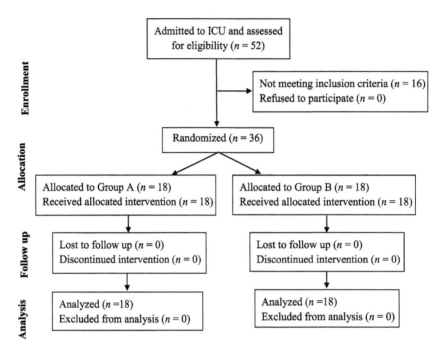

Figure 1. Study flowchart.

age (*p* = .39); ICU LOS (*p* = .54); specific medical conditions in terms of diabetes mellitus, hypertension, acute renal failure, chronic renal failure, cerebrovascular accident, leukemia, and hepatic cirrhosis (*p* = .35); diagnosis (*p* = .467); and illness severity based on APACHE III scale score (*p* = .37). The participants' medical and background data were combined to describe the population. Slightly more than half (54.1%) of the participants were male, the mean age was 53.64 ± 13.53 years (range: 23–65 years), the mean APACHE III scale score was 65.58 ± 14.08 (range: 32–109), the mean GRV was 56.69 ± 3.01, and the mean gavage volume was 150 ± 41.40 cc (range: 100–200 cc).

Interventional Positioning

No significant difference was found in the GRV between groups while in the supine position (*p* = .085), SR position (*p* = .106), or RL position (*p* = .059; Table 1). The mean

GRV was not significantly different either during Stage 2, which was measured after the second feeding (Group A in the SR position and Group B in the RL position; mean difference = −10.27, *t* = −1.74, *p* = .091), or during Stage 3, which was measured after the third feeding (Group A in the RL position and Group B in the SR position; mean difference = −10.94, *t* = 1.86, *p* = .071).

When comparing the GRV across position and group, although the main effect of position was found to be statistically significant (*F* = 21.89, *p* < .001), no significant interaction between position and group was found (*F* = 1.49, *p* = .232; Table 2).

The effect of group (A vs. B) and position (supine, SR, or RL) on GRV was statistically significant for both groups (both at *p* = .001; Table 1, Figure 2). For Group A, GRV was significantly lower than at the previous data collection point at each measurement point after the first. Moreover, GRV was significantly lower in the SR position compared

TABLE 1.

Comparison of Patient GRV Across Groups in the Three Interventional Positions

Position	Group A (*n* = 18)			Group B (*n* = 18)			Mean Difference	*t*	*p*
	M	*SD*	*SE*	*M*	*SD*	*SE*			
Supine	51.50	15.80	3.72	61.88	19.77	4.52	−10.38	−1.773	.085
Semirecumbent	49.50	15.50	3.65	59.38	19.94	4.64	−9.88	−1.661	.106
Right lateral	48.44	14.84	4.52	59.77	19.68	4.70	−11.33	−1.950	.059
Within group[a]	*F* = 11.34, *df* = 2, *p* < .001			*F* = 12.19, *df* = 2, *p* < .001					

Note. GRV = gastric residual volume.
[a]Repeated-measures analysis of variance.

TABLE 2.

Repeated-Measures ANOVA of the Effects of Position (Supine, SR, RL) and Group (A and B) on GRV

Source of Variation	Sum of Squares	df[a]	Mean Square	F	p
Position	142.16	2	71.08	21.89	< .001
Position × Group	220.81	2	4.84	1.49	.232

Note. ANOVA = analysis of variance; SR = semirecumbent; RL = right lateral; GRV = gastric residual volume.
[a]Epsilon correction with sphericity assumed.

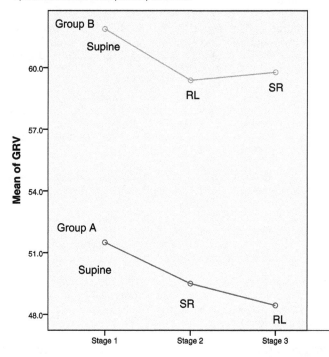

Figure 2. Comparison of gastric residual volume (GRV) by position (supine, semirecumbent [SR], and right lateral [RL]) and by group (A and B). Groups A and B were in the supine position in Stage 1. Group A was in the SR position in Stage 2 and in the RL position in Stage 3. Group B was in the RL position in Stage 2 and in the SR position in Stage 3.

with the supine position in both groups ($p < .05$), and GRV in the RL position was significantly lower than in the supine position in both groups ($p < .05$). Finally, GRVs in the SR and RL positions, although significantly and respectively different from the supine position, were not significantly different from each other ($p > .05$; Table 3).

Discussion

The hypothesis in this study was that, while in the SR position, participants would experience faster gastric emptying than while in other positions. The results of this study showed that altering body position effectively reduces GRV, with the SR and RL positions determined to be better at gastric emptying than the supine position. These findings suggest that positioning patients in either the RL or SR position accelerates the digestion of feedings. No significant difference between the SR and RL positions was identified in this study, although an increasing trend in GRV was identified for the RL position. No difference was found in terms of the order of positioning placement or of whether the patient was placed in the SR or RL position first. Similarly, Schallom, Dykeman, Metheny, Kirby, and Pierce (2015) found that elevating the head of the bed greater than 30° reduced oral secretion volume, reflux, and aspiration without inducing the development of pressure ulcers in gastric-fed adult patients receiving MV. In contrast, van der Voort and Zandstra (2001) showed that the GRV of mechanically ventilated adult patients in, respectively, prone and supine positions did not differ significantly. In addition, Hussein (2012) reported no significant difference between infants set, respectively, in RL and SR positions with regard to their mean GRV after feeding. Furthermore, Rezae et al. (2018) found an increase in gastric emptying in the RL position versus in the LL and supine positions in adults. Furthermore, Sanaka et al. (2013) showed that patients in the RL position experienced faster gastric emptying than their peers in the SR position. The use of the C-acetate breath test in this latter study to assess gastric emptying may have led to its divergent findings.

TABLE 3.

The Mean Difference in GRV by Groups by Position (Supine, SR, and RL)

Interventional Group		Position	Mean Difference	SE	p[a]
Group A	Supine	Semirecumbent	2.00	0.700	.033*
	Supine	Right lateral	3.05	0.563	.001*
	Semirecumbent	Right lateral	1.05	0.683	.423
Group B	Supine	Semirecumbent	2.50	0.506	.001*
	Supine	Right lateral	2.11	0.559	.005*
	Semirecumbent	Right lateral	−0.38	0.567	1.00

Note. GRV = gastric residual volume; SR = semirecumbent; RL = right lateral.
[a]Pairwise comparison with Bonferroni correction.
*$p < .05$.

Patients in the ICUs, although admitted for a variety of problems and injuries and receiving standard treatments, may experience adverse complications. Some complications such as DGE may cause other serious complications such as pneumonia and malnutrition. Therefore, the awareness of the healthcare providers regarding the methods available to control GRV, its prevalence, and its risk factors is necessary to improve the health and quality of patient care in the ICU.

Limitations

Several limitations affect this study. First, only the SR, RL, and supine positions were used. Future studies using additional positions such as the prone and right recumbent positions are suggested. Second, GRV was quantified as the volume aspirated via an NGT. This aspiration technique may be an unreliable method to assess GRV. Further studies using more-reliable techniques such as the C-acetate breath test are recommended to assess gastric emptying. Third, it should be assessed whether returning to the supine position makes a difference in terms of GRV or whether the movement alone decreases GRV. Fourth, only adults were assessed in this study, and previous research indicates that infants and young children may experience significantly different results than adults in terms of gastric emptying. Thus, conducting studies that include participants covering multiple age groups is recommended.

Conclusions

Overall, the findings of this study suggest that posing patients in either the RL or SR position is effective in accelerating the digestion of feedings. Understanding the best positioning for critically ill patients in ICUs may help decrease DGE and thus decrease other serious complications such as pneumonia and malnutrition. The results of this study contribute to a better understanding of the relationship among patient position, time, and GRV.

Acknowledgments

This study was adopted from an intensive care nursing master's thesis performed at Aja University of Medical Sciences, Tehran, Iran. The authors appreciate the Aja University of Medical Sciences for financial support (Grant No. 594260) as well as the valuable assistance of the participating patients and their families. We also sincerely thank the Chief of Bea'sat Hospital, Tehran, Iran, and the staff of the intensive care units at this hospital.

Author Contributions

Study conception and design: ZF, MK
Data collection: MK
Data analysis and interpretation: ZF, SB, AZ
Drafting of the article: ZF, MK, SB
Critical revision of the article: ZF

References

Aslani, M. A., Hanifi, N., Ahmadi, F., & Fallah, R. (2014). Effect of acupressure on amount of gastric emptying in mechanically ventilated patients hospitalized in intensive care units. *Journal of Hayat, 20*(2), 69–81. (Original work published in Persian)

Burn-Murdoch, R., Fisher, M. A., & Hunt, J. N. (1980). Does lying on the right side increase the rate of gastric emptying? *The Journal of Physiology, 302*, 395–398. https://doi.org/10.1113/jphysiol.1980.sp013251

Chen, S. S., Tzeng, Y. L., Gau, B. S., Kuo, P. C., & Chen, J. Y. (2013). Effects of prone and supine positioning on gastric residuals in preterm infants: A time series with cross-over study. *International Journal of Nursing Studies, 50*(11), 1459–1467. https://doi.org/10.1016/j.ijnurstu.2013.02.009

Chow, S. C., Shao, J., & Wang, H. (2008). *Sample size calculation in clinical research* (2nd ed.). Boca Raton, FL: Taylor & Francis Group.

DeLegge, M. H. (2011). Managing gastric residual volumes in the critically ill patient: An update. *Current Opinion in Clinical Nutrition & Metabolic Care, 14*(2), 193–196. https://doi.org/10.1097/MCO.0b013e328341ede7

Dietitians Association, Australia. (2015). *Enteral nutrition manual for adults in health care facilities.* Retrieved from http://daa.asn.au/wp-content/uploads/2011/11/enteral-nutrition-manual-oct-2010-pdf

Douglas, C. C., Lawrence, J. C., Bush, N. C., Oster, R. A., Gower, B. A., & Darnell, B. E. (2007). Ability of the Harris Benedict formula to predict energy requirements differs with weight history and ethnicity. *Nutrition Research, 27*(4), 194–199. https://doi.org/10.1016/j.nutres.2007.01.016

Dutch Dieticians Oncology Group. (2017). *Pancreatic cancer (nationwide guideline).* Retrieved from https://www.oncoline.nl/index.php?pagina=/richtlijn/item/pagina.php&id=40878&richtlijn_id=1061

Gattinoni, L., Tognoni, G., Pesenti, A., Taccone, P., Mascheroni, D., Labarta, V., ... Latini, R. (2001). Effect of prone positioning on the survival of patients with acute respiratory failure. *New England Journal Medicine, 345*(8), 568–573. https://doi.org/10.1056/NEJMoa010043

Gocze, I., Strenge, F., Zeman, F., Creutzenberg, M., Graf, B. M., Schlitt, H. J., ... Bein, T. (2013). The effects of the semirecumbent position on hemodynamic status in patients on invasive mechanical ventilation: Prospective randomized multivariable analysis. *Critical Care, 17*(2), R80. https://doi.org/10.1186/cc12694

Guerin, C., Gaillard, S., Lemasson, S., Ayzac, L., Girard, R., Beuret, P., ... Kaidomar, M. (2004). Effects of systematic prone positioning in hypoxemic acute respiratory failure: A randomized controlled trial. *JAMA, 292*(19), 2379–2387. https://doi.org/10.1001/jama.292.19.2379

Guo, B. (2015). Gastric residual volume management in critically ill mechanically ventilated patients: A literature review. *Proceedings of Singapore Healthcare, 24*(3), 171–180. https://doi.org/10.1177/2010105815598451

Heydari, A., & Emami Zeydi, A. (2014). Is gastric residual volume monitoring in critically ill patients receiving mechanical ventilation an evidence-based practice? *Indian Journal of Critical Care Medicine, 18*(4), 259–260. https://doi.org/10.4103/0972-5229.130588

Hussein, H. A. (2012). The difference between right side and semirecumbent positions after feeding on gastric residual volume among infant. *Journal of American Science, 8*(1), 127–132. Retrieved from http://www.jofamericanscience.org/journals/am-sci/am0801/019_7656am0801_127_132.pdf

Knaus, W. A., Wagner, D. P., Draper, E. A., Zimmerman, J. E., Bergner, M., Bastos, P. G., ... Harrell, F. E.Jr. (1991). The APACHE III prognostic system. Risk prediction of hospital mortality for critically ill hospitalized adults. *Chest, 100*(6), 1619–1636. https://doi.org/10.1378/chest.100.6.1619

Lord, L. M. (2018). Enteral access devices: Types, function, care, and challenges. *Nutrition in Clinical Practice, 33*(1), 16–38. https://doi.org/10.1002/ncp.10019

Montejo, J. C., Minambres, E., Bordeje, L., Mesejo, A., Acosta, J., Heras, A., ... Manzanedo, R. (2010). Gastric residual volume during enteral nutrition in ICU patients: The REGANE study. *Intensive Care Medicine, 36*(8), 1386–1393. https://doi.org/10.1007/s00134-010-1856-y

Nasiri, M., Farsi, Z., Ahangari, M., & Dadgari, F. (2017). Comparison of intermittent and bolus enteral feeding methods on enteral feeding intolerance of patients with sepsis: A triple-blind controlled trial in intensive care units. *Middle East Journal of Digestive Disease, 9*(4), 218–227. https://doi.org/10.15171/mejdd.2017.77

Nguyen, N. Q., Fraser, R. J., Bryant, L. K., Burgstad, C., Chapman, M. J., Bellon, M., ... Horowitz, M. (2008). The impact of delaying enteral feeding on gastric emptying, plasma cholecystokinin, and peptide YY concentrations in critically ill patients. *Critical Care Medicine, 36*(5), 1469–1474. https://doi.org/10.1097/CCM.0b013e31816fc457

Poveda, V. B., Castilho, A. C. B. A., Nogueira, L. S., Ferretti-Rebustini, R. E. L., & Silva, R. C. G. E. (2018). Assessing gastric residual volume: A description of nurses' clinical practice. *Revista da Escola de Enfermagem da USP, 52*, e03352. https://doi.org/10.1590/S1980-220X2017038803352

Reignier, J., Mercier, E., Le Gouge, A., Boulain, T., Desachy, A., Bellec, F., ... Lascarrou, B. (2013). Effect of not monitoring residual gastric volume on risk of ventilator-associated pneumonia in adults receiving mechanical ventilation and early enteral feeding: A randomized controlled trial. *JAMA, 309*(3), 249–256. https://doi.org/10.1001/jama.2012.196377

Rezae, J., Kadivarian, H., Abdi, A., Rezae, M., Karimpour, K., & Rezae, S. (2018). The effect of body position on gavage residual volume of gastric in intensive care units patients. *Iranian Journal of Nursing, 30*(110), 58–67. https://doi.org/10.29252/ijn.30.110.58 (Original work published in Persian)

Sanaka, M., Urita, Y., Yamamoto, T., Shirai, T., Kimura, S., Aoyagi, H., & Kuyama, Y. (2013). Right recumbent position on gastric emptying of water evidenced by (13) C breath testing. *World Journal of Gastroenterology, 19*(3), 362–365. https://doi.org/10.3748/wjg.v19.i3.362

Schallom, M., Dykeman, B., Metheny, N., Kirby, J., & Pierce, J. (2015). Head-of-bed elevation and early outcomes of gastric reflux, aspiration and pressure ulcers: A feasibility study. *American Journal of Critical Care, 24*(1), 57–66. https://doi.org/10.4037/ajcc2015781

Stewart, M. L. (2014). Interruptions in enteral nutrition delivery in critically ill patients and recommendations for clinical practice. *Critical Care Nurse, 34*(4), 14–21. https://doi.org/10.4037/ccn2014243

van der Voort, P. H. J., & Zandstra, D. F. (2001). Enteral feeding in the critically ill: Comparison between the supine and prone positions: A prospective crossover study in mechanically ventilated patients. *Critical Care, 5*(4), 216–220. https://doi.org/10.1186/cc1026

10

Translation, Adaptation and Validation of the Malay Version of the Cardiac Rehabilitation Barriers Scale

Li Sze CHAI[1] • Sidiah SIOP[2]* • Zabidah PUTIT[2] • Lily LIM[1] • Azylina GUNGGU[1] • Suk Fong TIE[3]

ABSTRACT

Background: The rate of cardiac rehabilitation attendance at the Sarawak Heart Centre was identified as very low, and the reason has not been investigated. A scale is needed to identify barriers to participation in cardiac rehabilitation among patients with heart disease in Sarawak, Malaysia.

Purpose: The purposes of this study were to translate, adapt, and evaluate the Malay-language version of the Cardiac Rehabilitation Barriers Scale (CRBS) and to measure the psychometric properties of the Malay-version CRBS to justify its use in Sarawak.

Methods: A forward and back-translation method was used. Content validity was assessed by three experts. Psychometric testing was conducted on a sample of 283 patients who were eligible to participate in cardiac rehabilitation. A construct validity test was performed using factor analysis. Cronbach's alpha was used to examine the internal consistency. The test–retest reliability was calculated using the intraclass correlation coefficient on 22 participants. Independent-samples t test and analysis of variance were conducted to assess the criterion validity. Mean scores for total barriers of the scale and each individual factor were compared among the different patient characteristics.

Results: The Malay-version CRBS showed an item level of content validity index of 1.00 for all of the items after improvements were made based on the experts' suggestions. The factor analysis, using principal component analysis with direct oblimin rotation, extracted four factors that differed from the original study. These four factors explained 52.50% of the cumulative percentage of variance. The Cronbach's alphas ranged from .74 to .81 for the obtained factors. Test–retest reliability was established using the intraclass correlation coefficient value of .78. Criterion validity was supported using the significant differences in the mean score for total barriers among educational level, driving distance, travel time to the hospital, and cardiac rehabilitation attendance.

Conclusions/Implications for Practice: This study found the Malay-version CRBS to be a valid and reliable instrument. It may be used with inpatients to identify barriers to participation in cardiac rehabilitation to promote rehabilitation attendance and improve patient care.

KEY WORDS:
translation, adaptation, psychometric testing, Cardiac Rehabilitation Barrier Scale, Malay.

Introduction

After in-hospital treatment, survivors of coronary heart disease (CHD) face substantial risks of recurrent cardiac event and death (Thune et al., 2011). Cardiac rehabilitation (CR) is an integral component in the management of CHD. The benefits of CR have been shown in a number of studies. Participation in CR has been associated with a 58% reduction in mortality (Beauchamp et al., 2013) and a significant reduction in hospital readmissions (Dunlay, Pack, Thomas, Killian, & Roger, 2014; Martin et al., 2012), which in turn may lower the overall costs of healthcare (Dendale, Hansen, Berger, & Lamotte, 2008). Despite these benefits, attendance rates as low as 7% and relatively high discontinuation rates of 8%–23% in CR programs have been reported (De Vos et al., 2013; Poh et al., 2015).

In an effort to improve CR attendance in Sarawak, a scale is necessary to address relevant patient and healthcare factor-related barriers. Sarawak, the largest state in Malaysia with an area of 124,450 km^2 and a population of 2.14 million, is located on Borneo Island (Department of Statistics Malaysia, 2017). Sarawak Heart Centre is the only government heart center in the state. Sarawak has a low catheterization laboratory to population ratio of 0.019 per 10,000, and the Sarawak Heart Centre manages about 7.2% of the total number of patients with heart disease in Malaysia (Wan Azman & Sim, 2015). The center is also the only government hospital in Sarawak to provide structured outpatient CR care at no cost to patients. However, an unpublished rehabilitation staff record from 2015 indicates suboptimal attendance in the outpatient CR program, with an attendance rate of 37.4% for all patients who were eligible to participate.

[1]MSc, RN, *Lecturer, Faculty of Medicine and Health Sciences, Department of Nursing, Universiti Malaysia Sarawak, Malaysia* • [2]PhD, RN, *Associate Professor, Faculty of Medicine and Health Sciences, Department of Nursing, Universiti Malaysia Sarawak, Malaysia* • [3]MSc, RN, *Matron, Sarawak Heart Centre, Malaysia.*

A review of the available scales was conducted that examined their constructs, dimensions, and appropriateness for use with patients with CHD who require CR. The Cardiac Rehabilitation Barriers Scale (CRBS) was chosen because it assesses patient, healthcare provider, and healthcare-system-related factors (Shanmugasegaram et al., 2012). The CRBS was developed in Canada based on literature review, feedback from cardiologists, and CR staffs. The first version of the CRBS has 19 items and was administered to two cardiac cohorts, including 272 inpatients, 1,497 outpatients, and 97 cardiologists. This version was subsequently revised into a 21-item scale and was psychometrically tested on 2,636 cardiac inpatients. Moreover, a Brazilian Portuguese version of the 21-item CRBS has been psychometrically validated (Ghisi et al., 2012), and the CRBS has been translated into the Colombian-Spanish, French, Punjabi, Korean, Indonesian, and Chinese languages. The CRBS may be administered to inpatients or outpatients to identify barriers to CR participation. The scale items are rated on a 5-point Likert-type scale that ranges from 1 (*strongly disagree*) to 5 (*strongly agree*). The four subscales in the CRBS are as follows: perceived needs and healthcare factors (nine items); logistical factors (five items) such as distance, cost, and transportation problems; work and time conflicts (three items); and comorbidities and functional status (four items). Higher scores indicate greater barriers to participation in a CR program.

It was necessary to translate the questionnaire into Malay, the official language of Sarawak State. Therefore, the purpose of this study was to translate, adapt, and evaluate the Malay-version CRBS. Furthermore, this study aimed to measure the psychometric properties of the translated CRBS to justify its use in Sarawak. The ultimate objective was to offer a translated instrument that may be used to provide information and facilitate research and that will improve patient care by improving CR attendance.

Methods

Translation and Cultural Adaptation

Before beginning the translation process, permission was obtained from the developer of the CRBS to adapt, translate, and use this scale. A forward translation method was used (Sousa & Rojjanasrirat, 2011), and the questionnaire was translated by two independent translators whose first language is Malay. One of the translators was a university nursing lecturer who had over 25 years of experience in lecturing in the English language and who had published books in both Malay and English. The other translator was a secondary school teacher who had taught subjects in both English and Malay for 18 years. The translated questionnaires from the two translators were compiled into a single translated questionnaire by the research team. During the compilation process, both translators were consulted using a group chat when two different words were chosen, with consultations continuing until consensus was reached on which word to

use. During this process, the research team and the translators decided to delete the word "severe" in Item 8 (…severe weather), as the word "severe" is not applicable to weather in the context of the research.

The translated questionnaire then underwent blind back-translation by a separate set of two translators. Neither of these translators, whose first language was English, knew about the original questionnaire. The first back-translator worked as a clinical physician who has used Malay and English in his clinical work for more than 10 years. The second back-translator was a secondary school teacher who had taught in both English and Malay for about 7 years. Next, the research team compared the back-translated questionnaires to the original questionnaire. The purpose of this comparison was to ensure that there was no difference in wording between the original items and the back-translated version. The meaning of all the items was found to be equivalent, except for Items 10 and 11. The research team then worked on rephrasing the items based on the suggestions from all of the four translators. For example, in Item 11, "…of time constraints" was rephrased to "I don't have enough time", as in the Malay language, "time constraints" is not commonly used and patients may have difficulties understanding the phrase. The preliminary version of Malay-version CRBS was then developed.

Subsequently, the research team worked to adapt the instructions and a few items on the original questionnaire. Five clinical CR nurses were invited to join the team for this adaptation process. Each had 7–15 years of experience in coronary care nursing and had experience with data collection in at least one research study or clinical trial. A half-day meeting was held, and each item was reviewed carefully. They were asked to contribute their knowledge and suggestions based on local information and context. The original instructions identified the barriers of patients who did not attend or who discontinued CR. For the Malay version, these instructions were adapted to examine respondents' view regarding their future attendance in CR programs, as the translated questionnaire was expected to be delivered before the respondents' CR appointment date. Phrases including "I have a problem with," "I must," and "I have" were added to Items 1, 2, and 8; Item 10; and Items 3, 4, 12, and 14, respectively. These adaptations did not affect the meaning of the original items.

The instrument was then emailed to three experts for quantification of content validity. The purpose of this step was to evaluate each item for content appropriateness and relevance. The experts included one physician who had experience working in cardiac care and was an investigator in clinical trials, one nursing educator who had more than 10 years of experience in cardiac care and was currently teaching coronary care nursing in a postbasic program, and one nursing matron in the CR unit who had more than 30 years of clinical experience in cardiac care nursing and was previously involved in clinical trials. The content validity scale developed by Davis (1992) was used. The experts rated each item in terms of clarity, appropriateness, and relevance to assess the barriers to CR on a 4-point scale (1 = *not relevant*, 2 = *somewhat relevant*, 3 = *quite relevant*, and 4 = *highly relevant*).

The content validity index (CVI) score was calculated for both the item level (I-CVI) and the scale level (S-CVI; Polit & Beck, 2006). The I-CVI was computed for each item by dichotomizing the 4-point scale, with items scored either 1 or 2 categorized into the "not relevant" category with 0 points each and items scored either 3 or 4 categorized into the "relevant" category with 1 point each. The points were later divided by the number of experts (3) to obtain the I-CVI value for each item. The S-CVI is the average of the I-CVIs for all of the scale items. As fewer than five experts were invited to rate the items, the I-CVI should be 1.00 for all items (Lynn, 1986), indicating that the S-CVI should be 1.00 as well (Polit & Beck, 2006). All of the invited experts responded within a week, and the calculated I-CVI value was 1.00 for all of the items except for Item 8, which scored a low value of .33. The S-CVI value was .97, which did not achieve the required CVI value. Examples in brackets were added to Item 8 to clarify the meaning of the statement "I have problems with weather." These examples were "too hot to be outside of the house or raining." After the revision to Item 8, the scale was emailed to the three experts again to once more quantify the content validity. All of them rated all items as 1.00, and thus, the scores for the I-CVI for all of the items and for the S-CVI were 1.00.

Psychometric Testing

Participants

Participants for the psychometric tests were recruited from the Sarawak Heart Centre using convenience sampling. Inclusion criteria were requiring CR and being eligible for CR program participation. Patients who had residual coronary stenosis or were assessed by healthcare providers to have limited ability to participate in the CR program because of stroke, physical impairment, or other reason were excluded. Data were collected between January and August 2017. Two hundred eighty-four inpatients were recruited, as the suggested sample size for performing factor analysis is at least 10 respondents for each item in the instrument being used (Nunnally, 1978). Questionnaires were administered to the patients before they were discharged from the hospital. The CR program involves eight sessions and requires attendance twice per week for a 1-month period. Participant attendance in the CR program was followed up by examining their attendance record. They were grouped into three categories, including "attended" if they attended all of the sessions; "discontinued" if they attended one or more, but not all, sessions; and "did not attend" if they were not present for any of the sessions. Twenty-two of those in the "attended" category were selected using a convenience sampling method for test–retest reliability, and the same scale was administered during their 6-week follow-up.

Ethical considerations

Ethical approval was obtained from the Medical Research and Ethic Committee, National Institutes of Health, Malaysia (Approval no. 5KKM/NIHSEC/P17-19). Informed consent was obtained from every participant. The participants were given full knowledge of the research process and could withdraw from the study at any time. They were assured that their personal data would remain confidential and that only the researcher would have full access to this data.

Psychometric validation

Data entry and data analysis were performed using SPSS Version 22.0 (IBM, Armonk, NY, USA). Returned questionnaires were examined for missing values. Percentage, pattern, and distribution of the missing values were analyzed before deciding on an approach to deal with these missing values.

A construct validity test was performed using factor analysis. The factorability of the 21 items was first assessed to determine the suitability of the data for use in factor analysis. This assessment included examining the correlation matrix, Kaiser–Meyer–Olkin measure of sampling adequacy, Bartlett's test of sphericity, diagonal of the anti-image correlation matrix, and communalities.

After confirming suitability, factor extraction was performed using principal component analysis (PCA), as the purpose was to identify the components underlying all of the 21 items. Number of components to retain was determined using the following tests: the rule of eigenvalue greater than 1, at least 50% of cumulative percentage of variance, scree test, and parallel analysis (Reise, Waller, & Comrey, 2000; Williams, Onsman, & Brown, 2010). The obtained factors were then rotated using varimax and direct oblimin rotations, with the factor loading significance set at .32 (Brown, 2009). Both rotations were examined before deciding on the final rotation method. Finally, the retained components were assessed to ensure that they had at least three items with loadings greater than .4 (Samuels, 2016).

Cronbach's alpha was used to estimate the internal consistency of the scale and subscales. The accepted minimum alpha value was set at .70, which confirms that correlations among items on the same subscale are acceptable (Tavakol & Dennick, 2011). The intraclass correlation coefficient (ICC) was used to assess the test–retest reliability of the scale. ICC estimates and their 95% confident intervals were calculated based on a mean-rating ($k = 2$), absolute-agreement, two-way mixed-effects model, with alpha values of more than .75 indicating good reliability (Koo & Li, 2016). The suggested sample size was a minimum of 15–20 to obtain an alpha value of .05 and a power of 80% and to detect a value of .70 for the ICC (Bujang & Baharum, 2017). Data were collected from the 22 participants in the "attended" category using the same scale 6 weeks later.

The Shapiro–Wilk test was performed, and the Q-Q plot was examined to confirm that data were normally distributed. Independent-samples *t* test and one-way analysis of variance (ANOVA) were then used to assess the criterion validity of the scale. The criteria that were chosen to test the criterion validity include gender, educational level, driving distance, travel time to the hospital, and CR attendance. These criteria were found to have barrier scores that differed significantly from previous CRBS studies (Ghisi et al., 2012; Shanmugasegaram, Oh, Reid, McCumber, & Grace, 2013). Mean scores for total barriers of the scale and of each individual factor were compared among these criteria.

Results

Data Screening

One questionnaire that was returned with 80.95% of the items unanswered was excluded from data analysis. The remaining 283 questionnaires contained an average of 0.54% missing values for all questionnaire items. Little's missing completely at random test resulted in a chi-square of 341.66 (df = 334, p = .38), indicating that the missing data were random. The missing data were thus replaced with a single imputation using the expectation–maximization algorithm, as this method preserves the relationship with other variables (Dong & Peng, 2013), which is an important basis for subsequent factor analysis.

Characteristics of the Participants

Table 1 shows the characteristics of the 283 participants. Mean age was 54.66 (SD = 10.48, range: 23–86) years. Most participants were male (83.75%) and had a nonuniversity level of education (88.34%); slightly over half (55.48%) reported a driving distance of more than 30 km to their CR program hospital, and 50.88% traveled over 1 hour to reach

TABLE 1.
Participant Characteristics (N = 283)

Category	n	%
Gender		
Male	237	83.75
Female	46	16.25
Educational level		
Nonuniversity	250	88.34
University	33	11.66
Driving distance, km		
≥ 30	157	55.48
< 30	126	44.52
Travel time, hour(s)		
≥ 1	144	50.88
< 1	139	49.12
CR attendance		
Did not attend	205	72.44
Discontinued	41	14.49
Attended	37	13.07

Note. CR = cardiac rehabilitation.

that hospital. Overall, CR attendance data showed that 72.44% did not attend the CR program and 14.49% discontinued CR after attending at least one but fewer than all sessions. Participants took 10–15 minutes to complete the questionnaire.

Content Validity

The Malay-version CRBS had I-CVI and S-CVI of 1.00. All of the items were retained in the final version of the instrument.

Construct Validity

Before performing factor analysis, the factorability of the data was examined. All of the items had a correlation of at least .30 with at least one other item in the correlation matrix, suggesting reasonable factorability. The Kaiser–Meyer–Olkin measure of sampling adequacy value was .73, which is above the recommended value of .60 and meets the "middling" criterion (Kaiser, 1974). Bartlett's test of sphericity was significant (χ^2[210] = 2072.62, p < .05). The diagonals of the anti-image correlation matrix were all above .60, and the communalities were all greater than .30. These results emphasize the appropriateness of proceeding with factor extraction.

Factor analysis was performed using PCA with all 21 items. Factor loading was set at .32 to suppress all loadings less than .32. Five components were identified with eigenvalues greater than 1, which explained 58.45% of the cumulative percentage of variance. The first component explained 21.46% of the variance, the second component explained 12.09% of the variance, and the third component explained 10.31% of the variance. The fourth and fifth components explained 5.96–8.64% of the variance. After varimax rotation, all of the components had at least three items with loadings greater than .40. However, four items (8, 16, 17, and 21) loaded on two components. Furthermore, the pattern matrix after direct oblimin rotation (delta = 0) showed that all of the components had at least three items with loadings greater than .40, but Item 8 loaded on two components.

The number of components retained was further examined using scree plot and parallel analysis. The scree plot showed a relatively large break after the fourth component, with the breaks between the subsequent components being all relatively small. The eigenvalues leveled off after the fourth or fifth component, a result that was rather ambiguous. The result of parallel analysis indicated that only four components of the original data produced an eigenvalue greater than the 95th percentile from the random data of 21 items, with 283 respondents. Thus, four components were retained for further analysis.

PCA was performed again with all 21 items by adding the commands to extract only four components. Varimax and direct oblimin rotations were conducted. The four components that were extracted explained 52.50% of the cumulative percentage of variance. Both rotations yielded very similar results, but the direct oblimin rotation provided the best-defined factor structure. The direct oblimin rotation showed that all items had primary loadings over .32 and that all components had at least three items with loadings greater than .40. The factors extracted were labeled as Factor 1, "perceived needs and functional status"; Factor 2, "personal and health problems"; Factor 3, "work and family commitments"; and Factor 4, "healthcare factors." The factor loading matrix for this final solution is presented in Table 2.

Internal Consistency

Cronbach's alpha was used to examine the internal consistency, and the overall value was calculated at .82. The alphas were moderate for each extracted factor: .79 for "perceived

needs and functional status" (nine items), .74 for "personal and health problems" (five items), .75 for "work and family commitments" (four items), and .81 for "healthcare factors" (three items). Alpha did not increase substantially for the scale or for individual factors if any item was deleted.

Reliability

Test–retest reliability was calculated using ICC with a mean-rating ($k = 2$), absolute-agreement, two-way mixed-effects model on 22 participants at a 6-week interval. The ICC value was .78.

TABLE 2.

Factor Loadings and Communalities Based on a Principal Component Analysis With Oblimin Rotation for 21 Items From the Malay-Version CRBS (N = 283)

Item	Factor 1	Factor 2	Factor 3	Factor 4	Variance Explained (%)	Eigen Value
Factor 1: perceived needs and functional status					21.46	4.51
7. I already exercise at home or in my community.	.864					
6. I don't need cardiac rehab (e.g., feel well, heart problem treated, not serious).	.813					
18. I can manage my heart problem on my own.	.681					
17. Many people with heart problems don't go, and they are fine.	.599					
16. My doctor did not feel that cardiac rehab is necessary.	.554					
13. I don't have the energy.	.471					
21. I prefer to take care of my health alone, not in a group.	.423					
15. I am too old.	.410					
9. I find exercise tiring or painful.	.377					
Factor 2: personal and health problems					12.09	2.54
3. I have transportation problems (e.g., access to a car, public transportation).		.842				
2. I have problem with cost (e.g., parking, gas).		.739				
1. I have problem with distance (e.g., not located in your area, too far to travel).		.711				
8. I have problem with weather (e.g., too hot to be outside of the house, raining).		.632				
14. I have other health problems that prevent me from going (specify: _____).		.460				
Factor 3: work and family commitments					10.31	2.17
4. I have family responsibilities (e.g., caregiving).			.858			
11. I don't have enough time (e.g., too busy, inconvenient class time).			.708			
12. I have work responsibilities.			.707			
10. I have to travel to other places (e.g., holiday trip, business trip).			.700			
Factor 4: healthcare factors					8.64	1.81
5. I don't know about cardiac rehab (e.g., doctor didn't tell me about it).				−.930		
20. It took too long to get referred and into the program.				−.797		
19. I think I was referred, but the rehab program didn't contact me.				−.788		

Note. Factor loadings < .32 were suppressed. CRBS = Cardiac Rehabilitation Barriers Scale.

Criterion Validity

Independent-samples t test and ANOVA were conducted to assess the criterion validity. Table 3 shows the mean score for total barrier of the scale and each individual factor among the different patient characteristics. The total barrier score ranged from 21 to 105. The mean score for total barrier was 54.02 (SD = 8.67) and ranged from 30 to 75. There were significant differences between educational level (p = .02), driving distance to the hospital, CR program location (p < .001), and travel time to the hospital (p < .001). Participants with a nonuniversity level of education had significantly higher barriers than respondents with a university level of education. Participants who needed to travel more than 30 km and who required a travel time of over 1 hour from their house to the hospital also faced higher barriers to attending CR programs. The mean score for total barriers did not differ between genders, although male participants reported significantly higher barriers in Factor 3 (work and family commitments).

One-way ANOVA showed a significant effect of the barriers score on CR attendance, $F(2, 280)$ = 34.68, p < .001. Post hoc analyses using Tukey's honestly significant difference test indicated that the mean score for total barriers was significantly higher for participants who did not attend the CR program than for those who did attend (p < .001). In addition, the mean score for total barriers was higher for respondents who did not attend the CR program than for those who discontinued CR after attending one but less than all sessions (p < .001). However, those who attended CR did not differ significantly from those who discontinued CR (p = .64). Furthermore, the barriers score for each individual factor showed significant effects on CR attendance. Table 4 shows the Tukey's honestly significant difference comparison between total barriers score and each individual factor.

Discussion

This study implemented the measures that were suggested in the literature in an attempt to develop a valid and reliable Malay-version CRBS. The questionnaire developed in Malay will be used to assess the barriers perceived by inpatients to CR program participation.

The translation and adaptation process followed the guidelines suggested by Sousa and Rojjanasrirat (2011). In comparing the back-translated questionnaires with the forward-translated questionnaires and the original version, Sousa and Rojjanasrirat suggested using a multidisciplinary committee composed of one methodologist, one healthcare professional, all four translators, and, if possible, the developer of the original instrument. The committee that was gathered for this study included a methodologist and healthcare professionals. Although the developer of the original scale was not invited, all of the identified discrepancies were resolved via discussion without affecting the meaning of the original items. The revised items achieved I-CVI and S-CVI scores of 1.00 after two rounds of expert reviews and item improvements based on the experts' suggestions.

Factor analyses using PCA with both varimax and direct oblimin rotations were conducted to extract the factors. This technique was used to assess the construct validity by examining the interrelationships among the variables in the Malay-version CRBS to identify the underlying structure of the variables. Rotated structure solutions are easier to interpret than the original extracted factors, and direct oblimin rotation may produce more accurate results for studies of human behavior (William et al., 2010). Direct oblimin rotation was chosen as the final rotation method in this study, as it provided the best-defined factor structure after the rotations.

No item was deleted during the process of translation and psychometric validation. The number of items is consistent with

TABLE 3.
Independent-Samples t-Test Scores

Characteristic	n	Factor 1 M	(SD)	p	Factor 2 M	(SD)	p	Factor 3 M	(SD)	p	Factor 4 M	(SD)	p	Total Score M	(SD)	p
Gender				.52			.05			.02[a]			.42			.15
Male	237	20.12	(4.12)		15.26	(4.14)		11.33	(3.30)		6.97	(1.87)		53.69	(8.73)	
Female	46	21.66	(4.94)		16.57	(4.11)		10.26	(2.57)		7.22	(1.86)		55.71	(8.19)	
Educational level				.08			.01[a]			.99			.35			.02[a]
Nonuniversity	250	20.54	(4.35)		15.71	(4.10)		11.16	(3.24)		7.05	(1.91)		54.46	(8.70)	
University	33	19.12	(3.66)		13.67	(4.23)		11.15	(2.96)		6.72	(1.42)		50.67	(7.73)	
Driving distance, km				.63			< .01[a]			.27			< .01[a]			< .01[a]
≥ 30	157	20.79	(4.54)		16.98	(3.90)		11.35	(3.29)		7.37	(2.02)		56.49	(8.53)	
< 30	126	19.85	(3.93)		13.59	(3.70)		10.92	(3.10)		6.57	(1.55)		50.94	(7.83)	
Travel time, hour(s)				< .01[a]			< .01[a]			.13			< .01[a]			< .01[a]
≥ 1	144	21.11	(4.72)		17.35	(3.69)		11.44	(3.27)		7.42	(2.01)		57.33	(8.16)	
< 1	139	19.61	(3.68)		13.53	(3.71)		10.86	(3.11)		6.59	(1.61)		50.59	(7.82)	

Note. Item range: Factor 1 = 9–45; Factor 2 = 5–25; Factor 3 = 4–20; Factor 4 = 3–15; total score = 21–105.
[a]Total mean scores differ between groups.

TABLE 4.
Tukey's HSD Comparison of Total Barrier Score and Each Individual Factor

Barriers Score (I)	Barriers Score (J)	Mean Difference (I–J)	SE	p	95% CI
Total barriers					
Attended	Did not attend	−9.41*	1.39	< .001	[−12.69, −6.14]
	Discontinued	−1.59	1.77	.639	[−5.75, 2.57]
Did not attend	Attended	9.41*	1.39	< .001	[6.14, 12.69]
	Discontinued	7.82*	1.33	< .001	[4.68, 10.96]
Discontinued	Attended	1.59	1.77	.639	[−2.57, 5.75]
	Did not attend	−7.82*	1.33	< .001	[−10.96, −4.68]
Factor 1: perceived needs and functional status					
Attended	Did not attend	−2.20*	0.75	.010	[−3.96, −0.43]
	Discontinued	0.10	0.95	.993	[−2.14, 2.34]
Did not attend	Attended	2.20*	0.75	.010	[0.43, 3.96]
	Discontinued	2.30*	0.72	.004	[0.61, 3.99]
Discontinued	Attended	−0.10	0.95	.993	[−2.34, 2.14]
	Did not attend	−2.30*	0.72	.004	[−3.99, −0.61]
Factor 2: personal and health problems					
Attended	Did not attend	−5.13*	0.66	< .001	[−6.69, −3.58]
	Discontinued	−1.79	0.84	.085	[−3.76, 0.19]
Did not attend	Attended	5.13*	0.66	< .001	[3.58, 6.69]
	Discontinued	3.34*	0.63	< .001	[1.85, 4.83]
Discontinued	Attended	1.79	0.84	.085	[−0.19, 3.76]
	Did not attend	−3.34*	0.63	< .001	[−4.83, −1.85]
Factor 3: work and family commitments					
Attended	Did not attend	−1.60*	0.56	.014	[−2.93, −0.27]
	Discontinued	−0.54	0.72	.728	[−2.23, 1.14]
Did not attend	Attended	1.60*	0.56	.014	[0.27, 2.93]
	Discontinued	1.06	0.54	.126	[−0.22, 2.33]
Discontinued	Attended	0.54	0.72	.728	[−1.14, 2.23]
	Did not attend	−1.06	0.54	.126	[−2.33, 0.22]
Factor 4: healthcare factors					
Attended	Did not attend	−0.48	0.33	.304	[−1.25, 0.29]
	Discontinued	0.63	0.41	.278	[−0.34, 1.61]
Did not attend	Attended	0.48	0.33	.304	[−0.29, 1.25]
	Discontinued	1.12*	0.31	.001	[0.38, 1.85]
Discontinued	Attended	−0.63	0.41	.278	[−1.61, 0.34]
	Did not attend	−1.12*	0.31	.001	[−1.85, −0.38]

Note. CI = confidence interval; HSD = honestly significant difference.
*p < .05.

the validation studies in the original version (Shanmugasegaram et al., 2012) and the Brazilian Portuguese version (Ghisi et al., 2012). Four factors were extracted from the PCA in this study, including perceived needs and functional status (nine items), personal and health problems (five items), work and family commitments (four items), and healthcare factors (three items). All of these factors were considered internally consistent, as each earned a Cronbach's alpha value greater

than .70 (Tavakol & Dennick, 2011). The reliability of the scale was also established with an ICC of .78.

Perceived needs and functional status were grouped together as the first factor in this study. This is different from the original structure, which grouped perceived needs and healthcare factors as the first factor. One plausible explanation is that patients in Sarawak interpret the barriers of perceived needs and of functional status as a single issue. The functional status items appear to relate to patients' perceived needs for CR. Moreover, the items related to perceived needs relate to the health status perception of patients—for example, "I don't need CR" and "I can manage my heart problem on my own." These perceptions on health status tend to affect the functional status of patients (Allahverdipour, AsghariJafarabadi, Heshmati, & Hashemiparast, 2013). Therefore, perceived needs and functional status were identified as two interconnected subscales and were combined into a single factor in this study.

Two items, Items 14 and 4, loaded on different factors in this study, which suggest different interpretations of these items in the Malaysian setting. Item 14 in the comorbidities subscale in the original CRBS loaded on four logistical factor items. A new factor, called "personal and health problems," was created for these items. One possible explanation for this difference from the original scale is that patients in Sarawak interpret the phrase "other health problems" in this item as personal problems that prevent them from participating in a CR program. Similarly, Item 4 in the logistical factors in the original CRBS loaded on all of the items in the work/time conflicts subscale. These items were combined in a new factor called "work and family commitments" in the Malay version. "Family responsibilities" in Item 4 may be interpreted by the patients as a commitment that acts as a barrier to CR participation.

In assessing criterion validity, the mean scores for total barriers and each individual factor were found to differ significantly among the groups of patients who attended CR, did not attend CR, and discontinued CR after attending at least one but fewer than all of the sessions. In addition, the scores were found to relate negatively to CR program attendance, with higher barrier scores associated with a higher likelihood of discontinuance or nonattendance. These findings are consistent with the findings of the original validation study (Shanmugasegaram et al., 2012).

The differences in the mean score for total barriers were also observed for educational level, driving distance, and travel time to the hospital. This is consistent with the barriers found in other studies to attending and utilizing CR programs. Higher educational level was shown to increase the likelihood of attending a CR program (Dunlay et al., 2009), whereas longer distance to the nearest CR provider was associated with lower CR uptake and attendance (van Engen-Verheul et al., 2012). It was also found that patients were significantly less likely to enroll in CR when travel time to attend a CR program was 60 minutes or more (Brual et al., 2010).

This study was affected by several limitations. First, there was high number of male patients, patients who did not attend the CR program, and patients with a relatively low level of education, which may reflect a selection bias. However, selection bias is unlikely, as a previous study also found the same differences in CRBS scores between the groups (Ghisi et al., 2012). Second, the Malay-version CRBS was administered to inpatients before hospital discharge. Patients may develop further or different barriers after hospital discharge.

Finally, as the study was conducted in Sarawak, the findings may only be generalizable to patients with a background similar to the participants in this study, especially in terms of similar healthcare system utilization patterns. Further studies on Malay-speaking patients are necessary to validate the findings in this study.

Implications

The Malay-version CRBS may be used with inpatients to identify barriers to CR program participation. The identified barriers should be modified to increase CR attendance and to further improve patient care.

Conclusions

The results of this study suggest that the Malay-version CRBS is a valid and reliable instrument. It may be used to identify the barriers to CR program participation and to suggest interventions to effectively increase CR program attendance.

Acknowledgments

This research was supported by Grant F05/SGS/1509/2016 from Universiti Malaysia Sarawak. We thank all of the participants in this study. We also extend our thanks to Dr. Asri and Dr. Ong Tiong Kiam for their permission to recruit patients in the Sarawak Heart Centre. Special thanks to Matron Saerah Wahet, Hu Chia Chia, Maria Udin, Siti Hasziah, Alice Semu, and Dayang Atikah for their support.

References

Allahverdipour, H., AsghariJafarabadi, M., Heshmati, R., & Hashemiparast, M. (2013). Functional status, anxiety, cardiac self-efficacy, and health beliefs of patients with coronary heart disease. *Health Promotion Perspectives, 3*(2), 217–229. https://doi.org/10.5681/hpp.2013.025

Beauchamp, A., Worcester, M., Ng, A., Murphy, B., Tatoulis, J., Grigg, L., ... Goble, A. (2013). Attendance at cardiac rehabilitation is associated with lower all-cause mortality after 14 years of follow-up. *Heart (British Cardiac Society), 99*(9), 620–625. https://doi.org/10.1136/heartjnl-2012-303022

Brown, J. D. (2009). Choosing the right type of rotation in PCA and EFA. *JALT Testing & Evaluation SIG Newsletter, 13*(3), 20–25.

Brual, J., Gravely-Witte, S., Suskin, N., Stewart, D. E., Macpherson, A., & Grace, S. L. (2010). Drive time to cardiac rehabilitation: At what point does it affect utilization? *International Journal of Health Geographics, 9*, 27. https://doi.org/10.1186/1476-072X-9-27

Bujang, M. A., & Baharum, N. (2017). A simplified guide to determination of sample size requirements for estimating the value of intraclass correlation coefficient: A review. *Archives of Orofacial Sciences, 12*(1), 1–11.

Davis, L. L. (1992). Instrument review: Getting the most from a panel of experts. *Applied Nursing Research, 5*(4), 194–197. https://doi.org/10.1016/S0897-1897(05)80008-4

De Vos, C., Li, X., Van Vlaenderen, I., Saka, O., Dendale, P., Eyssen, M., & Paulus, D. (2013). Participating or not in a cardiac rehabilitation programme: Factors influencing a patient's decision. *European Journal of Preventive Cardiology, 20*(2), 341–348. https://doi.org/10.1177/2047487312437057

Dendale, P., Hansen, D., Berger, J., & Lamotte, M. (2008). Long-term cost–benefit ratio of cardiac rehabilitation after percutaneous coronary intervention. *Acta Cardiologica, 63*(4), 451–456. https://doi.org/10.2143/AC.63.4.2033043

Department of Statistics Malaysia. (2017). Sarawak @ a glance. Retrieved from https://www.dosm.gov.my/v1/index.php?r=column/cone&menu_id=clJnWTITbWFHdmUwbmtSTE1EQStFZz09#

Dong, Y., & Peng, C. Y. J. (2013). Principled missing data methods for researchers. *Springerplus, 2*(1), 222. https://doi.org/10.1186/2193-1801-2-222

Dunlay, S. M., Pack, Q. R., Thomas, R. J., Killian, J. M., & Roger, V. L. (2014). Participation in cardiac rehabilitation, readmissions, and death after acute myocardial infarction. *The American Journal of Medicine, 127*(6), 538–546. https://doi.org/10.1016/j.amjmed.2014.02.008

Dunlay, S. M., Witt, B. J., Allison, T. G., Hayes, S. N., Weston, S. A., Koepsell, E., & Roger, V. L. (2009). Barriers to participation in cardiac rehabilitation. *American Heart Journal, 158*(5), 852–859. https://doi.org/10.1016/j.ahj.2009.08.010

Ghisi, G. L., Santos, R. Z., Schveitzer, V., Barros, A. L., Recchia, T. L., Oh, P., ... Grace, S. L. (2012). Development and validation of the Brazilian Portuguese version of the Cardiac Rehabilitation Barriers Scale. *Arquivos Brasileiros de Cardiologia, 98*(4), 344–352. https://doi.org/10.1590/S0066-782X2012005000025

Kaiser, H. F. (1974). An index of factorial simplicity. *Psychometrika, 39*(1), 31–36. https://doi.org/10.1007/BF02291575

Koo, T. K., & Li, M. Y. (2016). A guideline of selecting and reporting intraclass correlation coefficients for reliability research. *Journal of Chiropractic Medicine, 15*(2), 155–163. https://doi.org/10.1016/j.jcm.2016.02.012

Lynn, M. R. (1986). Determination and quantification of content validity. *Nursing Research, 35*(6), 382–386. https://doi.org/10.1097/00006199-198611000-00017

Martin, B. J., Hauer, T., Arena, R., Austford, L. D., Galbraith, P. D., Lewin, A. M., ... Aggarwal, S. G. (2012). Cardiac rehabilitation attendance and outcomes in coronary artery disease patients.

Circulation, 126(6), 677–687. https://doi.org/10.1161/CIRCULATIONAHA.111.066738

Nunnally, J. C. (1978). *Psychometric theory* (2nd ed.). New York, NY: McGraw-Hill.

Poh, R., Ng, H. N., Loo, G., Ooi, L. S., Yeo, T. J., Wong, R., & Lee, C. H. (2015). Cardiac rehabilitation after percutaneous coronary intervention in a multiethnic Asian country: Enrollment and barriers. *Archives of Physical Medicine and Rehabilitation, 96*(9), 1733–1738. https://doi.org/10.1016/j.apmr.2015.05.020

Polit, D. F., & Beck, C. T. (2006). The content validity index: Are you sure you know what's being reported? Critique and recommendations. *Research in Nursing & Health, 29*(5), 489–497. https://doi.org/10.1002/nur.20147

Reise, S. P., Waller, N. G., & Comrey, A. L. (2000). Factor analysis and scale revision. *Psychological Assessment, 12*(3), 287–297. https://doi.org/10.1037/1040-3590.12.3.287

Samuels, P. (2016). *Advice on exploratory factor analysis.* Centre for Academic Success, Birmingham City University, UK. https://doi.org/10.13140/RG.2.1.5013.9766

Shanmugasegaram, S., Gagliese, L., Oh, P., Stewart, D. E., Brister, S. J., Chan, V., & Grace, S. L. (2012). Psychometric validation of the Cardiac Rehabilitation Barriers Scale. *Clinical Rehabilitation, 26*(2), 152–164. https://doi.org/10.1177/0269215511410579

Shanmugasegaram, S., Oh, P., Reid, R. D., McCumber, T., & Grace, S. L. (2013). Cardiac rehabilitation barriers by rurality and socioeconomic status: A cross-sectional study. *International Journal for Equity in Health, 12*(1), 72. https://doi.org/10.1186/1475-9276-12-72

Sousa, V. D., & Rojjanasrirat, W. (2011). Translation, adaptation and validation of instruments or scales for use in cross-cultural health care research: A clear and user-friendly guideline. *Journal of Evaluation in Clinical Practice, 17*(2), 268–274. https://doi.org/10.1111/j.1365-2753.2010.01434.x

Tavakol, M., & Dennick, R. (2011). Making sense of Cronbach's alpha. *International Journal of Medical Education, 2*, 53–55. https://doi.org/10.5116/ijme.4dfb.8dfd

Thune, J. J., Signorovitch, J. E., Kober, L., McMurray, J. J., Swedberg, K., Rouleau, J., ... Solomon, S. D. (2011). Predictors and prognostic impact of recurrent myocardial infarction in patients with left ventricular dysfunction, heart failure, or both following a first myocardial infarction. *European Journal of Heart Failure, 13*(2), 148–153 https://doi.org/10.1093/eurjhf/hfq194

van Engen-Verheul, M., de Vries, H., Kemps, H., Kraaijenhagen, R., de Keizer, N., & Peek, N. (2012). Cardiac rehabilitation uptake and its determinants in the Netherlands. *European Journal of Preventive Cardiology, 20*(2), 349–356. https://doi.org/10.1177/2047487312439497

Wan Azman, W. A., & Sim, K. H. (Eds.). (2015). *Annual report of the NCVD-ACS registry, year 2011–2013.* Kuala Lumpur, Malaysia: National Cardiovascular Disease Database.

Williams, B., Onsman, A., & Brown, T. (2010). Exploratory factor analysis: A five-step guide for novices. *Journal of Emergency Primary Health Care, 8*(3), 1–11.

11

Chinese Immigrant Women's Experiences as Community Health Workers in Korea: A Focus Group Study

Jiyun KIM[1]* • Hyang KIM[2] • Hae-Ra HAN[3]

ABSTRACT

Background: The number of immigrant women in Korea is rapidly increasing. Immigrant women in Korea experience a host of health problems associated with living in a new country. Community health workers (CHWs) may be effective at delivering health promotion programs to vulnerable groups such as recent immigrants.

Purpose: Qualitative analysis was performed to identify the main themes characterizing the experiences of CHWs in recommending and guiding preventive screening tests for immigrant women.

Methods: This focus-group study was designed to investigate the experiences and perceptions of CHWs. We conducted interviews with 15 Chinese immigrant women who served as CHWs in a cancer screening program. We asked questions about the attitudes and perceptions that CHWs had from their research experiences. Each interview was audio-recorded and transcribed verbatim.

Results: Three main themes emerged: (a) recognizing the need for preventive healthcare, (b) becoming the CHWs who help people to be healthy, and (c) challenges to overcome to make CHWs more active. The CHWs in this study were willing to help other Chinese immigrant women and to improve their competency to help more effectively. However, they recognized limitations on their ability to address problems when delivering a breast and cervical cancer screening program.

Conclusions: When training CHWs for immigrants in Korea, frequent opportunities for consultation should be provided during program delivery to facilitate troubleshooting and help CHWs overcome challenges. A program that utilizes CHWs for various minority groups is needed.

KEY WORDS:
qualitative research, community health workers, cancer screening, focus groups, minority groups.

Introduction

As Korea became more urbanized, men in rural areas found it increasingly difficult to find marriage partners. To resolve this problem, the "Rural Bachelors Matching Drive" campaign began in the mid-1980s (Song, 2015). Rural bachelors were encouraged to seek spouses from abroad, facilitated by the Korean government (Kim-Bossard, 2018). Korean Chinese women first began to immigrate to Korea for marriage, followed by women from various Southeast Asian countries (Song, 2015). The number of women who have married Korean men and moved to Korea (so-called marriage-immigrant women or MIW) increased significantly from 82,828 in 2006 to 137,094 in 2019 (Korea Statistical Information Service, 2021a). The steady increase of MIW has brought about a change in the population structure of Korea, which had been a monocultural and monoethnic country for centuries, with multicultural families comprising a significant 10.3% of the total Korean population in 2019 (Korea Statistical Information Service, 2021b).

Despite their geographic closeness, MIW from China (CMIW) is quite distinct from Koreans in terms of language, political system, and healthcare system. In addition, CMIW often lack awareness of the healthcare services and healthcare delivery systems available in Korea (Koh & Koh, 2009). It is important for CMIW to stay healthy as they get older.

Our study team implemented a community health worker (CHW)-led randomized controlled intervention trial designed to promote breast and cervical cancer screening in CMIW. CHWs are trained paraprofessionals from the target community who work to ensure that immigrants receive appropriate health education and care (Verhagen et al., 2014). Health promotion programs facilitated by CHWs have been effective in addressing the unique healthcare needs of a variety of vulnerable populations, including immigrants with cultural and linguistic barriers (Han et al., 2017; Mock et al., 2007; Mojica et al., 2016). Particularly with regard to health checkups, CHW-delivered interventions are not only highly effective but also cost-effective (Mojica et al., 2016; Nimmons et al., 2017; Schuster et al., 2015).

[1]*PhD, RN, Associate Professor, School of Nursing, Gachon University, Incheon, Republic of Korea • [2]MSN, RN, Doctoral Student, College of Nursing, Seoul National University, Seoul, Republic of Korea • [3]PhD, RN, Professor, School of Nursing, Johns Hopkins University, Baltimore, Maryland, USA.

Upon completion of study activities, the CMIW who participated in the intervention trial as CHWs were interviewed and shared their experiences. By analyzing the experiences of these CHWs, the authors aimed to elucidate CMIW awareness of the activities of CHWs and to identify priorities for improving the CHW training program. The results of this study are expected to help promote effective CHW training by offering insights into how CHWs act as intermediaries between experts and CMIW in Korea. The authors hope that the results of this study may help promote effective CHW training by providing insight into how CHWs act as an intermediary between Korean experts and CMIW.

Methods

Research Design

Focus groups and one-on-one interviews were used in this qualitative study. A typical focus-group study involves three or four focus groups, each containing five to eight subjects (Krueger & Casey, 2014). One commonly cited guideline is that focus-group research requires at least two groups to define demographic characteristics, with three groups needed to find the most prevalent themes (Guest et al., 2017). As only a small number of participants and groups were available for this study, expert advice was sought during the design phase. The expert gave the opinion that individual interviews would be required to better understand the research concept during the research. In addition, using an individual interview approach would allow the study team to explore personal experiences, whereas focus group interviews would elicit shared opinions and perceptions (Lambert & Loiselle, 2008). Thus, in this study, two focus-group interviews were planned and the individual interviews were based on each focus group.

Ethical Considerations

The institutional review board at the university approved this study (IRB No. 1044396-201512-HR-060-01). Before the interviews, all the participants received an explanation of the study procedures and aims, which involved the experiences and perceptions about the activities performed by CHWs. The right of withdrawal, data privacy, and participants' feedback about the study results were also explained.

Participants

The research participants comprised CMIW who met the following inclusion criteria: (a) aged between 30 and 64 years, (b) able to communicate in Korean, and (c) agreed to participate in the interview.

To recruit study participants, the researcher approached the multicultural centers in two cities where many multicultural families live to identify women who had immigrated to Korea from China and who held leadership roles in their communities. These women were then asked to help recruit people who wanted to work as CHWs in the community. Ten women were recruited from City S, and seven were recruited from City A, both of which are in metropolitan areas and have a high number of multicultural couples.

Briefly, the parent study involved a randomized controlled trial in which 17 CMIW were trained as CHWs to deliver the study intervention, which consisted of education about breast and cervical cancer screening tests followed by monthly phone follow-ups and counseling for a period of 6 months. The CHWs received 6 hours of training to deliver the study intervention. CHW training was delivered by the bilingual research team at two community locations and addressed the following topics: cancers in women, recruitment, study questionnaire, education on breast and cervical cancers and related screening tests, phone counseling, and participation in meetings. Seventeen CHWs received training in June 2015. Upon completion of training, one CMIW decided not to work as a CHW, resulting in 16 CMIW working as CHWs during the study period. Once each month, CHWs and the research team gathered in groups and held roundtables to review the progress of the research.

For this qualitative study, 16 CHWs who participated in the parent study agreed to join. Each interview participant received 50,000 Korean won ($\cong$U.S. $45) from the research fund to compensate for their effort and time. The 16 CMIW in this study consisted of nine CHWs in City S and seven CHWs in City A. For the individual interview, one CHW was selected in each region. One CHW who was planned to do the individual interview in City A took a new job and was no longer available to participate in the interview. Thus, the two focus groups were composed of eight and six women, respectively, with one additional participant receiving a one-on-one interview. The mean age of the 15 participants was 37 years (range: 30–46 years). The characteristics of the participants are summarized in Table 1.

Setting and Data Collection

The interviews were conducted in a quiet room. All the participants signed informed consent after the study was explained to them. CHWs were seated around a rectangular table with their colleagues and the research team. Each interview was audio-recorded, and the research team also kept notes on the answers provided. Beverages and snacks were served during the interview to provide a relaxing and comfortable environment. The time taken to participate was 5 minutes to complete the brief demographics questionnaire and 50 minutes to complete the interview.

The principal investigator of the parent study served as the facilitator, and a trained research assistant operated the audio recorder and took notes. Each interview was mainly conducted in Korean. However, the participants were allowed to speak in Chinese when they found it difficult to express themselves in Korean. A bilingual member of the study team translated Chinese into Korean as needed. The facilitator encouraged the participants to speak freely to enhance group

Table 1

Demographic Characteristics of the Sample (N = 15)

Characteristic	n	%
Age (years)		
30–39	11	73.3
≥ 40	4	26.7
Residence in Korea (years)		
5–9	11	73.3
≥ 10	4	26.7
Education		
High school	9	60.0
College	6	40.0
Number of family members		
3	4	26.7
4	7	46.6
≥ 5	4	26.7
Perceived standard of living (1–11 [low–high])		
4 or 5	7	46.6
6 or 7	4	26.7
≥ 8	4	26.7
Perceived ability to speak Korean		
Moderate	12	80.0
Good	3	20.0

interactions. She made eye contact evenly while responding, listening to CHWs, and waiting for members of the focus group to vocalize what they wanted to express.

The focus group interviews for Group 1 were held on November 26, 2015; the focus group interviews for Group 2 were held on December 10, 2015; and the individual interview was held on February 26, 2016.

The interview guide consisted of open questions and provided a printed interview guide to all subjects and research teams. The interview guide was constructed in consultation with qualitative research experts. The questions included in the interview guide are presented below:

1. What do you think of CHWs?
2. How does this experience influence the service you deliver?
3. Please tell us how your life has changed by working as a CHW.
4. What do you think is needed to be a good CHW?
5. How did you feel while working as a CHW?

Data Analysis

Qualitative data were analyzed using the qualitative descriptive method. This method has the advantage of conveying a given situation vividly by describing the characteristics of the subject, lifestyle behaviors, and living situation in detail (Sandelowski, 2000). This methodology is the most appropriate for understanding the specific situation of women migrating to other countries for reasons of marriage. The focus-group and individual interviews were audio-recorded and subsequently transcribed verbatim. Trained research assistants listened to the audio recordings and read the transcriptions repeatedly to ensure familiarity, then coded the meaningful text, and grouped this text into categories. We then repeatedly discussed the main codes and main categories. In July 2016, it was confirmed by two researchers that the content of the manuscript material reflected the recorded content accurately. In September 2016, on the basis of the manuscript data, the summary of interviews by major question categories was reviewed by two focus group participants. Two researchers analyzed the data and exchanged opinions with each other 3 times. In June 2017, June 2018, and August 2018, the two researchers analyzed each other's analysis. A community nursing researcher who did not participate in the analysis reviewed this analysis in April 2019. ATLAS.ti software (Version 8) was used for data analysis.

Results

Each focus group and the individual interview resulted in similar themes, which allowed the data to be pooled. Three main themes with eight subthemes emerged from the interviews. The main themes included (a) recognizing the need for preventive healthcare, (b) becoming the CHWs who help people to be healthy, and (c) challenges to overcome to make CHWs more active. Subthemes included (a) obtaining regular health screening even if one is not sick, (b) looking back on one's own health management, (c) being trained to deliver a health program, (d) immersing in the CHW role as a health advocate, (e) women's limited understanding of CHW roles, (f) experiencing challenges while juggling multiple roles as a CHW, (g) worry about confidentiality and potential financial burdens, and (h) one-time activities as a CHW.

Theme 1: Recognizing the Need for Preventive Healthcare

At the beginning of this study, CHWs were unfamiliar with breast and cervical cancer screening tests. They came to recognize the importance of regular screening tests after being trained as CHWs. Two subthemes related to this theme included obtaining regular health screening even if one is not sick and looking back on one's own health management.

Obtaining regular health screening even if one is not sick

CHWs did not understand the necessity of health screening for disease prevention before they came to Korea. CHWs pointed out that if they had not come to Korea, they would not have sought health checkups while healthy. One middle-aged CHW who had been in Korea for 7 years and another participant relayed the perception of health management among Chinese:

> *Chinese people do not go to a hospital unless they get sick.* (Group 1)

Usually, women aged 30 years feel they are very healthy and don't go to hospitals. However, I learned that it is necessary to check my health even when I am healthy. (Group 2)

Looking back on one's own health management

When the CHWs learned about regular screening for cancer prevention and delivered cancer education, they thought about their own health management as well as the health of the clients (friends who were CMIW) in the program. One CHW expressed her perception about usual healthcare:

I do not usually care about my health. However, after I got [CHW] training, I came to consider my own health condition and usual health management. (Group 2)

Theme 2: Becoming the Community Health Workers Who Help People to Be Healthy

As CHWs gained new knowledge about screening for cancer prevention, they became appreciative of this health knowledge and information in maintaining personal health and of their role as health agents. When trained, CHWs found that new health information was not only relevant but also useful for their health and that of others. CHWs were eager to learn more medical knowledge as they wanted to help their friends. Two subthemes emerged related to this theme: being trained to deliver a health program and immersing in a CHW role as a health advocate.

Being trained to deliver a health program

CHWs expressed that the information they gained from CHW training and participating in the parent study offered them an opportunity to learn about diseases and the importance of breast and cervical cancer screening tests. They conveyed that they obtained useful information through the CHW training program:

As I participated in this program, I gained a lot of medical knowledge and learned about the process of breast and cervical cancer screening tests. (Group 1)

When I worked, I became active; I tried to find something out about the disease and the prevention test. (Group 2)

Immersing in the community health worker role as a health advocate

The CHWs unanimously agreed that the prevention program gave them feelings of vigor and enthusiasm. They actively searched for information about diseases, health management, screening tests, and navigation information (e.g., clinics) in Korea. CHWs expressed that they enjoyed the activities as CHWs and acknowledged that the activities were helpful to them and their friends. They described themselves as health advocates who help neighbors and friends in the immigrant

community. Often, changed behavior (i.e., uptaking cancer screening test for the first time) among them resulted in positive emotions about CHW roles, as expressed by one participant:

When I heard my friend got an exam, I was so happy! (Group 1)

I think the work of CHWs is helpful for my friend's health. (individual interviewer)

Theme 3: Challenges to Overcome to Make Community Health Workers More Active

CHWs often felt troubled about their roles and responsibilities and expressed a desire to overcome the related challenges to be good CHWs. They felt worthwhile working as CHWs and wanted to continue in this role. Four subthemes emerged related to this theme: women's limited understanding of CHW roles, experiencing challenges while juggling multiple roles as a CHW, worry about confidentiality and potential financial burden, and one-time activities as a CHW.

Women's limited understanding of community health worker roles

When the CHWs conducted phone follow-ups, some women asked them about what roles and responsibilities a CHW plays. Some CHWs shared that they had difficulty explaining their roles clearly. However, CHWs work to help ensure the health of CMIW, so they overcame their discomfort:

When I recommended this program, my client asked if I would get benefit from these activities. "Do you earn money in exchange for my information?" When I heard this, my mood got bad. (Group 1)

I keep calling, and it is burdensome when a friend doubts why I called and asks me why. (Group 2)

I explained that what I do is to help protect my friend's health. (Group 1)

My role as a CHWs is to help my friends, so I can do well without being uncomfortable with what I do. (Group 2)

Experiencing challenges while juggling multiple roles as a community health worker

As CHWs work to deliver health education and counseling about breast and cervical cancer and related screening tests, they must schedule their own work and receive questions from the clients. CHWs noted that they sometimes failed to give adequate answers to questions that they had not expected such as the types and methods of hysterectomy and the prognosis of cervical cancer. Some CHWs noted that they had felt burdened and overloaded by these activities. They also noted that they felt anxious when the women reported that they had yet received a screening test:

When I select a subject, I have a friend who was not selected because of the research criteria. It's hard to tell her that she can't participate in the study. (Group 2)

It was difficult for me because the period of time spent on recruiting and telephone counseling was too long. I have to make repeated phone calls. (Group 2)

We need to have knowledge about our activities. (Group 1)

My subject asked me something like what the doctor should answer. (Group 2)

Worry about confidentiality and potential financial burdens

CHWs expressed concern about certain questions on the study survey that were considered sensitive privacy. CHWs noted that the demographic question about income level was perceived by some CMIW as intrusive and unnecessary. Another source of concern for CHWs was the potential financial burden on women to have screening tests done. A CHW stated:

When I invited my friend to participate in the study and encouraged her to be tested [for breast and cervical cancers], I became worried that she would spend a lot of money on the test if there is any kind of disease. (Group 1)

One-time activities as a community health worker

CHWs' work was conducted in this study to promote screening tests to prevent breast cancer and cervical cancer and was separate from the public community health program in Korea. Thus, the funding for this program was limited, and the activities of the CHWs ended at the conclusion of the program. The CHWs expressed the opinion that it is necessary to retain the CHWs to do activities in various ways for the immigrants who need help with their health.

When immigrants come to Korea for the first time, they don't know much about the healthcare system, so I think it would be great if CHWs could help immigrants. (Group 1)

CHW activities were difficult, but I hope I can continue. I also want to learn about other diseases and health management. (Group 2)

Women from other countries also need help, and many have health problems. Therefore, CHWs like us are in a good position to help them. (Group 2)

Discussion

This study was performed to evaluate the experiences of CHWs who facilitate preventive screening tests for CMIW in Korea. The perceptions of CHWs regarding their activities and roles found in this study were similar to those found in a previous study (Glenton et al., 2013). The main themes and subthemes that emerged from the focus-group and individual interviews revealed that, although CHWs deliver preventive screening tests to the CMIW, they perceived various aspects of their experiences and realized the necessity of preventive healthcare.

The first theme, which highlighted the Chinese CHWs' recognition of the need for preventive healthcare, is consistent with the finding of a prior study that interviewed 19 CHWs recruited from four health centers conducting health promotion activities (Seutloali et al., 2018). CHWs, who were exposed to healthcare in China and more inclined to therapeutic services than preventive services (Meng et al., 2019), expressed that they had taken on a new awareness regarding the importance of using preventive services while healthy rather than only visiting hospitals when sick. When CHWs perceive a need for preventive health management, they also consider that their health management is important (Aseyo et al., 2018). Vietnamese MIW in Korea are more willing to take preventive tests if they have had experience receiving pap tests (F.-H. Lee et al., 2016). It is necessary to perform regular health screening tests and increase their interest in their personal health status. This makes them a role model, which is a key aspect of CHWs (Gale & Sidhu, 2019).

The second theme addressing the CHWs' perception of their role to help people remain or become healthier is also consistent with previous studies. The CHWs in this study expressed happiness with their overall activities, which seems to reflect their perceived empowerment as a "helper" or "health advocate" (Han et al., 2007). Moreover, learning new knowledge by doing CHW activities has been shown to serve as a motivating factor (George et al., 2017). In Korea, MIW work in government-funded multicultural centers to help their friends from other countries by providing translation and counseling services (J. Lee, 2021). Our evaluation of the activities of CHWs delivering health promotion programs revealed the need to implement and assess diverse types of programs using immigrants as CHWs.

MIW can easily obtain medical insurance in Korea. Korean health insurance is compulsory, and all Koreans (hereinafter referred to as "the insured") and their dependents are insured (National Health Insurance Act, 1999/2017). The insured pays medical insurance premiums depending on his or her income and assets (National Health Insurance Act, 1999/2016). Dependents are usually supported by their family, mainly by the insured, and do not receive other remunerations or income. The insured are categorized as either local subscribers or employees (National Health Insurance Act, 1999/2017). In the case of MIWs, if a Korean husband is the insured, then the MIW is registered as a dependent. If the MIV is an employee, then she can be the insured as an employee subscriber (National Health Insurance Act, 1999/2017). The insured and dependent may use medical services at a relatively low price if they are sick, give birth, or attend a regular medical checkup (National Health Insurance Act, 1999/2016). However, in a survey, 11.9% of MIW who were sick during a previous 1-year period reported not going to a hospital (Choi et al., 2019). MIW who are relatively new to Korea often do not speak Korean and do not know what kind of hospital to go to and so are unable to go to a hospital even when they are sick (Choi et al., 2019). CHWs may help facilitate MIW to successfully access healthcare services upon immigrated to Korea through helping them overcome language problems, facilitating mobility, aiding in decision making, and providing information about health issues (Simon et al., 2018).

The third theme addressed the challenges necessary to overcome to make CHWs more active. Although CHWs can effectively deliver interventions in the community, they had difficulty explaining their roles clearly because of program recipients' misconceptions about CHW roles (Austin-Evelyn et al., 2017). They also felt a burden of responsibility, a lack of knowledge, and concerns about the interventions they were delivering (Glenton et al., 2013). The CHWs perceived that their activities for CMIW were fruitful and necessary, but they felt burdened by their promises made to their friends and worried when the women chose not to participate. The findings of a recent study suggest that ambivalence may signal competence and act as a kind of adaptive function (Pillaud et al., 2018). Those authors explained that mixed feelings may be helpful in facilitating rapid adaptation to varying situations (Pillaud et al., 2018). This can involve achieving an equilibrium between the education provided in the intervention and their perception of it, and the study team can help them adapt to new activities by explaining the intervention program in more detail and giving feedback when difficult situations are encountered during program activities.

Although the present research team met regularly to check the progress of program delivery and to give feedback to the CHWs, the Chinese CHWs in this study expressed concern over their ability to disseminate health information. In addition to solving problems via face-to-face conversations with the research team and the CWHs, it may be helpful to provide feedback by observing the CHW in action and/or video recording during CHW activities (Parker et al., 2016). It may also be helpful to provide characteristics related to the health-related behavior of immigrants and appreciate that the information improves awareness among CHWs of promoting receiving cancer screening among immigrant women (Bhandari & Kim, 2016; F.-H. Lee, 2018). Similar to providing ongoing training to CHWs in low-income countries (O'Donovan et al., 2018), providing supportive supervision while CHWs perform interventions helps them be confident in their work.

The CHWs in this study expressed a desire to increase their competence. The CHWs wanted to continue their activities and wanted CHW activities to expand to other sectors. Besides, they said that immigrants from countries other than China also have CHW requirements. In the future, it will be possible to use CHWs in various fields related to multicultural families in Korea, and it will be possible to provide basic data from multicultural family support programs by closely examining the experiences of CHWs while they work.

CHWs are an important part of the healthcare system, especially for those who experience barriers to accessing adequate healthcare for cultural, linguistic, or other societal reasons (Herman, 2011). On the basis of the evidence that one-on-one training in concert with educational brochures is effective in increasing the cervical cancer screening rate (Kurt & Akyuz, 2019), teaching cancer screening promotion techniques to CHWs is recommended. The themes identified in this study may be used as components of educational programs for training immigrant CHWs who will promote health behaviors among the same ethnic group. Adequate training programs that utilize common elements for competency evaluation and ongoing support should be considered to establish CHWs as part of the healthcare system, which eventually should be considered a reimbursable workforce in communities (e.g., immigrant communities) with unique needs. Foreign caregivers face unexpected situations when working in other countries. Thus, providing appropriate support plays an important role in initial adaptation (Nursalam et al., 2020). In addition, supervision of their work and strategies to ensure the quality of their service need to be developed.

This study was affected by several limitations. First, obtaining qualitative descriptive results from a small number of immigrants from a single country limits the generalizability of the findings and conclusions. Immigrants from various countries and CHW activities in various fields should be considered in future studies. Second, the perspectives of Chinese CHWs living in metropolitan areas may differ from their peers living in rural areas because of potential differences in exposure to preventive care and in CHW burdens. Hence, further study needs to be done in rural areas to improve trustworthiness. Third, although the study team intended to enrich the data by combining individual interviews and focus groups in each region, one individual interviewee withdrew from the study because of personal reasons. With the limited chance of an interview, the facilitator created an atmosphere that allowed CHWs to express their opinions freely and responded well to help them fully represent both the experience and awareness of CHW that recommended and guided cancer screening in Korea. Despite its limitations, this study analyzed immigrant CHWs' experiences and perceptions related to healthcare-related activities in Korea and thus provides basic data on guidance that may be used to improve CHW training courses and activities in the future.

Conclusions

The focus group interviews conducted in this study provide information regarding the perceptions of CHWs among CMIW. Whereas the activities of CHWs increased the enthusiasm of the CMIW, the themes identified in this study reveal the necessity of improving the information provided and managing the ambivalence of CHWs. Therefore, health promotion programs involving CHWs should include training courses that increase the amounts of information and empowerment via the management of various cases.

Acknowledgments

The authors thank the Chinese Korean community health workers who participated in this study. This research was supported by the Basic Science Research Program through the National Research Foundation of Korea (NRF) funded by the Ministry of Education (Grant No. NRF-2013R1A1A2011804).

Author Contributions

Study conception and design: JK, HRH
Data collection: JK, HK
Data analysis and interpretation: JK, HK
Drafting of the article: All authors
Critical revision of article: JK, HRH

References

Aseyo, R. E., Mumma, J., Scott, K., Nelima, D., Davis, E., Baker, K. K., Cummimg, O., & Dreibelbis, R. (2018). Realities and experiences of community health volunteers as agents for behaviour change: Evidence from an informal urban settlement in Kisumu, Kenya. *Human Resources for Health, 16*, Article No. 53. https://doi.org/10.1186/s12960-018-0318-4

Austin-Evelyn, K., Rabkin, M., Macheka, T., Mutiti, A., Mwansa-Kambafwile, J., Dlamini, T., & El-Sadr, W. M. (2017). Community health worker perspectives on a new primary health care initiative in the Eastern Cape of South Africa. *PLOS ONE, 12*(3), Article e0173863. https://doi.org/10.1371/journal.pone.0173863

Bhandari, P., & Kim, M. (2016). Predictors of the health-promoting behaviors of Nepalese migrant workers. *The Journal of Nursing Research, 24*(3), 232–239. https://doi.org/10.1097/jnr.0000000000000120

Choi, Y., Kim, Y. S., Sun, B. Y., Dong, J. Y., Jung, H. S., Yang, K. M., Lee, E. A., & Hwang, J. M. (2019). *2018 Nationwide multicultural family survey*. Ministry of Gender Equity and Family. http://www.mogef.go.kr/io/lib/lib_v200.do?id=27536 (Original work published in Korean)

Gale, N. K., & Sidhu, M. S. (2019). Risk work or resilience work? A qualitative study with community health workers negotiating the tensions between biomedical and community-based forms of health promotion in the United Kingdom. *PLOS ONE, 14*(7), Article e0220109. https://doi.org/10.1371/journal.pone.0220109

George, M. S., Pant, S., Devasenapathy, N., Ghosh-Jerath, S., & Zodpey, S. P. (2017). Motivating and demotivating factors for community health workers: A qualitative study in urban slums of Delhi, India. *WHO South-East Asia Journal of Public Health, 6*(1), 82–89. https://doi.org/10.4103/2224-3151.206170

Glenton, C., Colvin, C., Carlsen, B., Swartz, A., Lewin, S., Noyes, J., & Rashidian, A. (2013). Barriers and facilitators to the implementation of lay health worker programmes to improve access to maternal and child health: Qualitative evidence synthesis. *Cochrane Database of Systematic Reviews, 2013*, Article No. CD010414. https://doi.org/10.1002/14651858.CD010414.pub2

Guest, G., Namey, E., & Mckenna, K. (2017). How many focus groups are enough? Building an evidence base for nonprobability sample sizes. *Field Methods, 29*(1), 3–22. https://doi.org/10.1177/1525822X16639015

Han, H.-R., Kim, K. B., & Kim, M. T. (2007). Evaluation of the training of Korean community health workers for chronic disease management. *Health Education Research, 22*(4), 513–521. https://doi.org/10.1093/her/cyl112

Han, H.-R., Song, Y., Kim, M., Hedlin, H. K., Kim, K., Ben Lee, H., & Roter, D. (2017). Breast and cervical cancer screening literacy among Korean American women: A community health worker–led intervention. *American Journal of Public Health, 107*(1), 159–165. https://doi.org/10.2105/AJPH.2016.303522

Herman, A. A. (2011). Community health workers and integrated primary health care teams in the 21st century. *Journal of Ambulatory Care Management, 34*(4), 354–361. https://doi.org/10.1097/JAC.0b013e31822cbcd0

Kim-Bossard, M. (2018). Challenging homogeneity in contemporary Korea—Immigrant women, immigrant laborers, and multicultural family. *Education About Asia, 23*(2), 38–41.

Koh, C.-K., & Koh, S.-K. (2009). Married female migrants' experiences of health care services. *The Journal of Korean Academic Society of Nursing Education, 15*(1), 89–99. https://doi.org/10.5977/JKASNE.2009.15.1.089 (Original work published in Korean)

Korea Statistical Information Service. (2021a). *Statistics of arrivals and departures: Status of marriage migrant by nationality/region*. https://kosis.kr/eng/search/searchList.do/

Korea Statistical Information Service. (2021b). *Vital statistics: Multicultural marriages by province, si (city), gun (county) and gu (borough)*. https://kosis.kr/eng/search/searchList.do/

Krueger, R. A., & Casey, M. A. (2014). *Focus groups: A practical guide for applied research* (5th ed.). Sage Publications.

Kurt, G., & Akyuz, A. (2019). Evaluating the effectiveness of interventions on increasing participation in cervical cancer screening. *The Journal of Nursing Research, 27*(5), Article e40. https://doi.org/10.1097/jnr.0000000000000317

Lambert, S. D., & Loiselle, C. G. (2008). Combining individual interviews and focus groups to enhance data richness. *Journal of Advanced Nursing, 62*(2), 228–237. https://doi.org/10.1111/j.1365-2648.2007.04559.x

Lee, F.-H. (2018). Intention to receive breast cancer screening and related factors of influence among Vietnamese women in transnational marriages. *The Journal of Nursing Research, 26*(2), 112–122. https://doi.org/10.1097/jnr.0000000000000210

Lee, F.-H., Wang, H.-H., Yang, Y.-M., Huang, J.-J., & Tsai, H.-M. (2016). Influencing factors of intention to receive Pap tests in Vietnamese women who immigrated to Taiwan for marriage. *Asian Nursing Research, 10*(3), 189–194. https://doi.org/10.1016/j.anr.2016.05.004

Lee, J. (2021). Supporting the social integration of migrant women in South Korea through language services: Roles of marriage migrant interpreters in multicultural family support centre counselling services. *The Translator*. Advance online publication. https://doi.org/10.1080/13556509.2021.1905208

Meng, Q., Mills, A., Wang, L., & Han, Q. (2019). What can we learn from China's health system reform? *BMJ, 365*, Article l2349. https://doi.org/10.1136/bmj.l2349

Mock, J., McPhee, S. J., Nguyen, T., Wong, C., Doan, H., Lai, K. Q., Nguyen, K. H., Nguyen, T. T., & Bui-Tong, N. (2007). Effective lay health worker outreach and media-based education for promoting cervical cancer screening among Vietnamese American women. *American Journal of Public Health, 97*(9), 1693–1700. https://doi.org/10.2105/AJPH.2006.086470

Mojica, C. M., Morales-Campos, D. Y., Carmona, C. M., Ouyang, Y., & Liang, Y. (2016). Breast, cervical, and colorectal cancer education and navigation. *Health Promotion Practice, 17*(3), 353–363. https://doi.org/10.1177/1524839915603362

National Health Insurance Act 1999, Ministry of Health § 2. (1999 & Rev. 2017). https://law.go.kr/LSW/eng/engLsSc.do?menuId= 2&query=NATIONAL%20HEALTH%20INSURANCE%20 ACT#liBgcolor32

National Health Insurance Act 1999, Ministry of Health § 41. (1999 & Rev. 2016). https://law.go.kr/LSW/eng/engLsSc.do?menuId= 2&query=NATIONAL%20HEALTH%20INSURANCE%20ACT #liBgcolor32

Nimmons, K., Beaudoin, C. E., & St. John, J. A. (2017). The outcome evaluation of a CHW cancer prevention intervention: Testing individual and multilevel predictors among Hispanics living along the Texas–Mexico border. *Journal of Cancer Education, 32*(1), 183–189. https://doi.org/10.1007/s13187-015-0930-0

Nursalam, N., Chen, C.-M., Efendi, F., Has, E. M. M., Hidayati, L., & Hadisuyatmana, S. (2020). The lived experiences of Indonesian nurses who worked as care workers in Taiwan. *The Journal of Nursing Research, 28*(2), Article e78. https://doi.org/10.1097/ jnr.0000000000000355

O'Donovan, J., O'Donovan, C., Kuhn, I., Sachs, S. E., & Winters, N. (2018). Ongoing training of community health workers in low-income and middle-income countries: A systematic scoping review of the literature. *BMJ Open, 8*(4), Article e021467. https://doi.org/10.1136/bmjopen-2017-021467

Parker, R., Jelsma, J., & Stein, D. J. (2016). Managing pain in women living with HIV/AIDS: A randomized controlled trial testing the effect of a six-week peer-led exercise and education intervention. *The Journal of Nervous and Mental Disease, 204*(9), 665–672. https://doi.org/10.1097/NMD.0000000000000506

Pillaud, V., Cavazza, N., & Butera, F. (2018). The social utility of ambivalence: Being ambivalent on controversial issues is recognized as competence. *Frontiers in Psychology, 9*, Article 961. https://doi.org/10.3389/fpsyg.2018.00961

Sandelowski, M. (2000). Whatever happened to qualitative description? *Research in Nursing & Health, 23*(4), 334–340. https://doi.org/10.1002/1098-240X(200008)23:4<334::AID-NUR9>3.0.CO;2-G

Schuster, A. L. R., Frick, K. D., Huh, B.-Y., Kim, K. B., Kim, M., & Han, H.-R. (2015). Economic evaluation of a community health worker-led health literacy intervention to promote cancer screening among Korean American women. *Journal of Health Care for the Poor and Underserved, 26*(2), 431–440. https://doi.org/10.1353/hpu.2015.0050

Seutloali, T., Napoles, L., & Bam, N. (2018). Community health workers in Lesotho: Experiences of health promotion activities. *African Journal of Primary Health Care & Family Medicine, 10*(1), Article 1558. https://doi.org/10.4102/phcfm.v10i1.1558

Simon, M. A., Tom, L. S., Leung, I., Taylor, S., Wong, E., Vicencio, D. P., & Dong, X. (2018). Chinese immigrant women's attitudes and beliefs about family involvement in women's health and healthcare: A qualitative study in Chicago's Chinatown. *Health Equity, 2*(1), 182–192. https://doi.org/10.1089/heq.2017.0062

Song, J. (2015). Five phases of brokered international marriages in South Korea: A complexity perspective. *Asian Studies, 1*(1), 147–176. https://doi.org/10.6551/AS.0101.07

Verhagen, I., Steunenberg, B., de Wit, N. J., & Ros, W. J. G. (2014). Community health worker interventions to improve access to health care services for older adults from ethnic minorities: A systematic review. *BMC Health Services Research, 14*, Article 497. https://doi.org/10.1186/s12913-014-0497-1

12

Home Coping Strategies for Fatigue Used by Patients with Lung Cancer Receiving Chemotherapy in Rural China

Xiaomeng DONG[1] • Jianying PENG[2] • Xingxing LI[3] • Qiyuan ZHAO[4] • Xiuwei ZHANG[5]*

ABSTRACT

Background: Cancer-related fatigue, a distressing symptom, is frequently reported by patients with lung cancer as increasing in severity with the number of rounds of chemotherapy. Yet, patients and healthcare providers are challenged to control this fatigue. Thus, healthcare providers must have interventions to effectively enhance coping engagement in patients with lung cancer.

Purpose: The aims of this study were to explore how patients with lung cancer in a rural area of China undergoing chemotherapy cope with the fatigue at home and to summarize their strategies.

Methods: A descriptive qualitative research approach was used, and data were collected using semistructured interviews. Sixteen patients with lung cancer with chemotherapy-related fatigue living in rural communities were recruited from a large, tertiary teaching hospital in Huzhou in eastern China. The transcripts of the interviews were analyzed using content analysis.

Results: Coping strategies for cancer-related fatigue were delineated into the three themes of (a) psychological adjustment, (b) efforts to change lifestyles and act as a Chinese health practitioner, and (c) relying on social support.

Conclusions/Implications for Practice: The participants in this study provided information on a variety of approaches to reducing/alleviating cancer-related fatigue that were influenced by Chinese culture. Healthcare providers and patients may work together in clinical settings to identify appropriate, effective coping solutions and then to incorporate these into the regular care regimen to help patients transition between hospital and home.

KEY WORDS:
coping, lung cancer, chemotherapy, cancer-related fatigue, qualitative research.

Introduction

Lung cancer (LC) is reported to be the most common cancer with the highest morbidity and mortality rate in China (Wang et al., 2019). The annual mortality rate of LC in China (626,000; Siegel et al., 2017) is considerably higher than that in the United States (155,870; Siegel et al., 2017) and the United Kingdom (over 46,000; Gemine et al., 2019). Recently, new LC treatment strategies, including surgery, combined chemotherapy and radiotherapy, and molecular targeted therapies, have been introduced (Kwon et al., 2020). The expansion of treatment opportunities in rural China has significantly improved survival rates in 5-year relative cases (J. Wu et al., 2020). Although chemotherapy treatment is a widely used treatment option for patients with LC, an estimated 80%–96% of patients undergoing this treatment experience cancer-related fatigue (CRF; Horneber et al., 2012). As defined by the National Comprehensive Cancer Network, CRF is a persistent and distressing subjective sense of physical, cognitive, and/or emotional tiredness or exhaustion related to cancer or its treatment that is not proportional to recent activities and that interferes with physical and psychosocial function, threatening patient health (Scott et al., 2011) and considerably impacting quality of life (H.-L. Chen et al., 2018).

Rural areas generally have higher rates of patients with final-stage LC than urban areas (Cao & Chen, 2019). Weaver found survivors of LC in rural areas to be more likely than their peers in urban areas to report distress (Andrykowski et al., 2017). In China, chemotherapy cancer centers are located primarily in large, urban hospitals that are difficult for residents of remote rural communities to access. Moreover, patients in rural communities often have insufficient access to health instructions from health professionals. Close monitoring and follow-up from healthcare providers have been shown to

[1]MSN, RN, School of Medicine, Huzhou University, Huzhou Central Hospital, Huzhou, China • [2]MSN, RN, Head Nurse, Department of Nursing, Xiangyang No. 1 People's Hospital, Hubei University of Medicine, Hubei, China • [3]MSN, RN, School of Medicine, Huzhou University, Huzhou Central Hospital, Huzhou, China • [4]MSN, RN, School of Medicine, Huzhou University, Huzhou Central Hospital, Huzhou, China; • [5]PhD, RN, Associate Professor, School of Medicine, Huzhou University, Huzhou Central Hospital, Huzhou, China.

promote the effective treatment of patients with LC (Can et al., 2004). Medical care services in China are disproportionally distributed among rural and urban populations (Zhang et al., 2017). Moreover, after hospital discharge, patients are largely in charge of managing their own illness and recovery to health. Some take proactive measures to reduce the effects of their disease and to cope with related fatigue and other symptoms (Bahrami et al., 2015). A systematic review highlighted the benefit of several nonpharmacological interventions, including physical activity, psychotherapy, and acupuncture, in overcoming fatigue (C. Wu et al., 2019). However, despite the known, negative effects of CRF, little is known about the subjective perceptions toward this type of fatigue among patients living in rural areas. Whether and how they cope with these symptoms between chemotherapy visits are also underestimated and undertreated by clinicians (Ebede et al., 2017).

Recently, researchers have focused increased attention to providing person-centered care in a people-centered way. Taking a person-centered approach helps healthcare providers better understand and assess the individual needs and preferences of patients (Lawford et al., 2018). Such individualized and holistic coping engagement has played an important and active role in reducing CRF and optimizing the health of patients with LC during their rehabilitation (Feldthusen & Mannerkorpi, 2019). However, little research has examined related coping strategies from the perspective of patients living in rural areas. It is crucial that healthcare providers promote the self-coping abilities of these patients to improve their continued recovery to health at home.

The purpose of this qualitative study was to explore the coping strategies of patients with LC experiencing symptoms of CRF during chemotherapy in rural China in the post-hospital-discharge recovery period.

Methods

Study Design

This descriptive qualitative study (Sandelowski, 2010) was designed to explore and gain a comprehensive overview of the strategies used by patients with LC to cope with CRF while undergoing chemotherapy. The descriptive qualitative research approach is a preferred method for studies that involve a series of descriptions of everyday terms including who, where, and what (Perry et al., 2020).

Participants and Setting

Maximum variation and snowball sampling (Saab et al., 2017) was the purposive sampling strategy used in this study to recruit a heterogeneous sample of patients with LC experiencing CRF from the oncology clinic of a university hospital in eastern China. The eligibility criteria included resident of a rural area, diagnosis of LC and CRF, age of 18 years or older, having received more than one cycle of chemotherapy, Brief Fatigue Inventory score of ≥ 4 (Mendoza et al., 1999), resident of a county, and having knowledge of their condition and the ability to express their fatigue-reduction experience. In the recruitment process, no restrictions were imposed on the type, site, or stage (except for Stage IV) of LC. The participants were required to meet the diagnosis of CRF outlined in the *International Statistical Classification of Diseases and Related Health Problems, 10th Revision* (Yeh et al., 2011), and fatigue was classified into three levels: mild (1–3), moderate (4–6), and severe (7–10; Lou et al., 2013). Individuals with moderate and severe fatigue experience multiple symptoms of distress and are generally the most well-informed individuals (Bastani et al., 2014). Finally, a demographic datasheet was used to collect gender, cancer stage, and chemotherapy treatment information.

Data Collection

In this study, the face-to-face interviews employed a semistructured approach and were conducted from November 2018 to January 2019. The first author had received extensive training in grounded theory research and phenomenology. She explained to each participant the purpose of the study and relevant details such as the interview method used and the need for voice recording. All collected information was kept confidential. Each interview lasted for about 1 hour, and most were conducted in the clinicians' office. Only two researchers and one participant were in the room during these interviews. Three of the 16 participants were interviewed twice because their first interviews were interrupted by their health problems or by unexpected visits from relatives. To better understand the participants' situations, after obtaining their written or verbal consent, the first author reviewed relevant information in their medical records. Instructions for the interview were provided by the corresponding author.

Participants were recruited and interviewed until no new information emerged, at which point data saturation was deemed to have been reached (Ryan & Noonan, 2019).

The interview guide included the following questions: (a) feelings and experiences after chemotherapy, (b) opinions regarding CRF, and (c) most beneficial/effective coping strategies for CRF used at home. The researcher adjusted the manner and sequence in which questions were asked based on the circumstances in each interview session. Every effort was made by the researcher to maximize the dialogue and maintain an empathetic understanding of the symptoms and feelings of the participants. During the interview, observational notes on the participants' affective responses (e.g., laughter, crying, sadness, impatience) and sensitive words were recorded to provided more sufficient contextual information in subsequent analysis (M. Wu et al., 2010). All of the participants were given psychological counseling by the first author (who was qualified as a professional counselor) after being interviewed.

Data Analysis

Qualitative content analysis was adopted to accurately summarize the participants' actual coping strategies for CRF during chemotherapy. This analysis approach is commonly used by researchers to discover and describe the focus of individual attention (Graneheim et al., 2017).

The content of each voice recording was transcribed verbatim and anonymized within 24 hours of each interview. Two of the researchers read and reread the transcribed text to become immersed in the data and gain a more complete understanding of the whole. They were reviewed and coded separately. The transcripts related to coping strategies were extracted from the whole and drawn together into one text. Two of the coders identified the important points extracted from participants' statements as potential meaning units (Ruan et al., 2020). Next, meaning units were condensed and labeled with a code that reflected participant statements abstractly. Similar codes may be gathered into a theme and then abstracted. The researchers identified the relationships and connections among all of the themes.

Trustworthiness

Credibility, transferability, dependability, and confirmability, as proposed by Lincoln and Guba, were examined to ensure the trustworthiness of the data (Denzin & Lincoln, 2018). Credibility was achieved by the researcher's prolonged engagement with the participants and by member check (Karlsson et al., 2019). Long interviews and repeated questions were conducted to resolve uncertainties and help the researchers gain authentic responses from the participants. Field notes were also used to increase the credibility of the data. Particularly, when the participants used indigenous or colloquial expressions, it was necessary to check how the expression was used in the original data and coding or to consult with the specialist and participants repeatedly and accurately. In addition, all of the participants received a copy of their interview transcripts and were asked to provide their feedback to the research team. To increase the transferability of the data, the demographic and clinical characteristics were explained carefully and thick descriptions of the context, setting, and equipment were provided for the readers to assess the transferability. To enhance dependability and confirmability, an audit trail was established and research meetings were arranged regularly for the team to discuss interpretations, codes, and themes. Furthermore, the decision making at every stage of the study was documented for later tracking and review.

Ethical Considerations

Ethics approval was obtained from the institutional review boards of Huzhou University and the hospital in which the study was conducted (2014-201). Patients meeting the inclusion criteria volunteered to participate in the study and provided written informed consent.

Results

Sixteen patients with LC who were currently undergoing chemotherapy and were diagnosed with CRF volunteered and were enrolled as participants. The participants included 12 men and four women, and all lived in rural communities in China. Their mean age was 66 years (range: 38–80 years), their mean number of chemotherapy cycles was 4 (range: 1–10 cycles), and their mean Brief Fatigue Inventory score was 7.9. Most were married and had a relatively low level of formal education. Four had been diagnosed with small cell LC, and 13 were at an advanced stage of cancer (≥ III). The data collected on participant characteristics are presented in Table 1, and on the basis of the results of content analysis, the three themes are summarized in Table 2.

Theme 1: Psychological Adjustment

This theme comprised the two subthemes of "adjust my thoughts and accept the fluctuating fatigue" and "reflect on what I have and seek satisfaction."

Adjust my thoughts and accept the fluctuating fatigue

Despite the fact that fatigue minimized their passion to engage in life activities, the participants felt that they had no alternative but to accept their fatigue. They expressed that they tended to be in a positive psychological state and believed that positive thoughts could lengthen their life.

> Sometimes I am nerveless and tired without any interest in anything. But sometimes, I am not too bad. I have no idea to overcome the fatigue. The only thing I can do is to persuade myself and adjust my thoughts to defeat the fatigue. What matters most is the attitude toward it. I have to accept. Think more positive aspects of my life, maybe I will live longer. (Patient 12)

Several of the participants seemed frightened and noted that their fatigue worsened when they were told that they had cancer. They tried to relax and cope with these troublesome and unbearable symptoms while falling into the plight.

> Actually, when I was told that fatigue is around me, I thought that the distress would defeat me. After a long duration, I gradually found that nothing will change when you are frightened to death. I do not know why I persuaded myself to accept the fatigue. The symptom is complicated and needs a long time to adapt or recover. Try to calm down. (Patient 8)

The participants described that it was difficult to understand why they became fatigued. Because of a lack of knowledge about CRF, they shifted their attention to avoid fatigue-related thoughts.

> I do not, do not want to think anything. I cannot control it. It is so overwhelming and I have no energy to do anything. Let it go. It is different from common tiredness. I really do not know its cause. Now that I cannot figure it out, stop thinking about it. Move on! (Patient 11)

Table 1

Patient Demographic and Clinical Characteristics

Patient Code	Age (Years)	Gender	Marital Status	Educational Level	Cycles of CT	Stages	Diagnosis	BFI Score
1	72	Male	Married	High school	2	IV	SCLC	8
2	68	Female	Married	Primary school	2	II	NSCLC	8
3	63	Male	Widowed	Primary school	2	IV	NSCLC	9
4	65	Male	Married	Primary school	8	IV	NSCLC	7
5	76	Male	Married	Primary school	1	II	NSCLC	8
6	80	Female	Married	Primary school	5	IV	NSCLC	6
7	75	Male	Divorced	High school	2	III	SCLC	8
8	78	Male	Married	Primary	10	IV	NSCLC	6
9	56	Male	Divorced	Bachelor	3	III	NSCLC	8
10	81	Male	Widowed	Primary school	6	IV	NSCLC	9
11	38	Male	Single	Postgraduate	1	III	NSCLC	8
12	45	Female	Married	Bachelor	1	III	NSCLC	9
13	66	Male	Married	High school	2	II	NSCLC	7
14	50	Male	Married	Primary	1	III	NSCLC	9
15	64	Male	Married	Primary	3	IV	SCLC	8
16	77	Female	Married	Primary	3	III	SCLC	8

Note. CT = chemotherapy; BFI = Brief Fatigue Inventory; SCLC = Small cell lung cancer; NSCLC = Non-Small cell lung cancer.

Stop overthinking. Just eat what you want to eat, laugh, and play. Repeatedly mentioning "tiredness, unhappiness" cannot change the reality of being fatigued. Try to think simply and you may live another year or two. (Patient 15)

Some of the participants even took their own fatigue experience as examples to encourage other patients to defeat their fatigue.

Table 2

Themes and Subthemes of Participant Coping Strategies

Theme	Subtheme
1. Psychological adjustment	(1) Adjust my thoughts and accept the fluctuating fatigue (2) Reflect on what I have and seek satisfaction
2. Efforts to change lifestyles and act as a Chinese health practitioner	(1) Eat nutritious food (2) Rest well (3) Take part in recreational activities (4) Take more exercise (5) Learn more knowledge about health management
3. Relying on social support	(1) Family support (2) Nurse support (3) Peer support

I persuaded my oldest sister, who was diagnosed with the same disease several times, to conquer her fear and fatigue. She lived to be 80 years old. I think she must have encountered many difficulties and frustration. Fatigue was just a small problem for her. She must have been able to defeat it. (Patient 1)

Several participants stated that their life was determined by their personal fate (*ming*). They noted that they had no alternative but to accept the fact that they would live with CRF and realized the importance of staying confident during their long-term struggle with CRF.

It is my fate. When I was born, my life was set by my "ming." Life is destined. I must encounter such distressing symptoms my whole life. I am ready for a long battle with fatigue. (Patient 15)

Reflect on what I have and seek satisfaction

During the process of revaluing what they have now and what they once had, the participants often compared themselves with other patients. They felt fortunate to live longer and to have a lower level of fatigue. They were content with their social status.

I am nearly 80 years old. It is enough for me to live another decade. Everyone will get older and it is an undeniable fact. I am so lucky that I was diagnosed with lung cancer when I was 75 years old, while others were diagnosed with lung cancer in their youth. (Patient 5)

I have gone through the toughest days in the past. I am proud of my social status. When I worked, I was a manager. (Patient 10)

Few people can live to 70, but I can. (Patient 1)

In addition, participants who held Buddhist beliefs shifted their focus from the future to the present to live in the moment.

Buddha told to me that all obstacles I encountered today are the result of what I did in the past. What I am doing now also influences my future. I should try my best to cherish what I have and seize the moment as much as I can.

Theme 2: Efforts to Change Lifestyles and Act as a Chinese Health Practitioner

This theme was further subdivided into five subthemes: eat nutritious food, rest well, take part in recreational activities, take more exercise, and learn more about health management.

Eat nutritious food

Nutritional intake is important for patients with CRF. The participants mentioned that having a poor appetite and having negative emotions may lead to poor immune system function and impair recovery. Three categories of food, including "nutritious food," "herbal tonics," and "Chinese herbal medicines," were introduced by the participants.

Some participants insisted that they should eat all kinds of nutritious foods to meet their nutritional demands. Patients themselves must determine which kinds of food are beneficial.

Eggs, seen as "yin," should not be eaten too much. I eat an egg each day and drink home-made soybean milk. We should eat more protein-rich foods, different vegetables, and cereal. I love seafood. It has high nutritional value. Vegetable juice is also a good choice. Cucumber juice and tomato juice are also rich in nutrients. (Patient 2)

Participants stated that, even if they were distressed and had no appetite, they always persuaded themselves to take in more food. One participant mentioned what to eat and how to eat:

We need to diversify our diet and eat multiple small meals. It is important to have a balanced diet. We should eat nutritious food but in moderation. Eating too much or too little is not good. Even if you have no appetite, you'd still better eat. If no nutrients are taken in, your condition will become worse. (Patient 13)

The participants were also very enthusiastic about herbal tonics.

It's good for health. I have eaten some dendrobium and Chinese caterpillar fungus (Chinese medicinal health products for nourishment) and they had a good effect. (Patient 3)

The participants showed their preference for Chinese herbal medicines but provided no detailed information. Although these herbal medicines work slower than Western medicine, they act to both prevent and cure disease (fatigue).

Persist in taking herbs more than 3 months and it will show good results without any major side-effects. Although it works slowly, the efficacy is apparent. (Patient 4)

Rest well

The participants in this study all lived at home and gradually became conscious of the importance of resting. In their opinion, resting helps distract from their troubles and things they are unable to do, while providing more time to think about how to live.

Go to the park and bask in the sun while drinking tea. I urge myself to spend a lot of time in the sunshine—about 7 ~ 8 hours a day. Lying around in the sun makes me warm and relaxed, and I never fear the cold. (Patient 14)

Take part in recreational activities

Participants described that they were fond of participating in leisure activities. Some expressed enjoying going to the temple to be surrounded by huge, centuries-old trees; playing Chinese chess and mahjong in community senior centers; and participating in farm tourism.

I always go to the temple and particularly love the shade under the huge trees. Buddha is looking at me and will guide me toward a better situation. (Patient 12)

All my friends like drinking tea. It is relaxing for me, a patient undergoing chemotherapy, to go out of the house and drink tea with friends. (Patient 13)

Some participants enjoyed where they lived and going outside to commune with nature.

I like going to the farmhouse in the mountains where the air is so fresh and clear that my lungs can be purified. Eating dinner, breathing clean air, walking along the windy, twisted mountain road.... (Patient 2)

Take more exercise

Exercise regimens were expanded gradually based on participant conditions. The participants mentioned two effective types of aerobic exercise: brisk walking and jogging. Some liked to exercise in the fresh air, starting slowly and gradually increasing their exercise intensity. Twenty minutes of exercise per session was enough, and most started out by doing 4 minutes of exercise only.

Usually, I get up early and go jogging. I take deep breaths while jogging. Four or five minutes of exercise was enough for me initially, and I increased the amount gradually. If I feel tired, I will sit down immediately to rest. It is important to choose a place where the air is fresh. (Patient 3)

Participants who have developed a jogging habit reported that jogging helped them reduce their fatigue.

I often felt tired in the past. But now, with the benefit of jogging, I can run several laps around the park. I feel my strength has improved. (Patient 9)

Learn more about health management

For the participants, knowledge about their disease and CRF was essential to beginning and sustaining coping practices. The participants gained important knowledge by watching TV, which is a major form of relaxation and a major source of health information. In addition, they developed their own methods to deal with CRF.

Good health shows are a resource. I pay attention to gathering and trusting health information seen on television shows. Sometimes I wrote down key information and then follow it. (Patient 4)

Theme 3: Relying on Social Support

This theme was divided into the three subthemes of family support, nurse support, and peer support. Participants sought emotional support from their families and relied on nurses' encouragement and their peers' disease (fatigue) narration.

Family support

Some of the participants reported that they perceived the caring from their family members. When they were experiencing loss of appetite, failings in their self-care, and fear of going out, they drew on the support of family members and other relatives to cope and to take in nutritional food, enhance their living abilities, and engage in social communications.

Gradually, I had no interest in food. I even felt that I lost the ability to smell the flavor of food. However, my husband always goes to the market and buys various kinds of vegetables to cook for me. Sometimes, I do not want to eat anything. He treats me as a baby and feeds me the food. Now I feel that I am stronger than before. I appreciate my husband. (Patient 2)

Sometimes I forget to take medicine, but my children remind me to take it. They often share something interesting with me and read the daily news for me. I know that they hope this makes me feel happy. I am becoming more and more dependent on my children. They often take time off from work to take care of me, including bathing and elimination. I am so lucky that my children are so thoughtful and dutiful. I have to admit that I am not strong. I

need their help. Gradually, it appears that I have grown a lot. (Patient 10)

I have experienced fatigue. I could not sleep well and the sleep disturbance made me become more and more haggard and worn out. I hated going out. I was afraid to meet people I knew. One day, I was surprised when many relatives came to visit me. I cried. I found that they were all my supporters. They gave me emotional support. I began to encourage myself and tried to move on and come out of my house. (Patient 12)

Nurse support

Participants noted that, even after they were discharged from the hospital, they still remembered what the nurses said and did for them. The warm words and touch of nurses bolstered their fighting spirit.

I cannot forget those days at the hospital. Nurses came to ask me how I was feeling every morning. Their warm words that "we all believe that you can overcome the fatigue" made me feel their caring and support. They also gave me some little notes to cheer me up. I put them on my desk and occasionally read and re-read them. When I am feeling particularly down, it is the encouragement from nurses that rescues me from my terrible headache. (Patient 8)

When I did not feel well, they always helped me resolve my symptoms of distress. They often patted me on the back and smiled at me. They made me feel as warm as at home. (Patient 7)

Peer support

A few of the participants were fortunate to have peers who were willing to share their experiences with reducing fatigue. They were inspired by these peers' fatigue stories and had greater hope for the future.

My neighbor was also a patient who has been fighting fatigue for many years. He told me that Job's tears seed had the potential to reduce fatigue. He also told me what he had experienced. I was touched by his life stories. He can overcome fatigue. I can too! (Patient 3)

Discussion

Three different types of home CRF coping strategies used by patients with LC undergoing chemotherapy, including psychological adjustment, efforts to change lifestyles, and relying on social support, were explored in this study.

Similar strategies for psychological adjustment such as coping by adapting and accepting CRF have been identified in previous studies (Bootsma et al., 2020). Keeping one's mind off negative things is a method of mental disengagement that helps people distance themselves from negative emotions (Ghodraty-Jabloo et al., 2016). Although all of the participants had dealt with emotional distress, it seemed that CRF indirectly influenced their reevaluation and potentially primed them to be willing to undergo an attitude transition from fear to bravery and optimism. The motivation for the changes is a strong desire to hold on to life. Natasha also reported that attitude plays an important role in patients' perceptions and helping patients cope with physical symptoms and side effects (Brown et al., 2015). Patients in one study who were triggered by fatigue were found to better appreciate what is worthwhile in life and to treasure life more (Tuominen et al., 2019). They tried not to dwell on the cause of CRF and focused on enjoying the present, which shows that the participants were attempting to control and reduce their fear and anxiety (Drageset et al., 2020). In addition, being self-motivated and seeking happiness are important for all people and particularly important to those confronting a life-threatening illness. Relatively high levels of self-recognition and positive thinking in the participants in this study were accompanied by the emergence of hope and inner growth. Within this process, they were better able to address their unmet needs and bothersome health issues and improve their coping strategies (Peng et al., 2019). Furthermore, the finding in this study that the participants encouraged themselves to achieve early recovery was also found in another study (Kang et al., 2017), which reported that patients who had a clear purpose in life were more likely to achieve happiness. Qualitative interviews are well suited to gaining insights into the inner world and health problems of patients (Abelson et al., 2019). Health professionals must be prepared to conduct interviews with patients before hospital discharge to explore their needs and help them set goals for improving their quality of life.

Some of the participants in this study expressed that their fate (*ming*) was determined by heaven and they were predestined to experience LC and CRF. This belief may be influenced by Chinese philosophy (Ruan et al., 2020). The ancient Chinese philosopher Wang Ch'ung posited that humanity was created by heaven and earth and believed that everyone had their individual fate (natural fatalism; Wei, 2017). However, in another study, fatalism was found to be a potential aggravator of patient anxiety and a negative influence on disease treatment (Zhao et al., 2014). Further studies on the relationship between fatalism and positive mental outlook are necessary to explore and identify the influence of this relationship on patient attitudes.

A traditional Chinese axiom is that prolonged illness transforms a patient into a doctor. With repeated hospitalizations, patients gradually realize they must rely on themselves in addition to medication to effectively control their fatigue. Thus, experiencing fatigue helps patients develop simple-but-effective lifestyle strategies, which leads them to act as practitioners in the struggle to reduce fatigue. Participant beliefs and values highlighted in this study included herbal treatments and diet therapies. According to the theory of "yin" and "yang," eggs are classified as a "yin" food.

Chinese hold that patients should limit their consumption of "yin" foods to avoid negatively impacting health (Y. C. Chen, 2001). Participants in this study acquired nutrients using "medicine and food homology" and Chinese herbal medicines. This strategy is rooted in Chinese traditional culture and dietotherapy. Many Chinese people believe certain foods to have unique medicinal tonic functions that allow their use as drugs, in line with the theory of medicine food homology (Gong et al., 2020). In a systematic review study, dietary interventions were found to be potentially effective in alleviating CRF and improving quality of life (Baguley et al., 2017). However, the dietary habits of patients should be respected and taken into consideration when healthcare providers develop dietary interventions. Several of the participants in this study expressed that they tried to act as doctors during their struggles with CRF. This finding highlights the active role that patients play in mitigating fatigue and may offer a reference for health professionals when providing culturally appropriate recommendations/guidance on medicine and diet. For example, the preferences of patients with fatigue with regard to traditional Chinese medicine versus Western medicine, vegetables versus meat, and refined grains versus whole grains should be assessed in the future.

In addition, participants in this study described that they frequently engaged in leisure activities such as hanging out in the park, breathing in fresh air, and drinking tea with friends. This finding is supported by another empirical study that reported self-care strategies to be moderately effective in patients with LC (O'Regan & Hegarty, 2017). Therefore, healthcare providers should encourage patients to try various relaxation strategies and help patients value their own self-relaxation strategies to build self-confidence in their ability to move on with life.

The participants in this study shared a belief that centuries-old trees held a spiritual connotation and represented longevity. Chinese culture has been greatly influenced by the philosophical and religious tenets of Confucianism, Taoism, and Buddhism (Ho & Brotherson, 2007). Some of the participants in this study expressed that they had entrusted their life to Buddha and received moral support from their religious faith to cope with their condition optimistically (Lui et al., 2009).

In the past, patients have been encouraged to limit their exercise and physical exertion. Today, an increasing number of trials have offered evidentiary support that exercise is safe and beneficial in preventing and controlling cancers; improving physical functions, cardiorespiratory fitness, and quality of life; and reducing CRF (Paramanandam & Dunn, 2015). The participants in this study mentioned engaging in two common types of physical activities: jogging and walking. The prevalence of these two activities may be associated with the participants' older age, limited types of physical activities available, physical condition, and capability. Simple ways that healthcare providers may help patients cope include providing appropriate exercise education and developing goal-setting exercises.

The participants in this study enjoyed staying at home, as they were cared for and actively supported by their families, neighbors, and friends. This study differs from Jane's study, which found that being housebound isolated patients from family members and friends (Scott et al., 2011). Echoing the finding of another qualitative study (Liao et al., 2018), families, friends, and peers accompanied participants in their fight against fatigue, which is extremely meaningful and supportive. A cross-sectional study of the supportive care needs of patients with LC found that 88.99% of participants reported the need to have family members or friends with them in the hospital (Zhang et al., 2019). In this study, the participants reported learning certain self-care strategies and obtaining health, psychological, and care-related information from family members. A previous correlational study reported that some patients with LC also experienced skin problems such as dry skin and pruritus that affected their quality of life (Chan et al., 2019). Family members and nurses, who are their main companions and supporters, should consider patients' personalized skin care needs. Social support helps strengthen patients and keeps them moving forward in their recovery. The participants in this study reported learning from the experiences and coping strategies of their peers. One previous study reported that patients in an exercise intervention not only gained access to resources from the exercise group but were more likely to manage fatigue effectively than before because of sharing with/learning from others in the same situation (Missel et al., 2019). None of the participants in this study were members of intervention groups. In fact, the long home-to-hospital distances, low level of formal education, and poor knowledge about CRF of the participants adversely impacted their compliance with home-care guidelines and made it difficult for healthcare providers to monitor and follow up. Therefore, group-based interventions in rural China is an issue that requires further consideration and development.

Limitations

Several limitations to this qualitative study need to be acknowledged, and the findings should be generalized with caution. First, the study focused on a small number of patients with LC over the age of 50 years undergoing chemotherapy in one hospital. Patients living in urban areas should also be explored. To increase the generalizability of findings and raise awareness of patient self-care issues, future studies may examine the coping strategies of patients with LC from various age groups and various locations using both qualitative and quantitative methods. In addition, information such as the current fatigue score, disease duration, and ethnicity data were not collected from participants. As these factors may influence the results, they should be controlled in future studies. Furthermore, as most researchers were not religious, they may have encountered difficulties in envisioning the influence of religion on patients' lives. Finally, some of the results were reflected in the context of Chinese culture, and further studies should be conducted in other countries and societies to examine cross-cultural commonalities and divergences.

Conclusions

In this qualitative study, the strategies for coping with chemotherapy-related fatigue used by patients with LC in home settings were explored. Three coping strategies were identified, including (a) psychological adjustment, (b) efforts to change lifestyles and act as a Chinese health practitioner, and (c) relying on social support. Chinese philosophical and religious tenets were found to strongly influence the strategies used by patients to cope with CRF at home. The insights gained from this study may be used to inform clinical practice and provide evidence for the further investigation of coping strategies and patient education related to fatigue in this population.

Implications for Practice

CRF is the most common symptom experienced by patients with cancer undergoing chemotherapy. However, little attention has been paid in clinical practice to this distressing and devastating symptom. Findings from this study have important implications for healthcare providers striving to develop targeted interventions to help patients relieve CRF symptoms in home settings. The various coping strategies described by the participants in this study provide sufficient details for healthcare providers to address CRF more comprehensively. In addition, healthcare providers should focus on exploring the inner world of patients while they are fatigued. Furthermore, the findings of this study provide significant insights into the influence of Chinese cultural beliefs on patients' cognitive resources and food choice preferences. This study suggests that healthcare providers should tailor plans to the beliefs and needs of their patients. Although some participants' solutions were specific to their personal situations, most of the solutions were universally applicable. Therefore, these responses may be adopted by healthcare providers as useful strategies to improve patient discharge instructions and assist patients with LC to transition from hospital to home.

Acknowledgments

The authors thank the patients for sharing their self-management experiences and the hospital staff for their help with recruitment.

Author Contributions

Study conception and design: XD, JP
Data collection: XD, XZ
Data analysis and interpretation: JP, XL
Drafting of the article: XD, JP
Critical revision of the article: QZ, XZ

References

Abelson, J. S., Chait, A., Shen, M. J., Charlson, M., Dickerman, A., & Yeo, H. (2019). Coping strategies among colorectal cancer patients undergoing surgery and the role of the surgeon in mitigating distress: A qualitative study. *Surgery, 165*(2), 461–468. https://doi.org/10.1016/j.surg.2018.06.005

Andrykowski, M. A., Steffens, R. F., Bush, H. M., & Tucker, T. C. (2017). Posttraumatic growth and benefit-finding in lung cancer survivors: The benefit of rural residence? *Journal of Health Psychology, 22*(7), 896–905. https://doi.org/10.1177/1359105315617820

Baguley, B. J., Bolam, K. A., Wright, O. R. L., & Skinner, T. L. (2017). The effect of nutrition therapy and exercise on cancer-related fatigue and quality of life in men with prostate cancer: A systematic review. *Nutrients, 9*(9), Article 1003. https://doi.org/10.3390/nu9091003

Bahrami, M., Shokrollahi, P., Kohan, S., Momeni, G., & Rivaz, M. (2015). Reaction to and coping with domestic violence by Iranian women victims: A qualitative approach. *Global Journal of Health Science, 8*(7), 100–109. https://doi.org/10.5539/gjhs.v8n7p100

Bastani, P., Abolhasani, N., & Shaarbafchizadeh, N. (2014). Electronic health in perspective of healthcare managers: A qualitative study in south of Iran. *Iranian Journal of Public Health, 43*(6), 809–820.

Bootsma, T. I., Schellekens, M. P. J., van Woezik, R. A. M., van der Lee, M. L., & Slatman, J. (2020). Experiencing and responding to chronic cancer-related fatigue: A meta-ethnography of qualitative research. *Psychooncology, 29*(2), 241–250. https://doi.org/10.1002/pon.5213

Brown, N. M., Lui, C. W., Robinson, P. C., & Boyle, F. M. (2015). Supportive care needs and preferences of lung cancer patients: A semi-structured qualitative interview study. *Supportive Care in Cancer, 23*(6), 1533–1539. https://doi.org/10.1007/s00520-014-2508-5

Can, G., Durna, Z., & Aydiner, A. (2004). Assessment of fatigue in and care needs of Turkish women with breast cancer. *Cancer Nursing, 27*(2), 153–161. https://doi.org/10.1097/00002820-200403000-00009

Cao, M., & Chen, W. (2019). Epidemiology of lung cancer in China. *Thoracic Cancer, 10*(1), 3–7. https://doi.org/10.1111/1759-7714.12916

Chan, J. C., Lee, Y. H., Liu, C. Y., Shih, H. H., Tsay, P. K., & Tang, W. R. (2019). A correlational study of skin toxicity and quality of life in patients with advanced lung cancer receiving targeted therapy. *The Journal of Nursing Research, 27*(6), Article e51. https://doi.org/10.1097/jnr.0000000000000339

Chen, H.-L., Liu, K., & You, Q.-S. (2018). Self-efficacy, cancer-related fatigue, and quality of life in patients with resected lung cancer. *European Journal of Cancer Care, 27*(6), Article e12934. https://doi.org/10.1111/ecc.12934

Chen, Y. C. (2001). Chinese values, health and nursing. *Journal of Advanced Nursing, 36*(2), 270–273. https://doi.org/10.1046/j.1365-2648.2001.01968.x

Denzin, N. K., & Lincoln, Y. S. (2018). *The Sage handbook of qualitative research* (5th ed.). Sage.

Drageset, S., Lindstrøm, T. C., & Ellingsen, S. (2020). "I have both lost and gained." Norwegian survivors' experiences of coping 9 years after primary breast cancer surgery. *Cancer Nursing, 43*(1), E30–E37. https://doi.org/10.1097/ncc.0000000000000656

Ebede, C. C., Jang, Y., & Escalante, C. P. (2017). Cancer-related fatigue in cancer survivorship. *Medical Clinics of North America, 101*(6), 1085–1097. https://doi.org/10.1016/j.mcna.2017.06.007

Feldthusen, C., & Mannerkorpi, K. (2019). Factors of importance for reducing fatigue in persons with rheumatoid arthritis: A qualitative interview study. *BMJ Open, 9*(5), Article e028719. https://doi.org/10.1136/bmjopen-2018-028719

Gemine, R. E., Ghosal, R., Collier, G., Parry, D., Campbell, I., Davies, G., Davies, K., Lewis, K. E., & LungCast Investigators. (2019). Longitudinal study to assess impact of smoking at diagnosis and quitting on 1-year survival for people with non-small cell lung cancer. *Lung Cancer, 129*, 1–7. https://doi.org/10.1016/j.lungcan.2018.12.028

Ghodraty-Jabloo, V., Alibhai, S. M. H., Breunis, H., & Puts, M. T. E. (2016). Keep your mind off negative things: Coping with long-term effects of acute myeloid leukemia (AML). *Supportive Care in Cancer, 24*(5), 2035–2045. https://doi.org/10.1007/s00520-015-3002-4

Gong, X., Ji, M., Xu, J., Zhang, C., & Li, M. (2020). Hypoglycemic effects of bioactive ingredients from medicine food homology and medicinal health food species used in China. *Critical Reviews in Food Science and Nutrition, 60*(14), 2303–2326. https://doi.org/10.1080/10408398.2019.1634517

Graneheim, U. H., Lindgren, B. M., & Lundman, B. (2017). Methodological challenges in qualitative content analysis: A discussion paper. *Nurse Education Today, 56*, 29–34. https://doi.org/10.1016/j.nedt.2017.06.002

Ho, S. W., & Brotherson, S. E. (2007). Cultural influences on parental bereavement in Chinese families. *OMEGA—Journal of Death and Dying, 55*(1), 1–25. https://doi.org/10.2190/4293-2021-5475-2161

Horneber, M., Fischer, I., Dimeo, F., Rüffer, J. U., & Weis, J. (2012). Cancer-related fatigue: Epidemiology, pathogenesis, diagnosis, and treatment. *Deutsches Ärzteblatt International, 109*(9), 161–171; quiz 172. https://doi.org/10.3238/arztebl.2012.0161

Kang, D., Kim, I.-R., Choi, E. K., Yoon, J. H., Lee, S. K., Lee, J. E., Nam, S. J., Han, W., Noh, D. Y., & Cho, J. (2017). Who are happy survivors? Physical, psychosocial, and spiritual factors associated with happiness of breast cancer survivors during the transition from cancer patient to survivor. *Psychooncology, 26*(11), 1922–1928. https://doi.org/10.1002/pon.4408

Karlsson, J., Eriksson, T., Lindahl, B., & Fridh, I. (2019). The patient's situation during interhospital intensive care unit-to-unit transfers: A hermeneutical observational study. *Qualitative Health Researchs, 29*(12), 1687–1698. https://doi.org/10.1177/1049732319831664

Kwon, C. Y., Lee, B., Kim, K. I., & Lee, B. J. (2020). Herbal medicine on cancer-related fatigue of lung cancer survivors: Protocol for a systematic review. *Medicine (Baltimore), 99*(5), Article e18968. https://doi.org/10.1097/md.0000000000018968

Lawford, B. J., Delany, C., Bennell, K. L., Bills, C., Gale, J., & Hinman, R. S. (2018). Training physical therapists in person-centered practice for people with osteo-arthritis: A qualitative case study. *Arthritis Care & Research, 70*(4), 558–570. https://doi.org/10.1002/acr.23314

Liao, Y. C., Liao, W. Y., Sun, J. L., Ko, J. C., & Yu, C. J. (2018). Psychological distress and coping strategies among women with incurable lung cancer: A qualitative study. *Supportive Care in Cancer, 26*(3), 989–996. https://doi.org/10.1007/s00520-017-3919-x

Lou, Y., Yates, P., McCarthy, A., & Wang, H. (2013). Fatigue self-management: A survey of Chinese cancer patients undergoing chemotherapy. *Journal of Clinical Nursing, 22*(7–8), 1053–1065. https://doi.org/10.1111/jocn.12174

Lui, C. W., Ip, D., & Chui, W. H. (2009). Ethnic experience of cancer: A qualitative study of Chinese-Australians in Brisbane, Queensland. *Social Work in Health Care, 48*(1), 14–37. https://doi.org/10.1080/00981380802440403

Mendoza, T. R., Wang, X. S., Cleeland, C. S., Morrissey, M., Johnson, B. A., Wendt, J. K., & Huber, S. L. (1999). The rapid assessment of fatigue severity in cancer patients: Use of the brief fatigue inventory. *Cancer, 85*(5), 1186–1196. https://doi.org/10.1002/(sici)1097-0142(19990301)85:5<1186::aid-cncr24>3.0.co;2-n

Missel, M., Borregaard, B., Schoenau, M. N., & Sommer, M. S. (2019). A sense of understanding and belonging when life is at stake—Operable lung cancer patients' lived experiences of participation in exercise. *European Journal of Cancer Care, 28*(5), Article e13126. https://doi.org/10.1111/ecc.13126

O'Regan, P., & Hegarty, J. (2017). The importance of self-care for fatigue amongst patients undergoing chemotherapy for primary cancer. *European Journal of Oncology Nursing, 28*, 47–55. https://doi.org/10.1016/j.ejon.2017.02.005

Paramanandam, V. S., & Dunn, V. (2015). Exercise for the management of cancer-related fatigue in lung cancer: A systematic review. *European Journal of Cancer Care, 24*(1), 4–14. https://doi.org/10.1111/ecc.12198

Peng, X., Su, Y., Huang, W., & Hu, X. (2019). Status and factors related to posttraumatic growth in patients with lung cancer: A STROBE-compliant article. *Medicine (Baltimore), 98*(7), Article e14314. https://doi.org/10.1097/md.0000000000014314

Perry, C. K., Ali, W., Solanki, E., & Winters-Stone, K. (2020). Attitudes and beliefs of older female breast cancer survivors and providers about exercise in cancer care. *Oncology Nursing Forum, 47*(1), 56–69. https://doi.org/10.1188/20.Onf.56-69

Ruan, J., Qian, Y., Zhuang, Y., & Zhou, Y. (2020). The illness experiences of Chinese patients living with lymphoma: A qualitative study. *Cancer Nursing, 43*(4), E229–E238. https://doi.org/10.1097/ncc.0000000000000717

Ryan, A., & Noonan, B. (2019). Exploring nurses' understanding of anticipatory nausea and vomiting in patients with cancer. *Oncology Nursing Forum, 46*(6), 738–745. https://doi.org/10.1188/19.Onf.738-745

Saab, M. M., Landers, M., & Hegarty, J. (2017). Exploring awareness and help-seeking intentions for testicular symptoms among heterosexual, gay, and bisexual men in Ireland: A qualitative descriptive study. *International Journal of Nursing Studies, 67*, 41–50. https://doi.org/10.1016/j.ijnurstu.2016.11.016

Sandelowski, M. (2010). What's in a name? Qualitative description revisited. *Research of Nursing and Health, 33*(1), 77–84. https://doi.org/10.1002/nur.20362

Scott, J. A., Lasch, K. E., Barsevick, A. M., & Piault-Louis, E. (2011). Patients' experiences with cancer-related fatigue: A review and synthesis of qualitative research. *Oncology Nursing Forum, 38*(3), E191–E203. https://doi.org/10.1188/11.Onf.E191-e203

Siegel, R. L., Miller, K. D., & Jemal, A. (2017). Cancer statistics, 2017. *CA: A Cancer Journal for Clinicians, 67*(1), 7–30. https://doi.org/10.3322/caac.21387

Tuominen, L., Stolt, M., Meretoja, R., & Leino-Kilpi, H. (2019). Effectiveness of nursing interventions among patients with cancer: An overview of systematic reviews. *Journal of Clinical Nursing, 28*(13–14), 2401–2419. https://doi.org/10.1111/jocn.14762

Wang, N., Mengersen, K., Tong, S., Kimlin, M., Zhou, M., Wang, L., & Hu, W. (2019). Lung cancer mortality in China: Spatial and temporal trends among subpopulations. *Chest, 156*(5), 972–983. https://doi.org/10.1016/j.chest.2019.07.023

Wei, Y. (2017). *The Chinese philosophy of fate*. Springer.

Wu, C., Zheng, Y., Duan, Y., Lai, X., Cui, S., Xu, N., Tang, C., & Lu, L. (2019). Nonpharmacological interventions for cancer-related fatigue: A systematic review and Bayesian network meta-analysis. *Worldviews in Evidence-Based Nursing, 16*(2), 102–110. https://doi.org/10.1111/wvn.12352

Wu, J., Bai, H. X., Chan, L., Su, C., Zhang, P. J., Yang, L., & Zhang, Z. (2020). Sublobar resection compared with stereotactic body radiation therapy and ablation for early stage non-small cell lung cancer: A National Cancer Database study. *The Journal of Thoracic and Cardiovascular Surgery, 160*(5), 1350–1357. E11. https://doi.org/10.1016/j.jtcvs.2019.11.132

Wu, M., Hsu, L., Zhang, B., Shen, N., Lu, H., & Li, S. (2010). The experiences of cancer-related fatigue among Chinese children with leukaemia: A phenomenological study. *International Journal of Nursing Studies, 47*(1), 49–59. https://doi.org/10.1016/j.ijnurstu.2009.05.026

Yeh, E.-T., Lau, S.-C., Su, W. J., Tsai, D. J., Tu, Y. Y., & Lai, Y. L. (2011). An examination of cancer-related fatigue through proposed diagnostic criteria in a sample of cancer patients in Taiwan. *BMC Cancer, 11*, Article No. 387. https://doi.org/10.1186/1471-2407-11-387

Zhang, T., He, H., Liu, Q., Lv, X., Song, Y., & Hong, J. (2019). Supportive care needs of patients with lung cancer in mainland China: A cross-sectional study. *The Journal of Nursing Research, 27*(6), Article e52. https://doi.org/10.1097/jnr.0000000000000338

Zhang, T., Xu, Y., Ren, J., Sun, L., & Liu, C. (2017). Inequality in the distribution of health resources and health services in China: Hospitals versus primary care institutions. *International Journal for Equity in Health, 16*(1), Article No. 42. https://doi.org/10.1186/s12939-017-0543-9

Zhao, Y., Wang, Y., Lian, J.-X., Chen, H., Liang, F., & Song, G.-M. (2014). Application of information–motivation–behavioral skills model in the early stage rehabilitation nursing of elderly patients with total hip replacement. *Chinese Journal of Nursing, 49*(8), 952–956.

13

Physical Activity and Cardiac Self-Efficacy Levels During Early Recovery After Acute Myocardial Infarction: A Jordanian Study

Abedalmajeed SHAJRAWI[1]* • Malcolm GRANAT[2] • Ian JONES[3] • Felicity ASTIN[4]

ABSTRACT

Background: Regular physical activity is important for patients with established coronary heart disease as it favorably influences their coronary risk profile. General self-efficacy is a powerful predictor of health behavior change that involves increases in physical activity levels. Few studies have simultaneously measured physical activity and self-efficacy during early recovery after a first acute myocardial infarction (AMI).

Purpose: The aims of this study were to assess changes in objectively measured physical activity levels at 2 weeks (T2) and 6 weeks (T3) and self-reported cardiac self-efficacy at hospital discharge (T1) and at T2 and T3 in patients recovering from AMI.

Methods: A repeated-measures design was used to recruit a purposive sample of patients from a single center in Jordan who were diagnosed with first AMI and who did not have access to cardiac rehabilitation. A body-worn activity monitor (activPAL) was used to objectively measure free-living physical activity levels for 7 consecutive days at two time points (T2 and T3). An Arabic version of the cardiac self-efficacy scale was administered at T1, T2, and T3. Paired *t* tests and analysis of variance were used to examine differences in physical activity levels and cardiac self-efficacy scores, respectively.

Results: A sample of 100 participants was recruited, of which 62% were male. The mean age of the sample was 54.5 ± 9.9 years. No statistically significant difference in physical activity levels was measured at 2 weeks (T2) and 6 weeks (T3). Cardiac self-efficacy scores improved significantly between T1, T2, and T3 across subscales and global cardiac self-efficacy.

Conclusions/Implications for Practice: Participants recovering from AMI in Jordan did not increase their physical activity levels during the early recovery phase, although cardiac self-efficacy scores improved. This may be because the increase in cardiac self-efficacy was not matched by the practical skills and knowledge required to translate this positive psychological construct into behavioral change. This study provides a first step toward understanding the complex relationship between cardiac self-efficacy and physical activity in this population. The authors hope that these findings support the design of culturally appropriate interventions to increase physical activity levels in this population.

KEY WORDS:
self-efficacy, acute myocardial infarction, physical activity, activPAL, accelerometer.

Introduction

Cardiovascular disease (CVD) is the most common cause of death worldwide, causing 31% of all deaths globally (total: 17.9 million per year; World Health Organization [WHO], 2017). This figure is much greater in low- and middle-income countries, where CVD is estimated to cause 82% of deaths (WHO, 2017). Cardiac rehabilitation is considered to be one of the most effective strategies to support secondary prevention in patients with CVD (Sumner et al., 2017). It has been recommended that patients recovering from acute myocardial infarction (AMI) should participate in cardiac rehabilitation within 10 days of leaving a hospital (Winzer et al., 2018). Other activities such as returning to work, driving, and sexual activity may be resumed after 6 weeks (Winzer et al., 2018).

Cardiac rehabilitation is a multifactorial intervention that is delivered in three phases by a multidisciplinary team. Cardiac rehabilitation programs aim to optimize psychosocial health, medical risk management, and lifestyle risk factor management (British Association for Cardiovascular Disease Prevention and Rehabilitation, 2017). When delivered as intended, cardiac rehabilitation can improve health-related quality of life and physiological parameters such as left ventricle ejection fraction, exercise tolerance, and coronary risk factor profile (Zhang et al., 2018).

Phase 2 of cardiac rehabilitation represents the early recovery phase that occurs between discharge from hospital and 6–8 weeks afterward (Bäck et al., 2017). From the patient perspective, research shows that the first 6 weeks after hospital discharge after AMI represent a particularly difficult

[1]PhD, RN, Assistant Professor, Faculty of Nursing, Applied Science Private University, Amman, Jordan • [2]PhD, Professor, Health and Rehabilitation Sciences, School of Health Sciences, University of Salford, Manchester, UK • [3]PhD, RN, Professor, School of Nursing and Allied Health, Liverpool John Moores University, UK • [4]PhD, RN, Professor, Centre for Applied Research in Health, University of Huddersfield; and Research and Development, Huddersfield Royal Infirmary, Acre Street, Huddersfield, UK.

transition period, often because of a fear of AMI recurrence linked to overexertion and physical activity (Astin et al., 2009).

People who undertake regular physical activity (PA) live longer and experience fewer cardiovascular events (Winzer et al., 2018). The European Society of Cardiology recommends that healthy adults should aim for at least 150 minutes a week of moderate-intensity PA, 75 minutes a week of vigorous-intensity PA, or an equivalent combination for 4–5 days a week (Ibanez et al., 2018).

Regular PA is also an important contributor to both primary and secondary cardiovascular prevention (Dibben et al., 2018). Patients with established CVD may slow the progression of coronary stenosis, improve endothelial function, and thereby improve their overall cardiovascular health and cardiorespiratory fitness by increasing their PA levels (Winzer et al., 2018). Improving cardiorespiratory fitness is a key factor to reducing the incidence of AMI complications and CVD mortality (Wasfy & Baggish, 2019). Several physiological benefits occur when sedentary time is replaced with PA such as stepping, standing, or light-intensity PA. These include an increase in high-density lipoprotein cholesterol and reductions in waist circumference and fasting insulin levels, which, in combination, reduce all-cause mortality (Del Pozo-Cruz et al., 2018). A cohort study conducted on over 30,000 patients with AMI reported that PA recorded at 6–10 weeks after AMI predicted mortality and readmissions at 1 year postdischarge (Ek et al., 2019). Data from a Swedish national registry (SWEDEHEART-registry) that studied a sample of 22,227 patients post-AMI for a mean follow-up time of 4.2 years found that increased levels of PA were related to reduced mortality post-AMI (Ekblom et al., 2018).

It is important to provide self-management support to patients recovering from AMI to help them make healthy lifestyle changes such as increasing PA levels (Dibao-Dina et al., 2018). Patients recovering from AMI need to be given tailored advice about PA on an individual basis to establish their baseline capacity (Bäck et al., 2017). This support is often provided as part of cardiac rehabilitation, and a recent review confirmed that attendees of a cardiac rehabilitation program had higher levels of PA than their control group peers (Dibben et al., 2018). However, this type of support is not routinely available.

A WHO report on CVD identified that the Middle East, which has a population of over 400 million, has a lower level of PA than other parts of the world (WHO, 2015). Approximately one third of the male adults and half of the female adults in the Middle East are physically inactive (WHO, 2015). The reasons for this are unclear.

In Jordan, conservative traditions, cultural norms, and beliefs regarding illness and recovery may contribute to low levels of PA among the general population (Barghouti et al., 2015). Moreover, Jordan lacks open spaces and parks, which Jordanian people prefer over sports facilities for engaging in PA (Barghouti et al., 2015). In Jordan, there are no cardiac rehabilitation or related structured education programs. Therefore, both the general Jordanian population and those recovering from AMI face potential obstacles to engaging in regular PA.

Cross-sectional surveys conducted in Europe have assessed self-reported PA levels in patients diagnosed with CHD. Data from over 15,000 participants showed that self-reported PA levels increased over time, with 20% of the sample reporting adequate levels of PA at follow-up (De Smedt et al., 2016). A more recent study showed similar findings (McKee et al., 2019). Self-reported PA levels in a sample of post-AMI patients improved significantly between baseline and 3 months after AMI, but almost half of the sample did not attain a PA level that matched guideline recommendations (McKee et al., 2019).

Self-report data on PA levels provide useful information about the context and types of PA but are limited because of variations in reporting and recall bias (Ekelund et al., 2011). Moreover, few studies have reported PA data on patients with AMI obtained objectively using accelerometers.

Cardiac rehabilitation has an impact on average step count. In two studies, an increase of 40% in number of steps was reported during rehabilitation compared with nonrehabilitation days (Jones et al., 2007; Savage & Ades, 2008). It is not clear if this improvement is able to be maintained after cardiac rehabilitation.

Primary outcomes of PA considered in prior research include step count, stepping time, standing time, upright time (the sum of standing and stepping time), and sedentary time (Granat, 2012; Ryan et al., 2006).

Step count per day has traditionally been measured using a pedometer. A guide to health intervention was developed to classify PA, with individuals who take fewer than 5,000 steps per day considered to have a sedentary life and individuals who take more than 10,000 steps per day considered to be active (Tudor-Locke et al., 2012). A previous study found that patients with acute coronary syndrome, heart failure, and coronary artery bypass grafting (CABG) or valve surgery after 1 year took approximately 6,000 steps per day (Thorup et al., 2016).

Time spent upright was assessed as 5.9 hours per day among an older healthy population in the United Kingdom (Fitzsimons et al., 2013) and 7.9 hours per day among healthy adults in the United States (Bassett et al., 2014). Standing time has been shown to have a dose–response association with all-cause mortality in adults, and increasing standing may alleviate the health risks of prolonged sitting (van der Ploeg et al., 2014).

Sedentary time is recognized as an independent coronary risk factor (Del Pozo-Cruz et al., 2018). Few studies have reported on this important PA parameter in patients recovering from AMI. An Australian study by Freene et al. (2018) showed that, although there was a significant improvement in exercise capacity and light-intensity PA, overall PA levels were low and sedentary behavior was high (Freene et al., 2018), indicating a need for greater emphasis on encouraging participants in cardiac rehabilitation programs to reduce their sedentary time. In addition, one report found that a healthy adult population in the United States spent an average of 16.1 hours per day sedentary (Bassett et al., 2014), whereas another report found that older adults in the United Kingdom spent an average of 18.06 hours per day sedentary (Fitzsimons et al., 2013).

Perceived self-efficacy (SE) is an important psychological construct known to influence engagement with PA among cardiac patients. General SE is defined by Bandura as "beliefs in one's capabilities to organize and execute the course of action required to produce given attainments" (Bandura, 1997, p. 3). Evidence indicates that SE is associated with increased PA levels in patients diagnosed with CVD and improved self-management, leading to positive health outcomes (Bergström et al., 2015). SE levels function in two ways in cardiac rehabilitation participants, namely, as a determinant of engagement in PA and as an outcome of participating in PA (Woodgate & Brawley, 2008).

Cardiac SE is a cardiac-specific measure of SE that reflects a person's belief in their ability to perform specific activities that form the foundation of secondary prevention such as healthy eating, maintaining physical functioning, and smoking cessation (Wang et al., 2016).

Limited research has reported on the PA levels of patients during the early stages of recovery from AMI. The increasing burden of CVD and low levels of PA in Middle Eastern populations provide a compelling rationale for the need to measure PA levels and cardiac SE in patients recovering from AMI. Thus, this study was designed to measure free-living PA levels and self-reported cardiac SE during early post-AMI recovery (6 weeks posthospital discharge) in patients with first AMI.

Purpose

The aims of this study were to
1. determine the PA levels (step count, stepping time, standing time, upright time [the sum of stepping time and standing time], and sedentary time) at T2 and T3; and
2. measure self-reported cardiac SE levels at T1, T2, and T3.

Methods

Design

A repeated-measures design was used, and data were collected at three time points: hospital discharge (T1), 2 weeks after discharge (T2), and 6 weeks after discharge (T3). These time points were selected because health behaviors established during early recovery after AMI are likely to influence long-term behaviors.

Setting

The study was carried out at Jordan University Hospital (JUH) in Amman, Jordan. JUH is a tertiary hospital with approximately 600 beds, including a 12-bed coronary care unit (CCU). JUH is one of four public cardiac centers in Jordan and conducts > 4,000 percutaneous coronary intervention (PCI) procedures per year. Patients from most cities in Jordan are referred based on contractual agreements with the Ministry of Health. JUH also receives private patients. This hospital holds 4.2% of the total number of hospital beds in Jordan and accounts for 4.1% of all hospital admissions (Ministry of Health in Jordan, 2019). In Jordan, patients with AMI are hospitalized for 3–5 days before discharge. There is no structured education or rehabilitation provided for patients during their hospital stay or after discharge.

Sampling and Participants

The target population was composed of all eligible patients admitted to the CCU with a clinically confirmed AMI (ST-elevation MI and non-ST-elevation MI). Participants were included in the study if they could read and understand the study information, were aged ≥ 18 years, were admitted to the CCU with a confirmed diagnosis of first AMI, and were clinically stable with an ejection fraction of > 35%. Patients with significant comorbidities that impede PA behaviors as well as patients treated by CABG were excluded. A sample of 100 participants was targeted, based on a power calculation performed in a previous study and on an assumed attrition rate of 20% (Cowie et al., 2011).

Ethical Approval

The University of Salford in the United Kingdom (HSCR14/120) and the institutional review board at JUH in Jordan (07/2015) granted ethical approval. The study was conducted according to the agreed protocol, and informed consent was sought before participation.

Data Collection Procedure

Data were collected between March and December 2015. A clinical nurse identified and screened all potential patients using hospital records. Eligible patients were approached in the CCU and provided with the participant information sheets. Twenty-four to 48 hours later, hemodynamically stable patients were transferred to the medical cardiac unit. At this time, the researcher discussed the study with eligible, interested patients and obtained informed consent. Demographic and clinical data were collected from patient questionnaires and medical records. The activPAL3 monitor (a body-worn PA monitor) was attached to the participants in the outpatient clinic. The participants revisited the clinic 2 and 6 weeks after hospital discharge. The participants were asked to wear the activPAL3 monitor at all times (24 hours/day, 7 days/week) but were told it could be removed temporarily when exposed to water. A paper version of the Arabic version of the cardiac SE questionnaire was administered at T1, T2, and T3.

Measures

Cardiac self-efficacy questionnaire

Cardiac SE was measured using the Cardiac Self-Efficacy Questionnaire (CSEQ; Sullivan et al., 1998), which is designed to evaluate specific aspects of SE relevant to coronary heart disease. This is important because SE has been strongly associated with changes in health behavior that may lead to beneficial health outcomes in patients diagnosed with CHD. This condition-specific measure, which reflects specific secondary prevention tasks, was chosen rather than a generic SE measure because there is evidence that SE beliefs that reflect specific tasks are stronger predictors of performance than generic SE beliefs (Rodgers et al., 2013). The CSEQ consists of 16 items divided into three sections: controlling symptoms (eight items), maintaining function (five items), and three items related to a healthy lifestyle (obesity, smoking, and dietary habits). Respondents are asked to rate how confident they feel on a 5-point Likert scale (0 = *not at all* to 4 = *completely confident*). The internal consistency of the CSEQ is .90 (Cronbach's alpha) for controlling symptoms and .87 for maintaining function (Sullivan et al., 1998).

To measure CSEQ in an Arabic population, this measure was translated and back-translated between English and Arabic. The forward translation into Arabic was performed independently by two Arabic-speaking researchers in the same field of research. An initial Arabic version of the CSEQ was produced based on a synthesis of these two translations. After that, a native-English-speaking researcher implemented the backward translation into English and resolved any inconsistencies. Some minor adaptations were made: Modern standard Arabic (Fusha) was used, gender applicability was changed, and the alternative response "Nonapplicable" was deleted. Face and content validity and reliability were examined, with the results showing the CSEQ as valid and reliable (Cronbach's alpha = .84).

Physical activity

The activPAL3 monitor is widely used to assess free-living PA, with previously established reliability and validity for step count, upright time, and sedentary time (Ryan et al., 2006). Free-living PA is defined as "the level of activity that the patients, within their physical limitations, at their own pace, and in their own environment, typically perform" (Moy et al., 2009). The activPAL3 has been cited as the gold standard for measuring sedentary behavior (Lyden et al., 2012) and has been validated in a wide range of populations such as older adults (Grant et al., 2008), in measuring posture and motion in adults (Godfrey et al., 2007), and in assessments of people with chronic heart failure (Cowie et al., 2011).

The activPAL3 is a lightweight (15 grams), small (53 × 35 × 7 mm), thigh-worn accelerometer-based device. It is attached to the skin at the midpoint of the anterior thigh using self-adhering, patented dual-layer hydrogels (PAL*stickies*). PA data are considered to be valid if data are available for a minimum of 3 days with at least 13 hours of measurement per day at each time point available for analysis (Edwardson et al., 2016).

Data Analysis

The activPAL3 data were downloaded using the manufacturer's software (ActivPAL Professional Software Version 7.2.32). Data were cleaned to remove nonwear periods (Edwardson et al., 2016). Data related to stepping, standing, and sedentary duration and number of steps were extracted. Upright time was calculated by adding standing and stepping time. All measures were reported as average per day. CSEQ questionnaire data were extracted from paper-based surveys. CSEQ data and activity outcome data were transferred to the IBM SPSS Version 22 (IBM, Inc., Armonk, NY, USA). Descriptive statistics, paired *t* tests, or Wilcoxon signed rank tests (if the necessary assumptions were not met) were used to compare mean scores at two time points, and a repeated-measures analysis of variance was used to compare three or more time points. An alpha of .05 was used as the cutoff for significance.

Results

An overview of the data collected at T1, T2, and T3 is presented in Figure 1. Of the 136 eligible patients, 36 declined to participate for personal reasons. Thus, 100 participants were initially enrolled in this study. The final sample was composed of 94 participants who were predominantly male (62%) with a mean age of 54.5 ± 9.9 years (*n* = 100) and an age range of 36–75 years (Table 1). The sample included 46 participants who had ST-elevation MI treated with primary PCI, 22 participants who were treated with thrombolytic agent (THROMB) and PCI, and 32 participants who were treated with PCI.

Self-Efficacy

Table 2 shows global and subscale cardiac SE scores. There was a statistically significant increase in mean self-reported global cardiac SE scores across the three time points (22.1 ± 8.2 vs. 35.0 ± 9.1 vs. 48.0 ± 8.5). This trend was replicated across the three subscales of control symptoms (11.1 ± 4.0 vs. 16.8 ± 4.9 vs. 23.6 ± 4.6), maintain function (6.8 ± 3.0 vs. 11.2 ± 3.0 vs. 15.5 ± 2.9), and healthy lifestyle (4.3 ± 2.3 vs. 7.0 ± 2.1 vs. 8.8 ± 2.0; Table 2). There was no difference found in SE by gender, educational level, marital status, or age (*p* > .05).

Physical Activity

Findings relating to PA level, including step count, stepping time, standing time, upright time, and sedentary time, are shown in Table 3. No statistically significant differences were found between T2 and T3 in terms of step count (6,819 ± 2,926 vs. 7,066 ± 2,580 steps/day) or stepping time (1.57 ± 0.64 vs. 1.62 ± 0.54 hours/day). There was a trend toward a decrease

Figure 1

Participant Flowchart

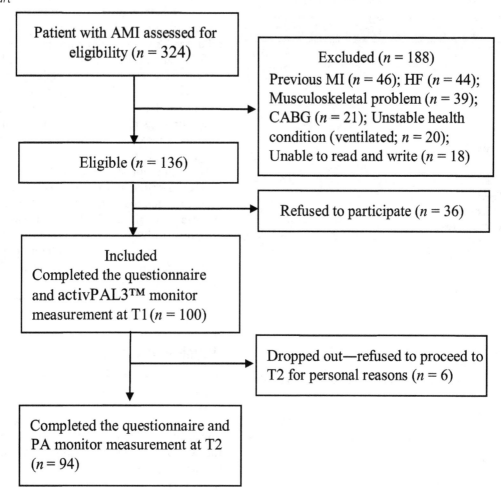

Note. AMI = acute myocardial infarction; MI = myocardial infarction; HF = heart failure; CABG = coronary artery bypass graft; T1 = hospital discharge; T2 = 2-weeks post discharge; T3 = 6-weeks post discharge.

in standing time (3.98 ± 1.69 vs. 3.84 ± 1.45 hours/day) and upright time (5.55 ± 2.1 vs. 5.46 ± 1.7 hours/day) and an increase in sedentary time (18.44 ± 2.1 vs. 18.53 ± 1.74 hours/day) recorded at T2 and T3, but these differences were not statistically significant.

Discussion

This was the first study to report on both self-reported cardiac SE and objectively measured free-living PA levels in patients with AMI during early recovery in Jordan. Mean global cardiac SE scores and associated subscale scores were found to increase significantly over time. However, this trend was not reflected in the objectively measured PA levels, which did not change significantly between T1 (2 weeks) and T2 (6 weeks).

Cardiac Self-Efficacy

Cardiac SE is considered to be an important factor associated with behavioral change in patients with CVD (Brouwer-Goossensen et al., 2018). There are few published studies available for comparison that measure SE levels during the early recovery period (up to 6 weeks postdischarge) in patients with CHD who are not offered cardiac rehabilitation. Most prior research has focused on long-term recovery.

In this study, patients with AMI who had not attended cardiac rehabilitation showed significant improvements in global, self-reported cardiac SE, and all subscales. This is consistent with one study conducted in the United States on a sample of patients with CHD that found a statistically significant improvement in general SE recorded 2 months post-AMI (Blanchard et al., 2006). However, Blanchard and his colleagues focused on gender-based differences in SE level among patients with CHD and patients recovering

Table 1

Sociodemographic and Clinical Characteristics (N = 100)

Variable	n	%
Age (years; *M* and *SD*)	54.5	9.9
Range	36–75	
Gender		
Male	62	62
Female	38	38
Marital status		
Single/widowed	26	26
Married	62	62
Divorced	12	12
Educational level		
Secondary school or less	13	33
Higher diploma or less	21	21
Bachelor's degree	39	39
Master's degree or higher	7	7
Employment		
Employed	31	31
Unemployed	11	11
Retired	22	22
Self-employed	36	36
Clinical data		
Type of treatment		
ST-elevation myocardial infarction treated by PCI	46	46
THROMB and PCI	22	22
PCI	32	32
Diagnosis date of coronary heart disease (months; *M* and *SD*)	65.3	37.3
Range	12–216	
Body mass index (*M* and *SD*)	25.6	1.61
Range	22.0–28.5	

Note. PCI = percutaneous coronary intervention; THROMB = Thrombolytic agent.

from CABG and did not measure changes in SE level between hospital discharge and 2 months postdischarge (Blanchard et al., 2006).

In addition, the degree of change in SE is affected by the measure that is used. In one U.S.-based study, exercise SE

levels were evaluated in 133 participants attending cardiac rehabilitation programs. Results showed that this construct was at its highest at the beginning of cardiac rehabilitation, decreased significantly 6 months later, and then had leveled off at the 18-month follow-up (Howarter et al., 2014).

Salari et al. (2016) measured cardiac SE and reported on patients recovering from angioplasty who had low cardiac SE levels at 6 months postoperation. The mean cardiac SE score was 8.43 ± 4.5, with scores ranging from 0 to 20. These findings diverge significantly from this study, which reported a mean cardiac SE score of 48.0 ± 8.5 and a score range from 0 to 64. Another study showed that post-CABG, angioplasty, and AMI patients reported lower and more-stable general SE levels over a 2-month period after cardiac rehabilitation than their control group peers (Poortaghi et al., 2013). However, this particular difference with this study may be because of the different SE measures used (Rodgers et al., 2013), different populations surveyed, and differences in measurement times. SE is a complex psychological construct that is influenced by other mechanisms that must be taken into account when comparing findings.

Physical Activity

This was the first study to report on objectively measured PA in patients with AMI recorded during the early recovery period. No significant differences were found in any of the five PA parameters between T2 (Week 2) and T3 (Week 6). The low levels of PA found in this study support the findings of the WHO regarding the rising prevalence of CVD risk factors and the low general level of PA in Middle Eastern countries (WHO, 2016).

The mean step count per day in this study was similar to the findings of other studies on patients with AMI and ACS (Houle et al., 2011; Izawa et al., 2006) that showed patients with AMI taking approximately 6,000 steps per day at 3–6 months after cardiac rehabilitation. Thorup et al. (2016) reported 8,000 steps per day as representative of the PA guidelines for patients with CHD. The population in this study tended toward the less-active end of this range at both T2 and T3, and mean step count per day was below the recommended PA level.

Table 2

Cardiac Self-Efficacy at Baseline, Week 2, and Week 6: Mean and SD Score

Questionnaire/Subscale	Baseline (*n* = 100)		Week 2 (*n* = 100)		Week 6 (*n* = 94)		F	p
	M	SD	M	SD	M	SD		
Global Cardiac Self-Efficacy Questionnaire (16 items overall)	22.1	8.2	35.0	9.1	48.0	8.5	268.5	< .001
Subscale 1 (control symptoms)	11.1	4.0	16.8	4.9	23.6	4.6	222.6	< .001
Subscale 2 (maintain function)	6.8	3.0	11.2	3.0	15.5	2.9	224.5	< .001
Subscale 3 (healthy lifestyle)	4.3	2.3	7.0	2.1	8.8	2.0	124.6	< .001

Table 3

Physical Activity Level Among Patients With AMI at Weeks 2–6

Physical Activity Measurement	Week 2 (*n* = 100)		Week 6 (*n* = 94)		*t*	*p*
	M	*SD*	*M*	*SD*		
Step count per day (average steps/day)	6,819	2,926	7,066	2,580	-0.55	.503
Stepping time (hours/day)	1.57	0.64	1.62	0.54	-0.54	.590
Standing time (hours/day)	3.98	1.69	3.84	1.45	0.51	.284
Upright time (hours/day)	5.55	2.10	5.46	1.70	0.30	.366
Sedentary time (sitting/lying time; hours/day)	18.44	2.10	18.53	1.74	-0.28	.380

Note. AMI = acute myocardial infarction.

Comparing objectively measured PA levels among healthy adults, patients with AMI, and older adult populations (> 65 years old), the step count in this study was below the step count of older adults reported in a previous study (7,066 steps/day vs. 8,493 steps/day), respectively. In addition, stepping time, standing time, and upright time in our sample were all below the results obtained from a sample of older, healthy adults (1.62 vs. 1.75 vs. 1.9 hours/day, 3.84 vs. 4.19 vs. 6.0 hours/day, and 5.46 vs. 5.94 vs. 7.9 hours/day, respectively). Moreover, sedentary time in the current study was higher than older adults and healthy adult populations (18.53 vs. 18.06 vs. 16.1 hours/day), respectively.

Standing time has a dose–response association with all-cause mortality in adults, and increasing standing may alleviate the health risks of prolonged sitting (van der Ploeg et al., 2014). This study found that mean upright time per day (5.46 hours) represented about 23% of the day of the participants, with sedentary time accounting for the remainder (77%, 18.53 hours). This was lower than the 32.9% reported for healthy adults in the United States (Bassett et al., 2014) and the 24.95% reported for older adults in the United Kingdom (Fitzsimons et al., 2013). Therefore, although the average age of the participants in this study was 54.5 years, their mean PA level was closer to that of the elderly population surveyed in Fitzsimons et al. (2013). Upright time did not change over the measured period.

Most time spent by the participants with AMI was sedentary, with 77% overall mean sedentary time reported at T2 and T3. Bassett et al. (2014) found that healthy adults spent 67% of their time in a sedentary state (sitting/lying time), whereas a similar study found that older adults (average: 68 years) spent 75% of their time in a sedentary state (Fitzsimons et al., 2013). This may be because of a lack of awareness of the importance of PA and a lack of structured education for patients with AMI in Jordan (Eshah, 2011). Excessive time spent in a sedentary state increases the risks of diabetes, obesity, dyslipidemia, and premature mortality (Winzer et al., 2018).

A study on the PA levels of healthy adults conducted in Jordan using a self-administered PA questionnaire provides an interesting comparison with the findings of this study (Barghouti et al., 2015), showing that PA levels were similarly low in both studies. The authors reported that a lack of awareness about the benefits of PA combined with barriers related to social and cultural norms may explain their findings (Barghouti et al., 2015). Another study conducted even more recently in the Middle East found that the healthy adult population spent most of their time either sedentary or at reduced levels of activity, finding that barriers to PA were social, cultural, and environmental as well as lack of motivation, lack of intention, and lack of awareness regarding the importance of PA (Sharara et al., 2018). These factors may help explain the lack of change in PA levels between T2 and T3 in this study. However, it has been shown that, even when interventions targeting behavioral change are introduced, obtaining meaningful and sustained changes in PA level is difficult (Greaves et al., 2011). Whatever the explanation, it is clear that there is an urgent need to increase PA levels in Middle Eastern populations.

Cardiac rehabilitation programs have been shown to increase the awareness and knowledge of patients regarding controlling CVD risk factors, improving self-management skills, and promoting PA (Dibben et al., 2018). In this study, the participants did not have access to a cardiac rehabilitation program. Thus, the findings show the need for an effective strategy to reduce sedentary time and increase PA. Therefore, patients with AMI must understand and appreciate that the need to promote their PA level is not optional but rather a necessary part of their recovery. In addition, establishing cardiac rehabilitation programs is essential for the current and future health of patients in Jordan.

This study aimed to measure the changes in SE and PA in the early recovery period. In this study, SE increased but PA did not change. However, behavioral change is a complex process that is affected by many factors, including motivation, opportunity, and capability, each of which may interact and influence the process (Michie et al., 2011). It might be that a lack of some of these factors was responsible for this observation.

This study was affected by several limitations. First, the research was conducted at a single center, which, although a major medical center with a countrywide catchment area, may limit the generalizability of the findings. Second, the sample was purposive, and > 50% of screened patients were ineligible because they had an ejection fraction < 35% and a previous AMI, were unable to read and write, or were treated with CABG. Moreover, 30% of the eligible patients with AMI refused to participate. A primary strength of this study is the objective measurement of a range of key PA parameters of a relatively large sample size with a high compliance rate, which has not been reported to date in this population.

Conclusions

Participants recovering from AMI in Jordan did not increase their PA levels during the early recovery phase, although cardiac SE scores improved. This may be because the increase in cardiac SE was not matched by the practical skills and knowledge required to translate this positive psychological construct into behavioral change. This study was conducted in a setting where there is an absence of cardiac rehabilitation facilities, limited lifestyle intervention options, barriers to PA, and a widespread lack of knowledge regarding recommended PA levels. This study provides a first step to understanding this complex relationship and, in combination with further research, may be used to support the design of culturally appropriate interventions to increase PA levels in the target population. Further studies to understand the mechanism that increases cardiac SE among patients with AMI after hospitalization in Jordan are warranted. In addition, replication of this study with long-term measurements in different populations to confirm the results is recommended.

Acknowledgments

Many thanks to the study participants and to the Jordan University Hospital staff team for all of their help with data collection.

Author Contributions

Study conception and design: All authors
Data collection: AS
Data analysis and interpretation: AS, MG
Drafting of the article: AS
Critical revision of the article: IJ, FA

References

Astin, F., Closs, S. J., McLenachan, J., Hunter, S., & Priestley, C. (2009). Primary angioplasty for heart attack: Mismatch between expectations and reality? *Journal of Advanced Nursing, 65*(1), 72–83. https://doi.org/10.1111/j.1365-2648.2008.04836.x

Bäck, M., Hansen, T. B., & Frederix, I. (2017). *Cardiac rehabilitation and exercise training recommendations, cardiac rehabilitation: Rationale, indications and core components.* Retrieved June 9, 2019, from https://www.escardio.org/Education/ESC-Prevention-of-CVD-Programme/Rehabilitation

Bandura, A. (1997). *Self-efficacy: The exercise of control* (illustrated, reprint ed.). Worth Publishers.

Barghouti, F., AbuRmaileh, N. N., Jallad, D. G., & Abd-Qudah, Y. (2015). Leisure time physical activity in Jordan: Knowledge and sociodemographic determinants. *International Medical Journal, 22*(4), 283–287.

Bassett, D. R. Jr., John, D., Conger, S. A., Rider, B. C., Passmore, R. M., & Clark, J. M. (2014). Detection of lying down, sitting, standing, and stepping using two activPAL monitors. *Medicine & Science in Sports & Exercise, 46*(10), 2025–2029. https://doi.org/10.1249/MSS.0000000000000326

Bergström, G., Börjesson, M., & Schmidt, C. (2015). Self-efficacy regarding physical activity is superior to self-assessed activity level, in long-term prediction of cardiovascular events in middle-aged men. *BMC Public Health, 15*(1), Article No. 820. https://doi.org/10.1186/s12889-015-2140-4

Blanchard, C. M., Reid, R. D., Morrin, L. I., Beaton, L. J., Pipe, A., Courneya, K. S., & Plotnikoff, R. C. (2006). Correlates of physical activity change in patients not attending cardiac rehabilitation. *Journal of Cardiopulmonary Rehabilitation and Prevention, 26*(6), 377–383.

British Association for Cardiovascular Disease Prevention and Rehabilitation. (2017). *2017 standards and core components for cardiovascular disease prevention and rehabilitation.* Retrieved August 26, 2018, from https://www.bacpr.com/pages/page_box_contents.asp?pageid=791

Brouwer-Goossensen, D., van Genugten, L., Lingsma, H. F., Dippel, D. W. J., Koudstaal, P. J., & den Hertog, H. M. (2018). Self-efficacy for health-related behaviour change in patients with TIA or minor ischemic stroke. *Psychology & Health, 33*(12), 1490–1501. https://doi.org/10.1080/08870446.2018.1508686

Cowie, A., Thow, M. K., Granat, M. H., & Mitchell, S. L. (2011). A comparison of home and hospital-based exercise training in heart failure: Immediate and long-term effects upon physical activity level. *European Journal of Cardiovascular Prevention & Rehabilitation, 18*(2), 158–166. https://doi.org/10.1177/1741826710389389

De Smedt, D., Clays, E., Prugger, C., De Sutter, J., Fras, Z., De Backer, G., Lovic, D., Baert, A., Kotseva, K., & De Bacquer, D. (2016). Physical activity status in patients with coronary heart disease: Results from the cross-sectional EUROASPIRE surveys. *Journal of Physical Activity and Health, 13*(12), 1378–1384. https://doi.org/10.1123/jpah.2016-0088

Del Pozo-Cruz, J., García-Hermoso, A., Alfonso-Rosa, R. M., Alvarez-Barbosa, F., Owen, N., Chastin, S., & Del Pozo-Cruz, B. (2018). Replacing sedentary time: Meta-analysis of objective-assessment studies. *American Journal of Preventive Medicine, 55*(3), 395–402. https://doi.org/10.1016/j.amepre.2018.04.042

Dibao-Dina, C., Angoulvant, D., Lebeau, J.-P., Peurois, J.-E., El Hirtsi, K. A., & Lehr-Drylewicz, A.-M. (2018). Patients' adherence to optimal therapeutic, lifestyle and risk factors recommendations after myocardial infarction: Six years follow-up in primary care. *PLOS ONE, 13*(9), Article e0202986. https://doi.org/10.1371/journal.pone.0202986

Dibben, G. O., Dalal, H. M., Taylor, R. S., Doherty, P., Tang, L. H., & Hillsdon, M. (2018). Cardiac rehabilitation and physical activity: Systematic review and meta-analysis. *Heart*, *104*(17), 1394–1402. https://doi.org/10.1136/heartjnl-2017-312832

Edwardson, C. L., Winkler, E. A. H., Bodicoat, D. H., Yates, T., Davies, M. J., Dunstan, D. W., & Healy, G. N. (2016). Considerations when using the activPAL monitor in field-based research with adult populations. *Journal of Sport and Health Science*, *6*(2), 162–178. https://doi.org/10.1016/j.jshs.2016.02.002

Ek, A., Ekblom, Ö., Hambraeus, K., Cider, Å., Kallings, L. V., & Börjesson, M. (2019). Physical inactivity and smoking after myocardial infarction as predictors for readmission and survival: Results from the SWEDEHEART-registry. *Clinical Research in Cardiology*, *108*(3), 324–332. https://doi.org/10.1007/s00392-018-1360-x

Ekblom, O., Ek, A., Cider, Å., Hambraeus, K., & Börjesson, M. (2018). Increased physical activity post–myocardial infarction is related to reduced mortality: Results from the SWEDEHEART registry. *Journal of the American Heart Association*, *7*, 24, Article e010108. https://doi.org/10.1161/JAHA.118.010

Ekelund, U., Tomkinson, G., & Armstrong, N. (2011). What proportion of youth are physically active? Measurement issues, levels and recent time trends. *British Journal of Sports Medicine*, *45*(11), 859–865. https://doi.org/10.1136/bjsports-2011-090190

Eshah, N. F. (2011). Jordanian acute coronary syndrome patients' learning needs: Implications for cardiac rehabilitation and secondary prevention programs. *Nursing & Health Sciences*, *13*(3), 238–245. https://doi.org/10.1111/j.1442-2018.2011.00608.x

Fitzsimons, C. F., Kirk, A., Baker, G., Michie, F., Kane, C., & Mutrie, N. (2013). Using an individualised consultation and activPAL™ feedback to reduce sedentary time in older Scottish adults: Results of a feasibility and pilot study. *Preventive Medicine*, *57*(5), 718–720. https://doi.org/10.1016/j.ypmed.2013.07.017

Freene, N., McManus, M., Mair, T., Tan, R., & Davey, R. (2018). Objectively measured changes in physical activity and sedentary behavior in cardiac rehabilitation: A prospective cohort study. *Journal of Cardiopulmonary Rehabilitation and Prevention*, *38*(6), E5–E8. https://doi.org/10.1097/HCR.0000000000000334

Godfrey, A., Culhane, K. M., & Lyons, G. M. (2007). Comparison of the performance of the activPAL professional physical activity logger to a discrete accelerometer-based activity monitor. *Medical Engineering & Physics*, *29*(8), 930–934. https://doi.org/10.1016/j.medengphy.2006.10.001

Granat, M. H. (2012). Event-based analysis of free-living behaviour. *Physiological Measurement*, *33*(11), 1785–1800. https://doi.org/10.1088/0967-3334/33/11/1785

Grant, P. M., Dall, P. M., Mitchell, S. L., & Granat, M. H. (2008). Activity-monitor accuracy in measuring step number and cadence in community-dwelling older adults. *Journal of Aging and Physical Activity*, *16*(2), 201–214. https://doi.org/10.1123/japa.16.2.201

Greaves, C. J., Sheppard, K. E., Abraham, C., Hardeman, W., Roden, M., Evans, P. H., Schwarz, P., & IMAGE Study Group (2011). Systematic review of reviews of intervention components associated with increased effectiveness in dietary and physical activity interventions. *BMC Public Health*, *11*, 119. https://doi.org/10.1186/1471-2458-11-119

Houle, J., Doyon, O., Vadeboncoeur, N., Turbide, G., Diaz, A., & Poirier, P. (2011). Innovative program to increase physical activity following an acute coronary syndrome: Randomized controlled trial. *Patient Education and Counseling*, *85*(3), e237–e244. https://doi.org/10.1016/j.pec.2011.03.018

Howarter, A. D., Bennett, K. K., Barber, C. E., Gessner, S. N., & Clark, J. M. R. (2014). Exercise self-efficacy and symptoms of depression after cardiac rehabilitation: Predicting changes over time using a piecewise growth curve analysis. *Journal of Cardiovascular Nursing*, *29*(2), 168–177. https://doi.org/10.1097/JCN.0b013e318282c8d6

Ibanez, B., James, S., Agewall, S., Antunes, M. J., Bucciarelli-Ducci, C., Bueno, H., Caforio, A. L. P., Crea, F., Goudevenos, J. A., Halvorsen, S., Hindricks, G., Kastrati, A., Lenzen, M. J., Prescott, E., Roffi, M., Valgimigli, M., Varenhorst, C., Vranckx, P., Widimský, P., & ESC Scientific Document Group. (2018). 2017 ESC guidelines for the management of acute myocardial infarction in patients presenting with ST-segment elevation: The task force for the management of acute myocardial infarction in patients presenting with ST-segment elevation of the European Society of Cardiology (ESC). *European Heart Journal*, *39*(2), 119–177. https://doi.org/10.1093/eurheartj/ehx393

Izawa, K. P., Watanabe, S., Oka, K., Osada, N., & Omiya, K. (2006). Effect of self-monitoring approach during cardiac rehabilitation on exercise maintenance, self-efficacy, and physical activity over a 1-year period after myocardial infarction. *Japanese Journal of Physical Fitness and Sports Medicine*, *55*(Suppl.), S113–S118. https://doi.org/10.7600/jspfsm.55.S113

Jones, N. L., Schneider, P. L., Kaminsky, L. A., Riggin, K., & Taylor, A. M. (2007). An assessment of the total amount of physical activity of patients participating in a phase III cardiac rehabilitation program. *Journal of Cardiopulmonary Rehabilitation and Prevention*, *27*(2), 81–85. https://doi.org/10.1097/01.HCR.0000265034.39404.07

Lyden, K., Kozey-Keadle, S. L., Staudenmayer, J. W., & Freedson, P. S. (2012). Validity of two wearable monitors to estimate breaks from sedentary time. *Medicine and Science in Sports and Exercise*, *44*(11), 2243–2252. https://doi.org/10.1249/MSS.0b013e318260c477

McKee, G., Mooney, M., O'Donnell, S., O'Brien, F., Biddle, M. J., & Moser, D. K. (2019). A cohort study examining the factors influencing changes in physical activity levels following an acute coronary syndrome event. *European Journal of Cardiovascular Nursing*, *18*(1), 57–66. https://doi.org/10.1177/1474515118786203

Michie, S., van Stralen, M. M., & West, R. (2011). The behaviour change wheel: A new method for characterising and designing behaviour change interventions. *Implementation Science*, *6*, 42. https://doi.org/10.1186/1748-5908-6-42

Ministry of Health in Jordan. (2019). *Ministry of Health annual statistical book 2019*. https://www.moh.gov.jo/Pages/viewpage.aspx?pageID=248

Moy, M. L., Matthess, K., Stolzmann, K., Reilly, J., & Garshick, E. (2009). Free-living physical activity in COPD: Assessment with accelerometer and activity checklist. *Journal of Rehabilitation Research & Development*, *46*(2), 277–286.

Poortaghi, S., Baghernia, A., Golzari, S. E., Safayian, A., & Atri, S. B. (2013). The effect of home-based cardiac rehabilitation program on self efficacy of patients referred to cardiac rehabilitation center. *BMC Research Notes*, *6*, 287. https://doi.org/10.1186/1756-0500-6-287

Rodgers, W. M., Murray, T. C., Selzler, A. M., & Norman, P. (2013). Development and impact of exercise self-efficacy types during and after cardiac rehabilitation. *Rehabilitation Psychology*, *58*(2), 178–184. https://doi.org/10.1037/a0032018

Ryan, C. G., Grant, P. M., Tigbe, W. W., & Granat, M. H. (2006). The validity and reliability of a novel activity monitor as a measure of walking. *British Journal of Sports Medicine, 40*(9), 779–784. https://doi.org/10.1136/bjsm.2006.027276

Salari, A., Balasi, L. R., Moaddab, F., Zaersabet, F., Saeed, A. N., & Nejad, S. H. (2016). Patients' cardiac self-efficacy after coronary artery angioplasty. *Jundishapur Journal of Chronic Disease Care, 5*(2), Article e60308. https://doi.org/10.17795/jjcdc-37251

Savage, P. D., & Ades, P. A. (2008). Pedometer step counts predict cardiac risk factors at entry to cardiac rehabilitation. *Journal of Cardiopulmonary Rehabilitation and Prevention, 28*(6), 370–377. https://doi.org/10.1097/HCR.0b013e31818c3b6d

Sharara, E., Akik, C., Ghattas, H., & Makhlouf Obermeyer, C. (2018). Physical inactivity, gender and culture in Arab countries: A systematic assessment of the literature. *BMC Public Health, 18*(1), 639. https://doi.org/10.1186/s12889-018-5472-z

Sullivan, M. D., LaCroix, A. Z., Russo, J., & Katon, W. J. (1998). Self-efficacy and self-reported functional status in coronary heart disease: A six-month prospective study. *Psychosomatic Medicine, 60*(4), 473–478. https://doi.org/10.1097/00006842-199807000-00014

Sumner, J., Harrison, A., & Doherty, P. (2017). The effectiveness of modern cardiac rehabilitation: A systematic review of recent observational studies in non-attenders versus attenders. *PLOS ONE, 12*(5), Article e0177658. https://doi.org/10.1371/journal.pone.0177658

Thorup, C., Hansen, J., Grønkjær, M., Andreasen, J. J., Nielsen, G., Sørensen, E. E., & Dinesen, B. I. (2016). Cardiac patients' walking activity determined by a step counter in cardiac telerehabilitation: Data from the intervention arm of a randomized controlled trial. *Journal of Medical Internet Research, 18*(4), Article e69. https://doi.org/10.2196/jmir.5191

Tudor-Locke, C., Craig, C. L., Thyfault, J. P., & Spence, J. C. (2012). A step-defined sedentary lifestyle index: <5000 steps/day. *Applied Physiology, Nutrition, and Metabolism, 38*(2), 100–114. https://doi.org/10.1139/apnm-2012-0235

van der Ploeg, H. P., Chey, T., Ding, D., Chau, J. Y., Stamatakis, E., & Bauman, A. E. (2014). Standing time and all-cause mortality in a large cohort of Australian adults. *Preventive Medicine, 69,* 187–191. https://doi.org/10.1016/j.ypmed.2014.10.004

Wang, W., Jiang, Y., & Lee, C.-H. (2016). Independent predictors of physical health in community-dwelling patients with coronary heart disease in Singapore. *Health and Quality of Life Outcomes, 14*(1), 113. https://doi.org/10.1186/s12955-016-0514-7

Wasfy, M. M., & Baggish, A. L. (2019). Truth about physical fitness and risk of acute myocardial infarction: The HUNT is on. *Journal of the American Heart Association, 8*(9), Article e012567. https://doi.org/10.1161/JAHA.119.012567

Winzer, E. B., Woitek, F., & Linke, A. (2018). Physical activity in the prevention and treatment of coronary artery disease. *Journal of the American Heart Association, 7*(4), Article e007725. https://doi.org/10.1161/JAHA.117.007725

Woodgate, J., & Brawley, L. R. (2008). Use of an efficacy-enhancing message to influence the self-regulatory efficacy of cardiac rehabilitation participants: A field experiment. *Rehabilitation Psychology, 53*(2), 153–161. https://doi.org/10.1037/0090-5550.53.2.153

World Health Organization. (2015). *Cardiovascular diseases.* Retrieved February 16, 2019, from http://www.emro.who.int/health-topics/cardiovascular-diseases/index.html

World Health Organization. (2016). *Health education and promotion: Physical activity and background.* Retrieved February 16, 2019, from http://www.emro.who.int/health-education/physical-activity/background.html

World Health Organization. (2017). *Cardiovascular diseases (CVDs).* Retrieved February 16, 2019, from https://www.who.int/en/news-room/fact-sheets/detail/cardiovascular-diseases-(cvds)

Zhang, Y., Cao, H., Jiang, P., & Tang, H. (2018). Cardiac rehabilitation in acute myocardial infarction patients after percutaneous coronary intervention: A community-based study. *Medicine, 97*(8), Article e9785. https://doi.org/10.1097/MD.0000000000009785

The Effects of Aromatherapy on Postpartum Women

Shuo-Shin TSAI[1] • Hsiu-Hung WANG[2]* • Fan-Hao CHOU[3]

ABSTRACT

Background: The postpartum period is the most crucial but also the most fragile stage of most pregnancies. The health benefits of aromatherapy have recently become more widely accepted among medical experts. Although a number of studies have examined these health benefits, no systematic reviews have been conducted to assess the effects of aromatherapy on the psychophysiological health of postpartum women.

Purpose: This systematic review was conducted to evaluate the effectiveness of aromatherapy interventions on the psychophysiological health of postpartum women, to determine the methods that were used to measure intervention effectiveness, and to identify the types of interventions that were used.

Methods: We searched for studies that evaluated the effects of aromatherapy on postpartum women published in the Chinese or English languages before March 2018. We used online databases such as the Taiwan Journal Index, Centre for European Policy Studies, Cumulative Index for Nursing and Allied Health Literature, Cochrane Library, PubMed, and Social Sciences Citation Index. The search keywords used were "women," AND "postpartum," OR "postnatal" AND "aromatherapy," OR "aroma," OR "essential oils." Only randomized controlled trials including humans as study participants were included. The methodological quality of the trials was assessed using the modified Jadad scale. The quality of the full-text studies was assessed by three reviewers.

Results: The 15 studies that were included in this systematic review were performed in Iran, England, and the United States and included 2,131 participants in total. The numbers of participants in each study ranged between 35 and 635. The review found that the effective duration of aromatherapy varied according to the essential oils that were selected. The visual analog scale was the most frequently used measure of postpartum pain. Most of the studies found that the aromatherapy intervention improved postpartum physiological and psychological health, with positive effects shown on anxiety, depression, distress, fatigue, mood, nipple fissure pain, physical pain, post-cesarean-delivery pain, post-cesarean-delivery nausea, postepisiotomy pain, postepisiotomy recovery, sleep quality, and stress. Most of the studies reported no serious intervention-related side effects.

Conclusions: This systematic review may serve as a reference for healthcare workers in caring for postpartum women. Aromatherapy may be applied as a noninvasive complementary intervention to promote physio-psychological comfort in postpartum women.

KEY WORDS:
aromatherapy, essential oils, postnatal, postpartum, systematic review.

Introduction

The postpartum or postnatal period is regarded as the fourth trimester of pregnancy and is defined as the time between giving birth and the recovery of a woman's reproductive organs to their prepregnancy state (Romano, Cacciatore, Giordano, & La Rosa, 2010; Sun, 2016). This is the most crucial but also the most fragile stage of pregnancy (World Health Organization, 2014). Women experience various changes in their physio-psychological state during the postpartum period and find it difficult to adapt to these changes, which may affect their role as mothers as well as their health-related quality of life. Therefore, postpartum women require timely assistance to adapt to postpartum life (Sun, 2016).

Aromatherapy, a complementary therapy frequently categorized under phytotherapy or botanical medicine, involves using essential oils (EOs) as therapeutic agents (Dunning, 2013; Gnatta, Kurebayashi, Turrini, & Silva, 2016). The use of EOs for mental, physical, and spiritual purposes traces back thousands of years to ancient Eastern and Western civilizations, including the Chinese, Egyptians, Greeks, Indians, and Romans, among others (Buckle, 2011; Chang, 2014). Aromatherapy is a compound noun that was reportedly first used by René Maurice Gattefossé in 1937 (as cited in Chang, 2014; Gattefosse, 1993). The experiments of Gattefossé confirmed the scientific argument that, because of their excellent permeability, EOs can enter the body via pathways such as inhalation (through the olfactory system) and absorption (through the surface of the skin; Buckle, 2011; Chang, 2014). EOs were applied to treat burns, wounds, gangrenosum, and other trauma

[1]MSN, RN, Doctoral Candidate, College of Nursing, Kaohsiung Medical University, and Lecturer, Department of Nursing, Chung-Jen Junior College of Nursing, Health Sciences and Management • [2]PhD, RN, FAAN, Professor, College of Nursing, Kaohsiung Medical University • [3]PhD, RN, Professor, College of Nursing, Kaohsiung Medical University.

injuries during World War I and World War II as well as to treat mental disorders in postwar society (Buckle, 2011; Chang, 2014). Aromatherapy is defined as the science and art of therapies that are applied intrinsically using smells and practical EOs (Lis-Balchin, 1999; Robins, 1999). EOs, known as volatile oils, are extracted from the stems, leaves, flowers, and fruits of certain plants and may be produced using distillation, enfleurage, chemical solvents, resin tapping, carbon dioxide (CO_2), and cold pressing (Ali et al., 2015; Buckle, 2011). The dozens of popular EOs in current use include rosemary, tea tree, cinnamon, bergamot, sage, ylang-ylang, chamomile, geranium, jasmine, lavender, lemon, and peppermint (Ali et al., 2015; Chang, 2014). Most EOs should not be applied to the skin undiluted (Dunning, 2013) and are therefore commonly administered through baths, local application, and inhalation to prevent or treat diseases, improve immune function, and protect human health (Ali et al., 2015; Buckle, 2011). The health benefits of aromatherapy are becoming more widely accepted among medical experts, and a number of studies have been conducted to evaluate these benefits (Ali et al., 2015). Gnatta et al. (2016) suggested that aromatherapy is practiced as a nursing intervention because it addresses psycho-physiological health and has been historically and widely practiced by nurses and that it is worth discussing aromatherapy within the context of nursing theory. However, no published articles have yet investigated the effects of aromatherapy on postpartum health. In addition, no clinical guidelines are currently available for the application of aromatherapy on postpartum women. Using an alternative, noninvasive therapeutic approach such as aromatherapy to address psychosomatic discomfort during the postpartum period may highlight the independence of nursing care while increasing comfort and relaxation and beneficial treatment outcomes among postpartum women. The objectives of this article are to (a) review the evidence from clinical trials that have assessed the benefits and safety of aromatherapy on the psycho-physiological health of postpartum women, (b) determine the methods used to measure the effectiveness of aromatherapy, and (c) identify the intervention approaches that were used. The Preferred Reporting Items for Systematic Reviews and Meta-Analyses guidelines (Moher, Liberati, Tetzlaff, Altman, & The PRISMA Group, 2009) were used during the review process to ensure a high level of quality and transparency in data selection and reporting.

Methods

Eligibility Criteria

Aromatherapy studies meeting the following criteria were included in this systematic review: (a) described the intervention, its implementation, and the aromatherapy medium (menthol, peppermint, lavender, orange peel, and *Citrus aurantium*); (b) examined physiological and psychological health of postpartum participants; that is, physiological health factors included nipple fissures, postepisiotomy perineal discomfort,

postepisiotomy pain, postepisiotomy recovery, physical pain, fatigue, post-cesarean-section (CS) delivery pain, post-CS-delivery nausea, and sleep quality, and psychological health factors included mood, anxiety, stress, depression, and distress; (c) were designed as randomized controlled trials (RCTs); (d) reported results in a full article that was published in either Chinese or English; and (e) used humans as study participants. Studies that used combined therapies, case reports, case series, descriptive studies, letters to editors, or reviews were excluded. The target populations were all postpartum women, and the studies were all conducted for a period of 8 weeks or less.

Information Sources

We searched online databases for Chinese- and English-language studies evaluating the effects of aromatherapy on postpartum women that were published before March 2018. The online databases that were used included the Taiwan Journal Index (Index to Taiwan Periodical Literature System, $n = 35$), Chinese Electronic Periodicals Service ($n = 37$), Cumulative Index for Nursing and Allied Health Literature ($n = 25$), Cochrane Library ($n = 156$), PubMed ($n = 395$), and Social Sciences Citation Index ($n = 45$). The search keywords that were used included "women," AND "postpartum," OR "postnatal" AND "aromatherapy," OR "aroma," OR "essential oils." As noted, only RCTs that examined humans as study participants were included in this review. In addition, the literature was carefully searched for references and citations to articles included in this study to avoid repetition and to include as many relevant original studies as possible.

Study Selection

Titles and structured summaries were reviewed independently by three researchers to identify potentially relevant articles. Next, the full texts of these articles were reviewed to confirm that the eligibility criteria were met and to extract the requisite information, which included study characteristics (author, year, country, design, participants, and risk of bias), intervention characteristics (type of aromatherapy, aromatherapy dose, treatment frequency, administration method, duration per session, total number of sessions, and total duration of intervention), and main outcomes. Data extraction was performed by three independent researchers, and any differences in opinion were resolved through mutual discussion and agreement.

Data Items

The modified Jadad scale is frequently used to assess the quality of trial reports that are candidates for inclusion in systematic reviews. This scale has an interrater reliability of .9, indicating that it is a useful tool (Oremus et al., 2001). The methodological quality of the included trials was assessed using the modified Jadad scale (Oremus et al., 2001). It is highly reliable and easily used. Thus, it is feasible to appraise the quality of the original studies (Dimitriou, Mavridou, Manataki, & Damigos, 2017; Oremus et al., 2001). The quality of the trials was analyzed using an eight-item scale (randomization, blinding, withdrawals and dropouts, inclusion and exclusion criteria, adverse effects, and statistical analysis), and "high" quality was determined by a score of equal to or greater than 4 (Table 1). All of the items were assessed by three researchers, and concurrence among all three was achieved through discussion.

Risk of Bias

The validity of the eligible RCTs was ascertained by evaluating the frequency and duration of the aromatherapy interventions, determining the methods that were used to measure intervention effectiveness, and identifying the intervention approaches that were used. Three researchers provided validity ratings independently, and the rating scores given by each matched completely.

Results

Study Selection

The initial search strategy identified 693 potentially relevant articles. After removing duplicates, 557 studies remained.

TABLE 1.
Modified Jadad Scale

Eight Items of the Modified Jadad Scale	Score
1. Was the study described as randomized?	
Yes	+ 1
No	0
2. Was the method of randomization appropriate?	
Yes	+ 1
No	− 1
Not described	0
3. Was the study described as blinded?	
Yes	+ 1
No	0
4. Was the method of blinding appropriate?	
Yes	+ 1
No	− 1
Not described	0
5. Was there a description of withdrawals and dropouts?	
Yes	+ 1
No	0
6. Was there a clear description of the inclusion and exclusion criteria?	
Yes	+ 1
No	0
7. Was the method used to assess adverse effects described?	
Yes	+ 1
No	0
8. Was the method of statistical analysis described?	
Yes	+ 1
No	0

Afterward, 540 studies were excluded because of their use of combined therapies, being a review article, not using EOs in the intervention, not including postpartum participants, and not including human participants. After screening the titles and abstracts of the remaining articles, 17 remained for full-text screening. Three studies were excluded in this stage because of being either a pilot study (2) or a qualitative study (1). In addition, one study was subsequently obtained from a reference. Thus, 15 RCTs were included in this review. A detailed flowchart for the study selection process is presented in Figure 1. The included studies were conducted in Iran, England, and the United States, with 2,131 participants and the number of participants per study ranging from 35 to 635. The participants in these studies were all postpartum women. Two of the included studies evaluated the effectiveness of aromatherapy in alleviating nipple fissure pain, five evaluated the alleviation of discomfort and pain and the effect on episiotomy recovery outcomes, three evaluated the alleviation of pain and nausea after CS, two evaluated improvements in sleep quality, and five evaluated the effect on psychological health.

Trial Quality

Information on the participants, design, intervention, follow-up, main outcome, and modified Jadad scale scores for the studies are presented in Table 2, and the main results of each study are compared numerically. All 15 of the RCTs met stringent standards for quality. The method of randomization was appropriate in eight of the studies (Study nos. 1, 7–9, and 11–14), seven studies used no blinding (Study nos. 1, 5–7, and 11–13), single blinding was used in four studies (Study nos. 3, 4, 14, and 15), and double blinding (Study nos. 2 and 9) and triple blinding (Study nos. 8 and 10) were used in two studies each. An appropriate blinding procedure was used in five studies (Study nos. 2, 3, 10, 14, and 15). There were descriptions of withdrawals and dropouts in eight studies (Study nos. 1–3, 5, 6, 12, 13, and 15). All of the studies presented clear descriptions of inclusion and exclusion criteria and applied appropriate statistical analysis. Six articles described adverse effects of the intervention (Study nos. 3, 4, 8, 9, 13, and 14). All of the studies received scores between 4 and 6.5, indicating high quality.

Effects of Aromatherapy on Physiological Health

Effect of aromatherapy on nipple fissures

Many lactating mothers experienced varying degrees of nipple trauma and that most followed poor breastfeeding-related practices (Ahmed, Mohamed, & Abu-Talib, 2015). Two Iranian studies evaluated improvements in nipple fissures in breastfeeding women, with one using an aromatherapy intervention on 110 primiparous lactating women. This intervention applied four drops of menthol essence on the nipple and areola after each feeding for 2 weeks. The visual analog

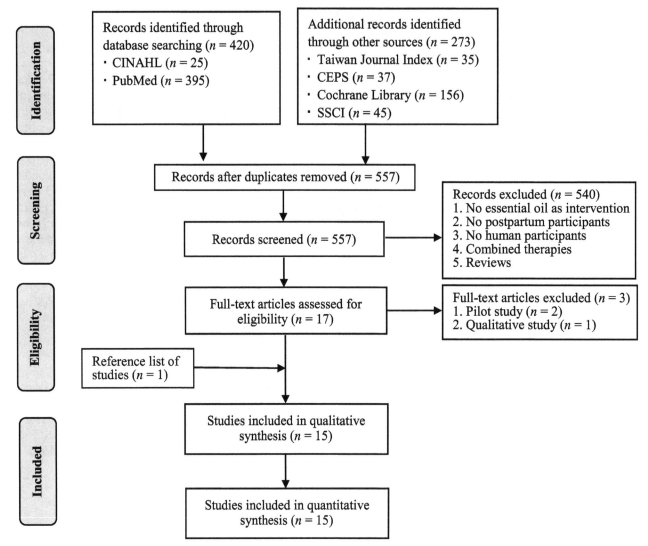

Figure 1. Flowchart for study selection. CINAHL = Cumulative Index to Nursing and Allied Health Literature; CEPS = Chinese Electronic Periodicals Service; SSCI = Social Sciences Citation Index.

scale (VAS; 0–10 cm) and Amir Scale (1–10 mm) were used to measure intensity of pain and severity of damage, respectively. In addition, the presence of nipple discharge was observed (Study no. 1). Other studies were conducted to assess the effects of peppermint water in alleviating nipple cracks. Peppermint water was produced by introducing peppermint EO gradually into 1 liter of distilled water. After every feeding from Day 1 to Day 14, the nipples were washed with water and then the nipple and areola were covered with peppermint-water-saturated cotton. The nipple and areola were washed again before the next feeding (Study no. 12).

The results of these studies were consistent in their findings that menthol essence and peppermint water were respectively effective in preventing and alleviating nipple pain, fissures, and damage in primiparous breastfeeding women when the aromatherapy intervention was conducted after each feeding for 2 weeks postpartum. These studies indicate that menthol and peppermint aromatherapy may be used in nursing practice to alleviate nipple fissures in breastfeeding mothers.

Effect of aromatherapy after episiotomy

Episiotomies are performed to expand the diameter of the outlet pelvis during normal spontaneous delivery (Masoumi, Keramat, & Hajiaghaee, 2011). Five of the included articles examined the effectiveness of aromatherapy in alleviating discomfort and pain and in facilitating recovery after episiotomy. One study that was conducted in England used lavender oil aromatherapy. Subjects in this study took a daily, half-hour bath into which six drops of lavender oil had been added. After each bath, they completed a VAS to measure degree of discomfort experienced. Moreover, the condition of the perineum was assessed as part of the midwife's normal daily examination of the subjects. There was some consistency in the results between the third and fifth days, with a reduction in mean discomfort scores. However, aromatherapy did not reduce perineum daily discomfort (Study no. 3). In Iran, four studies were conducted to assess the effectiveness of aromatherapy in reducing discomfort and pain and in facilitating recovery after episiotomy. Three of these

TABLE 2.

Summary of the 15 RCTs Evaluating Aromatherapy Effects on Postpartum Women

Study	Participant	Design	Intervention	Follow-Up	Main Outcome	Score
1. Akbari, Alamolhoda, Baghban, & Mirabi (2014) Iran	110 primiparous lactating women IG = 55, CG = 55	RCT	Four drops of menthol essence on the nipple and areola after each feeding CG = four drops of their own milk	3, 10, and 14 days	Nipple fissure pain VAS ($p < .001$), nipple fissure damage Amir Scale ($p < .001$), and nipple fissure discharge Amir Scale ($p < .001$)	5
2. Behmanesh et al. (2011) Iran	89 episiotomy in primiparous women, aged 17–34 years IG = 30, G2 = 30, G3 = 29	RCT/double blind	Ten drops of 2% lavender-EO-based olive oil added to 5 L of bathwater, twice a day G2 = olive oil, G3 = distilled water	2 hours, 5 and 10 days	1. Postepisiotomy pain VAS ($p = .030$) 2. Perineum REEDA score ($p = .001$)	6
3. Dale & Cornwell (1994) England	635 episiotomy in women IG = 217, G2 = 213, G3 = 205	RCT/single blind	Six drops of pure lavender oil added to bathwater for 30 minutes daily G2 = synthetic EO G3 = inert substance	10 days	1. Daily discomfort VAS: no significance 2. Daily mood VAS: no significance	6.5
4. Hadi & Hanid (2011) Iran	200 women who underwent CS IG = 100, PG = 100	RCT/single blind	• Two drops of 2% lavender essence through oxygen mask for 3 minutes • Placebo was a similar, clinically neutral aromatic material	Half, 8 and 16 hours	Post-CS-delivery pain VAS ($p < .001$)	4.5
5. Keshavarz Afshar et al. (2015) Iran	158 primiparous women who received vaginal delivery, aged 18–35 years IG = 79, PG = 79	RCT	• A cotton ball containing four drops of 10% lavender EO and sesame carrier oil placed inside a cylindrical container. They inhaled 10 deep breaths from a distance of 20 cm, four times a week. • Placebo was sesame carrier oil.	4 and 8 weeks	PSQI (1) 4 weeks: no significance (2) 8 weeks ($p < .05$)	4
6. Kianpour, Mansouri, Mehrabi, & Asghari (2016) Iran	140 postpartum women IG = 70, SG = 70	RCT	Three drops of lavender EO on their palms, rubbed them together. They inhaled it, three times a day for 4 weeks	2 weeks, 1 and 3 months	DASS-21 and the Edinburgh Stress, Anxiety, and Depression Scale for stress, anxiety, and depression: 2 weeks ($p = .012$, $p = .001$, and $p = .003$, respectively), 1 M ($p = .001$), 3 M ($p = .001$)	4
7. Lane et al. (2012) United States	35 women who deliver by CS IG = 22, PG = 8, SG = 5	RCT	• A cotton ball containing spirits of peppermint placed inside a small ziplock bag. They inhaled three deep breaths. • Placebo was sterile water with green food coloring.	2 and 5 minutes	Post-CS-delivery nausea, an ordinal nausea scale: 2 minutes ($p < .001$), 5 minutes ($p = .005$)	4
8. Mirghafourvand, Charandabi, Hakimi, Khodaie, & Galeshi (2016) Iran	96 postpartum women IG = 48, PG = 48	RCT/triple blind	• Ten drops of orange peel EO added to a glass of water. They drank it after meals, three times a day. • Placebo was water, propylene glycol, and 1–2 drops of orange edible EO.	8 weeks	PSQI ($p < .05$)	6

(continues)

TABLE 2.

Summary of the 15 RCTs Evaluating Aromatherapy Effects on Postpartum Women, Continued

Study	Participant	Design	Intervention	Follow-Up	Main Outcome	Score
9. Mirghafourvand, Mohammad Alizadeh Charandabi, Hakimi, Khodaie, & Galeshi (2017) Iran	96 postpartum women IG = 48, PG = 48	RCT/double blind	• Ten drops of orange peel EO added to a glass of water. They drank it after meals, three times a day. • Placebo was water, propylene glycol, and 1–2 drops of orange edible EO.	8 weeks	Edinburgh Postnatal Depression Questionnaire: no significance STAI: no significance	6
10. Olapour et al. (2013) Iran	60 women who deliver by CS IG = 30, PG = 30	RCT/triple blind	• Three drops of 10% lavender oil essence were poured on cotton in cast containers. They inhaled it for 5 minutes from a distance of 10 cm. • Placebo was a base of aromatherapy blend without lavender essence.	4, 8, and 12 hours	Post-CS-delivery pain VAS: 4 hours ($p = .008$), 8 hours ($p = .024$), 12 hours ($p = .011$)	5
11. Sheikhan et al, (2012) Iran	60 episiotomy in primiparous women IG = 30, SG = 30	RCT	Sitz baths (0.25 ml of lavender oil essence per 5 L of water) for 30 minutes, twice a day	4 and 12 hours, 5 days	Postepisiotomy pain VAS: 4 hours ($p = .001$), 12 hours: no significance, 5 days ($p < .001$) Perineum REEDA score: 5 days ($p = .000$)	4
12. Sayyah Melli et al. (2007) Iran	196 lactating primiparous women IG = 98, CG = 98	RCT	Peppermint water was poured on cotton. They put it on their nipple and areola after the nipple was washed with water after every feeding.	14 days	1. Nipple and areola cracks Amir Scale ($p < .01$) 2. Cracked nipple (relative risk = 3.6, 95% CI [2.9, 4.3]) 3. Nipple pain rating scales (odds ratio = 5.6, 95% CI [2.2, 14.6]; $p < .005$)	5
13. Sharifipour, Bakhteh, & Mirmohammad (2015) Iran	80 women who deliver by CS, aged 18–35 years IG = 40, PG = 40	RCT	• Three drops of *Citrus aurantium* essence were poured on cotton. They inhaled it for 5 minutes from a distance of 10 cm. • Placebo was normal saline.	12 hours	STAI ($p < .001$)	6
14. Vakilian, Atarha, Bekhradi, & Chaman (2011) Iran	120 episiotomy in primiparous women IG = 60, SG = 60	RCT/single blind	Sitz baths (five to seven drops of 1.5% lavender EO per 4 L of water), twice a day	10 days	1. Postepisiotomy pain VAS: no significance 2. Perineum edema: no significance 3. Perineum leaved suture: no significance 4. Perineum redness ($p = .001$) 5. Perineum dehiscence: no significance	6.5

(continues)

TABLE 2.

Summary of the 15 RCTs Evaluating Aromatherapy Effects on Postpartum Women, Continued

Study	Participant	Design	Intervention	Follow-Up	Main Outcome	Score
15. Vaziri et al. (2017) Iran	56 episiotomy in primiparous women, aged 18–35 years IG = 29, PG = 27	RCT/single blind	• Five drops of 1% lavender oil essence were poured on cotton. They inhaled it for 10–15 minutes from a distance of 20 cm. • Placebo was sesame oil.	1 hour and tomorrow morning	1. Perineal pain VAS ($p = .004$, $p < .001$) 2. Physical pain VAS ($p < .001$) 3. Fatigue VAS ($p = .02$, $p < .001$) 4. Distress VAS ($p < .001$) 5. PANAS: positive moods ($p < .001$), negative moods ($p = .007$, $p < .001$)	5.5

Note. RCTs = randomized controlled trials; IG = intervention group; CG = comparison group; PG = placebo group; SG = standard therapy group; CS = cesarean section; EO = essential oil; PSQI = Pittsburgh Sleep Quality Index; STAI = State-Trait Anxiety Inventory; VAS = visual analog scale; REEDA = Redness, Edema, Ecchymosis, Discharge, and Approximation; DASS-21 = 21-item Depression, Anxiety, and Stress Scale; CI = confidence interval; PANAS = Positive and Negative Affect Schedule.

studies asked the subjects to bathe in lavender oil twice a day to reduce pain, dehiscence, the number of sutures, infection, and Redness, Edema, Ecchymosis, Discharge, and Approximation (REEDA) score (Study nos. 2, 11, and 14). Lavender oil baths reduced redness (Study no. 14) and pain and REEDA scores (Study nos. 2 and 11). Furthermore, the effectiveness of lavender oil inhalation on perineal pain, physical pain, and fatigue was assessed in one of the included studies. The intervention with lavender oil was repeated 6 hours after the first intervention and at bedtime in three doses during the first 24 hours after delivery. Lavender oil inhalation was found to be effective in reducing pain and fatigue (Study no. 15). Two of five studies did not find significant side effects (Study nos. 3 and 14), with cases finding minor irritation (Study no. 14) and the others reporting no side effects at all (Study nos. 2, 11, and 15).

These results suggest that aromatherapy using five to 10 drops of lavender oil added to 4–5 liters of bathwater twice a day for 5–10 days (Study nos. 2, 11, and 14) or five drops of lavender oil inhalation for 10–15 minutes (Study no. 15) may have beneficial effects on wound care (Study nos. 2, 11, 14, and 15) and physical pain and fatigue (Study no. 15) in women after perineal episiotomy.

Effect of aromatherapy after cesarean section delivery

CS delivery, the most widely performed surgery worldwide, is continuing to increase in prevalence (Masoumi et al., 2011). Three studies examined the effectiveness of aromatherapy in alleviating nausea (Study no. 7) and pain (Study nos. 4 and 10) after CS delivery. In Iran, two studies asked subjects to inhale lavender essence for 3 and 5 minutes, respectively, to reduce pain (Study nos. 4 and 10) after CS delivery. Lavender aromatherapy was found to be effective in reducing post-cesarean-delivery pain (Study nos. 4 and 10). The results of a study conducted in the United States support the use of a spirit of peppermint (82% ethyl alcohol, peppermint oil,

purified water, peppermint leaf extract) aromatherapy intervention as a useful adjunct treatment for postoperative nausea after CS delivery (Study no. 7). One of three studies did not find side effects (Study no. 4), whereas the others did not mention side effects (Study nos. 7 and 10).

On the basis of these findings, lavender (Study nos. 4 and 10) and peppermint (Study no. 7) aromatherapies may be used as an effective complementary therapy for controlling nausea (Study no. 7) and pain (Study nos. 4 and 10) after CS.

Effect of aromatherapy on sleep

Two studies in Iran examined the effectiveness of aromatherapy in improving sleep quality in postpartum women. In one of these studies, 158 primiparous women received a cylindrical container in which a cotton ball infused with four drops of 10% lavender EO and sesame carrier oil had been placed. These women were instructed to inhale 10 deep breaths and then to place the container beside their pillow until morning (Study no. 5). The other Iranian study asked the 96 postpartum women participants to drink one glass of water into which 10 drops of orange peel EO had been added three times a day after each meal for 8 weeks (Study no. 8). One of these two studies found side effects, including dizziness (6.3%) and increased urination (10.4%; Study no. 8), and the other did not mention side effects (Study no. 5).

These results support the positive effects of lavender (Study no. 5) and orange peel (Study no. 8) aromatherapies on the sleep quality of women at 8 weeks postpartum.

Effect of Aromatherapy on Psychological Health

Five studies examined the effectiveness of aromatherapy on psychological health. The effects of lavender oil bath on daily mood have been assessed in England (Study no. 3), with the results indicating that lavender oil has no effect on daily mood. However, another study (Study no. 15) reported better mood status and distress scores in the lavender oil essence inhalation group than in the control group. A clinical trial (Study no. 13) investigated the effectiveness of *Citrus aurantium* essence in improving anxiety in 80 Iranian women. The intervention involved applying three drops of *Citrus aurantium* essence and asking the participants to inhale for 5 minutes. The results support using this intervention as an effective complementary therapy to help control anxiety. This result is in line with another study (Study no. 6) that reported significant reductions in stress, anxiety, and depression in postpartum women who had undergone an aromatherapy with lavender intervention. However, a further study (Study no. 9) reported a nonsignificant reduction in depression and anxiety levels during the postpartum period after aromatherapy with orange EO.

In summary, three of these five studies indicate that inhalation aromatherapy, either with lavender oil (Study nos. 6 and 15) or *Citrus aurantium* essence (Study no. 13), improves psychological health in postpartum women, whereas the studies that used bath (Study no. 3) and drink (Study no. 9) interventions found no significant effects.

Summary of Aromatherapy Outcomes

The EOs described in the included articles included pure, diluted, and mixtures of multiple EOs. The identified effects on the psycho-physiological health of the postpartum women subjects are presented in Tables 2 and 3. Lavender was the EO that had the greatest effect on psycho-physiological health (n = 9; Study nos. 2–6, 10, 11, 14, and 15).

Summary Measures

The primary outcome measurement was relief of pain, including nipple fissure pain, physical pain, postepisiotomy pain, and post-CS pain, measured using either the VAS or the Pain Rating Scale. Moreover, severity of nipple fissure discharge and nipple fissure damage were assessed using the Amir Scale; distress was assessed using the distress VAS; fatigue was assessed using the fatigue VAS; perineal discomfort was assessed using either the daily discomfort VAS or the daily mood VAS; mood status was assessed using the Positive and Negative Affect Schedule; depression was assessed using either the Edinburgh Postnatal Depression Questionnaire or the 21-item Depression, Anxiety, and Stress Scale (DASS-21); anxiety was assessed using the Spielberger State-Trait Anxiety Inventory, DASS-21, or the Edinburgh Stress, Anxiety, and Depression Scale; stress was assessed using either DASS-21 or the Edinburgh Stress, Anxiety, and Depression Scale; quality of sleep was assessed using the Pittsburgh Sleep Quality Index; post-CS nausea was assessed using the Ordinal Nausea Scale; and episiotomy

TABLE 3.
Outcomes of Aromatherapy

Outcome	No. of Studies	Aromatherapy	No. of Effects
Physiological health			
Nipple fissures	2	Menthol (1) and peppermint (1)	2
After episiotomy	5	Lavender	
1. Pain	4		3
2. REEDA			
(1) Redness	3		3
(2) Edema	3		2
(3) Ecchymosis	2		2
(4) Discharge	2		2
(5) Approximation	2		2
3. Leaved suture	1		0
4. Dehiscence	1		0
5. Daily discomfort	1		0
After CS delivery	3		
1. Pain	2	Lavender	2
2. Nausea	1	Peppermint	1
Sleep	2	Lavender (1) and orange peel (1)	2
Physical pain	1	Lavender	1
Fatigue	1	Lavender	1
Psychological health	5		
Mood	2	Lavender	1
Stress	1	Lavender	1
Depression	2	Lavender (1) and orange peel (1)	1 (lavender)
Anxiety	3	Lavender (1), orange peel (1), and *Citrus aurantium* (1)	2 (lavender and *Citrus aurantium*)
Distress	1	Lavender	1

Note. CS = caesarean section; REEDA = Redness, Edema, Ecchymosis, Discharge, and Approximation.

wound was assessed using the REEDA score. The VAS was the most frequently used measure of postpartum pain.

Discussion

EOs may be combined with usual care to improve health status, providing a natural and noninvasive option for care (Ali et al., 2015). Twelve of the 15 RCTs evaluated mainly reported on the effectiveness of aromatherapy in improving physiological health outcomes in postpartum women. Most of the included studies found positive effects of the interventions on physiological health in postpartum women. Aromatherapy was found to reduce nipple fissure pain, nipple fissure damage severity, nipple fissure discharge, post-CS-delivery pain, post-CS-delivery nausea, physical pain, fatigue, postepisiotomy pain, and perineum REEDA scores and to improve sleep quality. Although only five of the included studies examined the effect of aromatherapy on psychological health outcomes in the postpartum period, two of these showed nonsignificant outcomes (Dale & Cornwell, 1994; Mirghafourvand, Mohammad-Alizadeh-Charandabi, Hakimi, Khodaie, & Galeshi, 2017). Although most of the included studies indicated positive effects of interventions in terms of improving postpartum physio-psychological health, few of these studies assessed health effects such as nausea, physical pain, fatigue, stress, and distress. Therefore, additional studies evaluating the effects of aromatherapy on physiological and psychological health in postpartum women are warranted.

The most common modes of aromatherapy during the postpartum period were the addition of lavender oil to bathwater, lavender oil inhalation, and menthol oil application to the skin. However, lavender oil application caused a skin reaction. Overall, aromatherapy in these studies was administered using various methods, including baths, drinking, inhalation, and topical treatment for external use. The methods differed based on the health requirements of the postpartum women and the EO that was selected for use. Aromatherapy intervention for 30 minutes in baths relieved discomfort and pain and improved recovery after episiotomy. The effective duration of aromatherapy varied by the EO that was used.

Although we reviewed all of the RCTs that included humans as study participants, this systematic review was affected by methodological limitations. Six electronic databases were searched, and the review was restricted to published articles only. However, it was encouraging that the RCTs were available for review and that the methodological quality of the included trials was high. Another limitation is the small number of countries in which the included studies were conducted. Most were conducted in Iran. This may be because of two reasons: (a) Aromatherapy is an accessible and convenient method for improving health in Iran (Akbari et al., 2014; Behmanesh et al., 2011; Hadi & Hanid, 2011; Keshavarz Afshar et al., 2015; Kianpour et al., 2016; Mirghafourvand, Mohammad-Alizadeh-Charandabi, Hakimi, Khodaie, & Galeshi, 2016, 2017; Olapour et al., 2013; Sayyah Melli et al., 2007; Sharifipour et al., 2015; Sheikhan et al., 2012; Vakilian et al., 2011; Vaziri et al., 2017), and (b) only RCTs

that studied human participants were considered. Complementary and alternative therapy is integral to the culture of the Iranian people (Fahimi, Hrgovic, El-Safadi, & Münstedt, 2011), and aromatherapy is one of the most widely used types of complementary and alternative therapies (Lis-Balchin, 1999). Moreover, the large majority of studies that were conducted outside Iran were not RCTs. For instance, one study used a nonequivalent control group pretest–posttest design to examine the effects of EOs on labor stress, labor anxiety, and postpartum anxiety in Korea (Hur, Cheong, Yun, Lee, & Song, 2005). Another used a quasi-experimental between-groups design to investigate the effects of aromatherapy massage on psychological health in postpartum women in Japan (Imura, Misao, & Ushijima, 2006).

Because of the nature of aromatherapy intervention, it may be difficult to conduct single-, double-, and triple-blinded studies. However, eight of the included studies attempted to blind the outcome assessors to minimize potential methodological bias (Behmanesh et al., 2011; Dale & Cornwell, 1994; Hadi & Hanid, 2011; Mirghafourvand et al., 2016, 2017; Olapour et al., 2013; Vakilian et al., 2011; Vaziri et al., 2017). Moreover, because the other seven included studies were not blinded (Akbari et al., 2014; Keshavarz Afshar et al., 2015; Kianpour et al., 2016; Lane et al., 2012; Sayyah Melli et al., 2007; Sharifipour et al., 2015; Sheikhan et al., 2012), bias may have occurred and influenced the study results. To supply further evidence in support of aromatherapy as a valid therapy in postpartum women, studies with rigorous blinding procedures should be conducted. Additional systematic review studies evaluating more RCTs should be conducted to better understand the impact of aromatherapy on postpartum women.

Furthermore, three studies described the adverse effects of applying aromatherapy interventions that use lavender (Dale & Cornwell, 1994; Hadi & Hanid, 2011; Vakilian et al., 2011). An RCT involving 120 subjects evaluated postepisiotomy healing in a lavender EO treatment group and a povidone–iodine sitz bath group, which both received treatment twice a day for 10 days, and found no significant difference between the two groups in terms of pain intensity, edema, leaved suture, and dehiscence and a significant difference in terms of redness. No side effects were found with the exception of slight irritation in two of the studies (Vakilian et al., 2011). Two studies reported side effects (dizziness and increased urination) associated with applying aromatherapy using orange peel EO. A glass of water with 10 drops of orange peel EO was consumed three times a day for 8 weeks by the experimental group, with significantly lower levels of dizziness and urination reported in the control group, which received routine care (Mirghafourvand et al., 2016, 2017). One study revealed no side effects in the *Citrus aurantium* essence oil group (Sharifipour et al., 2015), whereas the other nine studies did not describe adverse effects (Akbari et al., 2014; Behmanesh et al., 2011; Keshavarz Afshar et al., 2015; Kianpour et al., 2016; Lane et al., 2012; Olapour et al., 2013; Sayyah Melli et al., 2007; Sheikhan et al., 2012; Vaziri et al., 2017). According to the findings of this systematic review regarding side effects, lavender and *Citrus aurantium* aromatherapies are likely safe applications for postpartum women.

Conclusions

The number of RCTs in the literature evaluating the effects of aromatherapy on postpartum women has increased in recent years. The articles included in this systematic review addressed the effectiveness of aromatherapy on the physiological and psychological health of subjects in terms of nipple fissures, episiotomy, CS delivery, sleep, mood, stress, anxiety, distress, and depression. The methods used to measure this effectiveness included the VAS; Amir Scale; REEDA; Pittsburgh Sleep Quality Index; DASS-21; Edinburgh Stress, Anxiety, and Depression Scale; Ordinal Nausea Scale; Edinburgh Postnatal Depression Questionnaire; Pain Rating Scale; and Positive and Negative Affect Schedule. The interventions used included bathing, inhalation, drinking, and swabbing.

Aromatherapy may be considered for women during the postpartum period. Lavender was found to be the most widely applied intervention. Few of the included studies examined specific health effects with, for example, only one article examining effects on fatigue. Thus, there may be insufficient clinical evidence to support the practical application of these aromatherapies on postpartum women. Further studies using larger samples and better quality in terms of methodology and end points are necessary to build on current findings.

Acknowledgments

The authors thank the College of Nursing, Kaohsiung Medical University, for providing access to online databases for searching.

Author Contributions

Study conception and design: SST
Data collection: All authors
Data analysis and interpretation: All authors
Drafting of the article: SST
Critical revision of the article: SST, HHW

References

Ahmed, E. M. S., Mohamed, H. A. E. F., & Abu-Talib, Y. M. (2015). Evidence based guideline using to alleviate traumatic nipple among nursing mothers. *World Journal of Nursing Sciences*, *1*(3), 35–44. https://doi.org/10.5829/idosi.wjns.2015.1.3.93201

Akbari, S. A., Alamolhoda, S. H., Baghban, A. A., & Mirabi, P. (2014). Effects of menthol essence and breast milk on the improvement of nipple fissures in breastfeeding women. *Journal of Research in Medical Sciences*, *19*(7), 629–633.

Ali, B., Al-Wabel, N. A., Shams, S., Ahamad, A., Khan, S. A., & Anwar, F. (2015). Essential oils used in aromatherapy: A systemic review. *Asian Pacific Journal of Tropical Biomedicine*, *5*(8), 601–611. https://doi.org/10.1016/j.apjtb.2015.05.007

Behmanesh, F., Tofighi, M., Delavar, M. A., Zeinalzadeh, M., Moghadamnia, A. A., & Khafri, S. (2011). A clinical trial to compare the effectiveness of lavender essential oil and olive oil at healing postpartum mother's perinea. *HealthMED*, *5*(6), 1512–1516.

Buckle, J. (2011). *Clinical aromatherapy essential oils in practice, 2nd ed.* (T. Y. Hung, Trans.). Taipei City, Taiwan, ROC: Elsevier. (Original work published 2003)

Chang, P. J. (2014). *Application and practice of aroma therapy*. Taipei City, Taiwan, ROC: Open Learning Culture. (Original work published in Chinese)

Dale, A., & Cornwell, S. (1994). The role of lavender oil in relieving perineal discomfort following childbirth: A blind randomized clinical trial. *Journal of Advanced Nursing*, *19*(1), 89–96. https://doi.org/10.1111/j.1365-2648.1994.tb01056.x

Dimitriou, V., Mavridou, P., Manataki, A., & Damigos, D. (2017). The use of aromatherapy for postoperative pain management: A systematic review of randomized controlled trials. *Journal of Perianesthesia Nursing*, *32*(6), 530–541. https://doi.org/10.1016/j.jopan.2016.12.003

Dunning, T. (2013). Aromatherapy: Overview, safety and quality issues. *OA Alternative Medicine*, *1*(1), 1–6. https://doi.org/10.13172/2052-7845-1-1-518

Fahimi, F., Hrgovic, I., El-Safadi, S., & Münstedt, K. (2011). Complementary and alternative medicine in obstetrics: A survey from Iran. *Archives of Gynecology and Obstetrics*, *284*(2), 361–364. https://doi.org/10.1007/s00404-010-1641-8

Gattefosse, R. M. (1993). *Gattefosse's aromatherapy*. Essex, England: CW Daniel.

Gnatta, J. R., Kurebayashi, L. F. S., Turrini, R. N. T., & Silva, M. J. P. (2016). Aromatherapy and nursing: Historical and theoretical conception. *Revista da Escola de Enfermagem da USP*, *50*(1), 130–136. https://doi.org/10.1590/S0080-623420160000100017

Hadi, N., & Hanid, A. A. (2011). Lavender essence for post-cesarean pain. *Pakistan Journal of Biological Sciences*, *14*(11), 664–667. https://doi.org/10.3923/pjbs.2011.664.667

Hur, M. H., Cheong, N. Y., Yun, H. S., Lee, M. K., & Song, Y. (2005). Effects of delivery nursing care using essential oils on delivery stress response, anxiety during labor, and postpartum status anxiety. *Journal of Korean Academy of Nursing*, *35*(7), 1277–1284. https://doi.org/10.4040/jkan.2005.35.7.1277

Imura, M., Misao, H., & Ushijima, H. (2006). The psychological effects of aromatherapy-massage in healthy postpartum mothers. *Journal of Midwifery and Women's Health*, *51*(2), e21–e27. https://doi.org/10.1016/j.jmwh.2005.08.009

Keshavarz Afshar, M., Behboodi Moghadam, Z., Taghizadeh, Z., Bekhradi, R., Montazeri, A., & Mokhtari, P. (2015). Lavender fragrance essential oil and the quality of sleep in postpartum women. *Iranian Red Crescent Medical Journal*, *17*(4), e25880. https://doi.org/10.5812/ircmj.17(4)2015.25880

Kianpour, M., Mansouri, A., Mehrabi, T., & Asghari, G. (2016). Effect of lavender scent inhalation on prevention of stress, anxiety and depression in the postpartum period. *Iranian Journal of Nursing and Midwifery Research, 21*(2), 197–201. https://doi.org/10.4103/1735-9066.178248

Lane, B., Cannella, K., Bowen, C., Copelan, D., Nteff, G., Barnes, K., ... Lawson, J. (2012). Examination of the effectiveness of peppermint aromatherapy on nausea in women post C-section. *Journal of Holistic Nursing, 30*(2), 90–104; quiz 105–106. https://doi.org/10.1177/0898010111423419

Lis-Balchin, M. (1999). Possible health and safety problems in the use of novel plant essential oils and extracts in aromatherapy. *Journal of the Royal Society for the Promotion of Health, 119*(4), 240–243. https://doi.org/10.1177/146642409911900407

Masoumi, Z., Keramat, A., & Hajiaghaee, R. (2011). Systemic review on effect of herbal medicine on pain after perineal episiotomy and cesarean cutting. *Journal of Medicinal Plants, 4*(40), 1–16.

Mirghafourvand, M., Mohammad-Alizadeh-Charandabi, S., Hakimi, S., Khodaie, L., & Galeshi, M. (2016). Effect of orange peel essential oil on postpartum sleep quality: A randomized controlled clinical trial. *European Journal of Integrative Medicine, 8*(1), 62–66. https://doi.org/10.1016/j.eujim.2015.07.044

Mirghafourvand, M., Mohammad-Alizadeh-Charandabi, S., Hakimi, S., Khodaie, L., & Galeshi, M. (2017). The effect of orange peel essential oil on postpartum depression and anxiety: A randomized controlled clinical trial. *Iranian Red Crescent Medical Journal, 19*(2), e30298. https://doi.org/10.5812/ircmj.30298

Moher, D., Liberati, A., Tetzlaff, J., Altman, D. G., & The PRISMA Group. (2009). Preferred reporting items for systematic reviews and meta-analyses: The PRISMA statement. *PLoS Medicine, 6*(7), e1000097. https://doi.org/10.1371/journal.pmed.1000097

Olapour, A., Behaeen, K., Akhondzadeh, R., Soltani, F., al Sadat Razavi, F., & Bekhradi, R. (2013). The effect of inhalation of aromatherapy blend containing lavender essential oil on cesarean postoperative pain. *Anesthesiology and Pain Medicine, 3*(1), 203–207. https://doi.org/10.5812/aapm.9570

Oremus, M., Wolfson, C., Perrault, A., Demers, L., Momoli, F., & Moride, Y. (2001). Interrater reliability of the modified Jadad quality scale for systematic reviews of Alzheimer's disease drug trials. *Dementia and Geriatric Cognitive Disorders, 12*(3), 232–236. https://doi.org/10.1159/000051263

Robins, J. L. W. (1999). The science and art of aromatherapy. *Journal of Holistic Nursing, 17*(1), 5–17. https://doi.org/10.1177/089801019901700102

Romano, M., Cacciatore, A., Giordano, R., & La Rosa, B. (2010). Postpartum period: Three distinct but continuous phases. *Journal of Prenatal Medicine, 4*(2), 22–25.

Sayyah Melli, M., Rashidi, M. R., Delazar, A., Madarek, E., Kargar Maher, M. H., Ghasemzadeh, A., ... Tahmasebi, Z. (2007). Effect of peppermint water on prevention of nipple cracks in lactating primiparous women: A randomized controlled trial. *International Breastfeeding Journal, 2*, 7. https://doi.org/10.1186/1746-4358-2-7

Sharifipour, F., Bakhteh, A., & Mirmohammad, A. (2015). Effects of Citrus aurantium aroma on post-cesarean anxiety (in Persian). *Iranian Journal of Obstetrics, Gynecology and Infertility, 18*(169), 12–20.

Sheikhan, F., Jahdi, F., Khoei, E. M., Shamsalizadeh, N., Sheikhan, M., & Haghani, H. (2012). Episiotomy pain relief: Use of lavender oil essence in primiparous Iranian women. *Complementary Therapies in Clinical Practice, 18*(1), 66–70. https://doi.org/10.1016/j.ctcp.2011.02.003

Sun, J. C. (2016). Nursing care of puerperium period. In Y. M. Yu, (Ed.), *Maternal–newborn nursing* (8th ed., pp. 360–419). New Taipei City, Taiwan, ROC: New Wun Ching. (Original work published in Chinese)

Vakilian, K., Atarha, M., Bekhradi, R., & Chaman, R. (2011). Healing advantages of lavender essential oil during episiotomy recovery: A clinical trial. *Complementary Therapies in Clinical Practice, 17*(1), 50–53. https://doi.org/10.1016/j.ctcp.2010.05.006

Vaziri, F., Shiravani, M., Najib, F. S., Pourahmad, S., Salehi, A., & Yazdanpanahi, Z. (2017). Effect of lavender oil aroma in the early hours of postpartum period on maternal pains, fatigue, and mood: A randomized clinical trial. *International Journal of Preventive Medicine, 8*, 29. https://doi.org/10.4103/ijpvm.IJPVM_137_16

World Health Organization. (2014). *WHO recommendations on postnatal care of the mother and newborn*. Retrieved from http://www.who.int/iris/handle/10665/97603

15

Effect of a Breathing Exercise on Respiratory Function and 6-Minute Walking Distance in Patients Under Hemodialysis

Tajmohammad ARAZI[1] • Mansooreh ALIASGHARPOUR[2] • Sepideh MOHAMMADI[3]* •
Nooredin MOHAMMADI[4] • Anoushirvan KAZEMNEJAD[5]

ABSTRACT

Background: Pulmonary disorders and poor functional capacity are common complications in patients under hemodialysis. Although breathing exercise is frequently prescribed to improve respiratory function, its efficacy in this patient community is not well established.

Purpose: Our study was designed to determine the effectiveness of a breathing exercise on respiratory function and 6-minute walk (6MW) distance in patients under hemodialysis.

Methods: A randomized controlled trial approach was used. The sample consisted of 52 patients under hemodialysis from a university teaching hospital in Iran. The experimental group (n = 26) received the breathing exercise program and was encouraged to perform incentive spirometry for 2 months. The control group (n = 26) received only routine hospital care. The respiratory function test and 6MW test were performed at baseline and at 2 months after the intervention (posttest).

Results: The two groups were homogeneous in terms of respiratory function parameters, 6MW distance, and demographic characteristics at baseline. Forced expiratory volume in 1 second and forced vital capacity were significantly better in the experimental group compared with the control group at 2 months after intervention. No significant difference was found in 6MW distance between the groups at the 2-month posttest.

Conclusions/Implications for Practice: The 2-month breathing exercise effectively improved pulmonary function parameters (forced vital capacity, forced expiratory volume in 1 second) in patients under hemodialysis but did not affect 6MW distance. Hemodialysis nurses should strengthen their clinical health education and apply breathing exercise programs to reduce the pulmonary complications experienced by patients under hemodialysis.

KEY WORDS:
hemodialysis, respiratory function tests, breathing exercise, incentive spirometry, six-minute walk test.

Introduction

Chronic kidney disease (CKD), an increasing concern worldwide, is characterized by irreversible destruction of nephrons (De Nicola & Zoccali, 2016; Lin et al., 2013). CKD is a complicated and progressive disorder that affects most important organ systems, including the cardiovascular, musculoskeletal, metabolic, and respiratory systems (Webster et al., 2017). Pulmonary complications are important and prevalent disorders in patients with CKD, with prominent complications including pleural effusion, pulmonary edema, pulmonary hypertension, and acute respiratory distress syndrome (Hsieh et al., 2016; Palamidas et al., 2014). Hemodialysis is the most common method used to treat kidney failure in patients with CKD (de Almeida et al., 2019). Although hemodialysis reduces some CKD complications, impaired pulmonary function is a prevalent complication that leads to severe problems in patients under hemodialysis (Cho et al., 2018; Unal et al., 2010). Pulmonary disorders in these patients may be the result of fluid overload, high blood pressure, permeability of the capillaries, or circulating uremic toxins (Yılmaz et al., 2016). Respiratory disorders are common complications among Iranian patients under hemodialysis, and a high prevalence of pulmonary hypertension has been shown in this population (Mousavi et al., 2008). Breathing exercises are frequently a

[1]MSN, Nursing Educator, Department of Nursing and Operating Room, Neyshabur University of Medical Sciences, Neyshabur, Iran • [2]MSN, Nursing Educator, Faculty of Nursing and Midwifery, Department of Medical Surgical Nursing, Tehran University of Medical Sciences, Tehran, Iran • [3]PhD, Assistant Professor, Department of Nursing, Nursing Care Research Center, Health Research Institute, Babol University of Medical Sciences, Babol, Iran • [4]PhD, Associate Professor, Department of Nursing, School of Nursing and Midwifery, Iran University of Medical Sciences, Tehran, Iran • [5]PhD, Professor, Department of Biostatistics, School of Medicine, Tarbiat Modares University, Tehran, Iran.

convenient and simple strategy to improve lung efficiency, and the incentive spirometer (IS) is a device that is widely used in these exercises (Alaparthi et al., 2016). IS works to expand the user's lungs by allowing deeper breathing and is used to help patients improve lung functioning (Restrepo et al., 2011). Although medical evidence indicates that IS device may be useful in preventing pulmonary complications, the degree of benefit in different populations such as patients under hemodialysis, patients undergoing coronary artery bypass graft surgery, and patients with lung cancer is uncertain, and there are significant discrepancies among physicians in terms of the medical efficacy of using IS (Haeffener et al., 2008; Liu et al., 2019; Silva et al., 2011). Moreover, patients with CKD experience reduced physical performance, and studies have shown that patients under hemodialysis experience significantly lower physical functional capacity, as evaluated by the 6-minute walk (6MW) test, than their healthy adult peers (Bučar Pajek et al., 2016). Pulmonary complication is one of the reasons that patients under hemodialysis experience poor functional exercise capacities (Smith & Burton, 2012). The 6MW test is a well-tolerated submaximal exercise test that aids in the assessment of functional capacity and provides valuable information about physical performance and response to therapy in cases of chronic cardiopulmonary disease such as chronic pulmonary hypertension (Ghofraniha et al., 2015). Therefore, this study was designed to determine the effectiveness of a breathing exercise on respiratory function and 6MW distance in patients under hemodialysis.

Methods

Design

This study used a randomized, nonblinded controlled trial approach with two groups (experimental and control).

Setting and Participant

This study was conducted at Shahid Hasheminejad Kidney Center, which is the national referral center for urology and nephrology in Iran. The participants were patients undergoing hemodialysis in the dialysis ward. Data were collected from November 2018 to March 2019. Study inclusion criteria included (a) ≥18 years old; (b) forced vital capacity (FVC) and forced expiratory volume in 1 second (FEV_1) values at least 15% below the normal ranges, based on age and height; (c) having normal thoracic and vertebral column and legs; (d) being able to perform the breathing exercise and the 6MW test; (e) currently receiving hemodialysis three times a week; and (f) under hemodialysis for at least 6 months. Otherwise eligible patients were excluded from this study if they had an acute respiratory disease or respiratory infections during the study period or if they were unable or unwilling to participate.

Sampling

This study followed a similar study (Haeffener et al., 2008) in targeting 99% power and 95% confidence interval and aiming to find a minimum 4% difference in FVC and FEV_1 among the two groups. Thus, a minimum of 17 patients was required in each group. Fifty-two patients (26 per group) participated in the study, accounting for a possible sample loss up to 50%.

One hundred eighty patients visited the target hospital for hemodialysis three times per week. Of these, 87 visited the hospital on even-numbered days of the week, and 93 visited the hospital on odd-numbered days of the week. Cluster randomization was initially advocated to minimize treatment contamination between the two groups. Days of the week were randomly assigned to the experimental (even-numbered days) and control (odd-numbered days) arms by flipping a coin. Subsequently, 87 patients in the even-day pool and 93 patients in the odd-day pool were assessed for eligibility. Thirty-four and 32 patients, respectively, in the two pools failed to meet the inclusion criteria and were excluded from the randomization list. Finally, 26 eligible patients in each cluster ($n = 53$ in the experimental arm and $n = 61$ in the control arm) were assigned randomly to the study by a random number generator application. All 52 patients (26 per group) completed the study program, and all completed the posttest questionnaire at 2 months after program completion (Figure 1).

Intervention

The experimental group received the breathing exercise program in addition to routine hospital care. The breathing exercise program included use of the IS device. The experimental group participants were instructed in how to use the IS and were asked to (a) "hold the IS in an upright position"; (b) "put the mouthpiece spirometer in your mouth"; (c) "after quiet expiration, inhale deeply and slowly"; (d) "hold your breath for as long as possible and then exhale normally"; and (e) "repeat each of these steps 10 times every hour after you wake up for a period of 2 months." The researcher provided each patient with one IS device and an associated pictorial educational booklet. All of the IS devices used in this study were similar and of the same brand. Compliance with the breathing exercise was assessed via telephone calls every week. All of the participants in the experimental group adhered to the breathing exercise program, and no complaints were reported by these participants regarding using the IS device. The remaining 26 patients (control group) received only routine hospital care, which included connecting the patient to the hemodialysis machine, performing weight control, and providing education on fluid imbalance, hypertension, nutritional diet, and the prevention of hemodialysis complications such as muscle cramps and peripheral edema.

Outcome Measures

Respiratory function parameters and 6MW distance, assessed using the FVC and FEV_1 test and the 6MW test, were the primary end point measures used in this study. The respiratory function tests, including the FVC, FEV1, and 6MW tests, were performed in both groups at baseline as well as 2

Figure 1
Study Design Flowchart

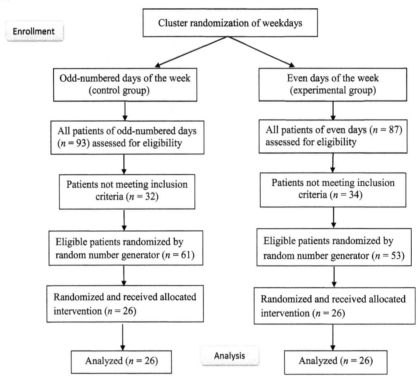

months after study enrollment. One standard spirometer model (model: Flowhandy ZAN Type 3.1) was used during the study. The reliability of this spirometer was assessed using the test–retest method. To assess reliability, the respiratory function test was measured in 15 subjects twice within 5 minutes under the same conditions. The obtained correlation coefficient was 95%.

The 6MW test was performed in accordance with the comprehensive guidelines developed by the American Thoracic Society (ATS Committee on Proficiency Standards for Clinical Pulmonary Function Laboratories, 2002). All of the participants performed the 6MW test along a 30-meter-long, flat and comfortable surface in the hospital (marked with meter tacks). They were instructed to (a) wear comfortable shoes and clothes, (b) rest for 10 minutes before doing the test (during which time heart rate and blood pressure were measured and potential contraindications were assessed by the researcher), and (c) walk for 6 minutes. All necessary information was given to the participants, including walking speed, stop time, and advice regarding potential adverse feelings such as fatigue, cramps, chest pain, and dyspnea. The supervisor used standard phrases of encouragement (e.g., you are doing fine) recommended by the American Thoracic Society.

Data Analysis

The SPSS Version 16.0 (SPSS, Inc., Chicago, IL, USA) was used to examine the data. Descriptive statistics such as mean, standard deviation, and percentage were used to describe the

baseline characteristics of the patients. Statistical analyses to identify the differences among the groups included unpaired t tests and chi-square test.

Ethical Approval

The ethical research committee of Tehran University of Medical Sciences reviewed and approved this study (approval number: 91-02-28-18230), and the study was registered in the Iranian Registry of Clinical Trials under Registration Code IRCT2012080522226N10. All of the participants provided informed consent and were assured that their participation was voluntary and that their data would be anonymized and kept confidential. Furthermore, the participants were informed that they could withdraw from the study at any time without any negative impact to their regular treatment.

Results

Experimental and control group demographic characteristics are compared in Table 1. This study found no significant differences in baseline characteristics between the groups. Most of the participants in both groups were middle-aged women. No significant intergroup differences were found in terms of gender ($p = .57$), age ($p = .08$), weight ($p = .68$), or time since diagnosis ($p = .59$).

Respiratory function tests and 6MW distance were compared between the two groups at baseline, with results

Table 1

Baseline Characteristics of the Research Sample

Parameter	Experimental Group (n = 26)			Control Group (n = 26)			χ^2/t	p
	n (%)	M	SD	n (%)	M	SD		
Gender							0.31	.57
Male	12 (46.2)			10 (38.5)				
Female	14 (53.8)			16 (61.5)				
Age (years)		45.76	2.11		48.12	3.01	1.76	.08
Weight (kg)		67.65	3.17		70.14	2.96	4.03	.68
Height (cm)		165.00	1.89		168.00	4.78	0.67	.59

shown in Table 2. No significant intergroup difference was found at baseline in terms of FEV_1 ($p = .54$), FVC ($p = .33$), and 6MW distance ($p = .68$). At the 2-month posttest, the experimental group earned significantly better values in terms of FEV_1 ($p = .02$) and FVC ($p = .04$) than the control group. However, no significant intergroup difference was found in terms of 6MW distance at the 2-month posttest ($p = .43$; Table 2).

Discussion

This study investigated the efficacy of a breathing exercise on respiratory function and 6MW distance in patients under hemodialysis. Although the use of IS as a breathing exercise has increased in recent years and IS is now frequently prescribed to improve respiratory function, there is limited evidence supporting its benefits. Moreover, no clear evidence establishing the effectiveness of IS in improving respiratory function and functional capacity in patients under hemodialysis has been published (Eltorai et al., 2018).

In this study of patients under hemodialysis, the data analysis showed a positive effect of using IS on respiratory function test results (FVC, FEV_1). These findings are congruent with the finding of a previous study that practicing a breathing exercise with IS (IS training for 2 months, three sessions per week) improved diaphragmatic excursion in patients under hemodialysis (Mansour et al., 2018). In addition, a systematic review showed that inspiratory muscle training with a load ranging from 30% to 60% of the maximal inspiratory pressure and lasting from 2 to 6 months has the potential to improve respiratory muscle strength, functional capacity, and lung function in patients with CKD (de Medeiros et al., 2017). Despite the above, some studies have recommended against adding IS to the common standard of treatment (Tyson et al., 2015). Martin et al. cited patients' nonadherence to IS protocols as an important factor behind patients failing to achieve the positive effect of IS. They mentioned that patient perspectives on the potential benefits of IS, multimedia patient education, and previous use of the device may improve the rate of correct IS usage and increase compliance during IS implementation (Martin et al., 2018). Analysis of a systematic review study (Narayanan et al., 2016) revealed an inconsistency in the evidence related to IS compliance. Therefore, comprehensive research in these areas is needed to help obtain valid inferences regarding the effectiveness of using IS.

Table 2

Comparison of Outcomes Between the Experimental and Control Groups at Baseline and at 2 Months After the Intervention (Posttest)

Time	Experimental Group (n = 26)		Control Group (n = 26)		t	p
	M	SD	M	SD		
Baseline						
FEV_1 (L)	2.12	0.54	2.04	0.39	0.60	.54
FVC (L)	2.81	0.58	2.66	0.53	0.97	.33
6MW distance (meters)	349.00	57.55	359.88	65.04	−0.63	.68
2 months after intervention						
FEV_1 (L)	2.31	0.48	2.03	0.40	2.28	.03*
FVC (L)	2.98	0.61	2.66	0.53	2.04	.05*
6MW distance (meters)	359.65	54.75	360.65	67.26	−0.05	.43

Note. FEV_1 = forced expiratory volume in 1 second; FVC = forced vital capacity; MW = minute walk; L = liters.
*$p < .05$.

Respiratory disorders are a leading cause of poor exercise capacities in patients under hemodialysis, with these patients experiencing significantly poorer exercise capacities, as evaluated using the 6MW test, than healthy adults (Bučar Pajek et al., 2016; Watanabe et al., 2016). This study was designed to investigate the effect of a breathing exercise on 6MW distance in patients under hemodialysis. Although the mean walking distance of the experimental group had improved by about 10 meters at the 2-month posttest, no significant difference was found between the two groups at the 2-month posttest. The results of this study echo the findings of Aliasgharpour and Hadiyan (2011), which showed that, although the 6MW distance of patients under hemodialysis in the intervention group increased after doing the exercise, the increase did not result in a statistically significant posttest difference between the intervention and control groups. Contrary to our results, Silva et al. (2011) found that inspiratory muscle training for 2 months significantly increased 6MW distance scores in patients under hemodialysis but no did not affect pulmonary function.

In addition to respiratory complications, other factors such as uremic myopathy, anemia, and malnutrition are known to affect the results of the 6MW distance test in patients under hemodialysis. The breathing exercise program did not affect these factors, which may be a reason why the participants in this study exhibited effectively improved pulmonary function parameters but no significant change in 6MW distance.

A review of related articles found inconsistent evidence regarding a positive effect for breathing exercises on functional capacity and endurance as measured using the 6MW test in patients. Further prospective studies should be conducted to evaluate the use of IS in this context and to compare results with respiratory physical therapeutic techniques and other respiratory devices.

Research Limitations

During this study, patient follow-up was conducted by telephone call only (no home visits). To remedy this limitation, this intervention should be repeated using home visits, observational follow-up, or hourly, audible reminders for IS implementation.

Conclusions/Implication for Practice

The findings of the study showed that the use of IS improves pulmonary function parameters (FVC, FEV_1) and does not significantly change 6MW distance. An IS is a convenient and inexpensive breathing exercise device that may easily be used by patients under hemodialysis to improve their respiratory functions.

Hemodialysis nurses spend far more time with patients than other healthcare workers and are responsible for teaching patients about preventing and managing hemodialysis complications. Therefore, teaching breathing exercises to patients under hemodialysis as a safe way to reduce pulmonary

complications may play an important role in improving pulmonary outcomes in these patients.

Acknowledgments

Our research was supported by the Tehran University of Medical Sciences. We would like to thank all of the respectful staff and patients of the Hashemi Nejad Hospital in Tehran who helped us in this study.

Author Contributions

Study conception and design: SM, MA, TA.
Data collection: SM, TA.
Data analysis and interpretation: AK, NM.
Drafting of the article: SM, TA, NM, AK.
Critical revision of the article: SM, TA, NM.

References

Alaparthi, G. K., Augustine, A. J., Anand, R., & Mahale, A. (2016). Comparison of diaphragmatic breathing exercise, volume and flow incentive spirometry, on diaphragm excursion and pulmonary function in patients undergoing laparoscopic surgery: A randomized controlled trial. *Minimally Invasive Surgery, 2016*, Article ID 1967532. https://doi.org/10.1155/2016/1967532

Aliasgharpour, M., & Hadiyan, Z. (2011). Assessment of a designed exercise program on physical capacity using six-minute walking test (6MWT) in hemodialysis patients. *Journal of Hayat, 17*(3), 59–68. (Original work published in Persian)

ATS Committee on Proficiency Standards for Clinical Pulmonary Function Laboratories. (2002). ATS statement: Guidelines for the six-minute walk test. *American Journal of Respiratory and Critical Care Medicine, 166*, 111–117. https://doi.org/10.1164/ajrccm.166.1.at1102

Bučar Pajek, M., Čuk, I., Leskošek, B., Mlinšek, G., Buturović Ponikvar, J., & Pajek, J. (2016). Six-minute walk test in renal failure patients: Representative results, performance analysis and perceived dyspnea predictors. *PLOS ONE, 11*(3), Article ID e0150414. https://doi.org/10.1371/journal.pone.0150414

Cho, M.-K., Kim, S. Y., & Shim, H. Y. (2018). Validity and reliability of the Korean version of the dialysis symptom index for hemodialysis patients. *The Journal of Nursing Research, 26*(6), 399–410. https://doi.org/10.1097/jnr.0000000000000267

de Almeida, C. P., Ponce, D., & Balbi, A. L. (2019). Effect of hemodialysis on respiratory mechanics in acute kidney injury patients. *Hemodialysis International, 23*(1), 101–105. https://doi.org/10.1111/hdi.12684

de Medeiros, A. I. C., Fuzari, H. K. B., Rattesa, C., Brandão, D. C., & de Melo Marinho, P. É. (2017). Inspiratory muscle training improves respiratory muscle strength, functional capacity and quality of life in patients with chronic kidney disease: A systematic review. *Journal of Physiotherapy, 63*(2), 76–83. https://doi.org/10.1016/j.jphys.2017.02.016

De Nicola, L., & Zoccali, C. (2016). Chronic kidney disease prevalence in the general population: Heterogeneity and concerns. *Nephrology, Dialysis, Transplantation, 31*(3), 331–335. https://doi.org/10.1093/ndt/gfv427

Eltorai, A. E. M., Szabo, A. L., Antoci, V. Jr., Ventetuolo, C. E., Elias, J. A., Daniels, A. H., & Hess, D. R. (2018). Clinical effectiveness of incentive spirometry for the prevention of postoperative pulmonary complications. *Respiratory Care, 63*(3), 347–352. https://doi.org/10.4187/respcare.05679

Ghofraniha, L., Dalir Sani, Z., Vakilian, F., Khajedalooyi, M., & Arabshahi, Z. J. (2015). The six-minute walk test (6MWT) for the evaluation of pulmonary diseases. *Journal of Cardio-Thoracic Medicine, 3*(2), 284–287. https://doi.org/10.22038/JCTM.2015.4374

Haeffener, M. P., Ferreira, G. M., Barreto, S. S. M., Arena, R., & Dall'Ago, P. (2008). Incentive spirometry with expiratory positive airway pressure reduces pulmonary complications, improves pulmonary function and 6-minute walk distance in patients undergoing coronary artery bypass graft surgery. *American Heart Journal, 156*(5), 900.e1–900.e8. https://doi.org/10.1016/j.ahj.2008.08.006

Hsieh, C. W., Lee, C. T., Chen, C. C., Hsu, L. P., Hu, H. H., & Wu, J. C. (2016). Pulmonary hypertension in patients on chronic hemodialysis and with heart failure. *Hemodialysis International, 20*(2), 208–217. https://doi.org/10.1111/hdi.12380

Lin, C. C., Chen, M. C., Hsieh, H. F., & Chang, S. C. (2013). Illness representations and coping processes of Taiwanese patients with early-stage chronic kidney disease. *The Journal of Nursing Research, 21*(2), 120–128. https://doi.org/10.1097/jnr.0b013e3182921fb8

Liu, C.-J., Tsai, W.-C., Chu, C.-C., Muo, C.-H., & Chung, W.-S. (2019). Is incentive spirometry beneficial for patients with lung cancer receiving video-assisted thoracic surgery? *BMC Pulmonary Medicine, 19*(1), Article No. 121. https://doi.org/10.1186/s12890-019-0885-8

Mansour, H. S., El-Dein, H. M. E., Mohamed, F. A., & Ahmed, T. F. (2018). Efficacy of incentive spirometer training on diaphragmatic excursion and quality of life in hemodialysis patients. *The Medical Journal of Cairo University, 86*, 3997–4002. https://doi.org/10.21608/MJCU.2018.62195

Martin, T. J., Patel, S. A., Tran, M., Eltorai, A. S., Daniels, A. H., & Eltorai, A. E. M. (2018). Patient factors associated with successful incentive spirometry. *Rhode Island Medical Journal, 101*(9), 14–18.

Mousavi, S. A., Mahdavi-Mazdeh, M., Yahyazadeh, H., Azadi, M., Rahimzadeh, N., Yoosefnejad, H., & Ataiipoor, Y. (2008). Pulmonary hypertension and predisposing factors in patients receiving hemodialysis. *Iranian Journal of Kidney Diseases, 2*(1), 29–33.

Narayanan, A. L., Hamid, S. R., & Supriyanto, E. (2016). Evidence regarding patient compliance with incentive spirometry interventions after cardiac, thoracic and abdominal surgeries: A systematic literature review. *CJRT: Canadian Journal of Respiratory Therapy, 52*(1), 17–26.

Palamidas, A. F., Gennimata, S. A., Karakontaki, F., Kaltsakas, G., Papantoniou, I., Koutsoukou, A., Milic-Emili, J., Vlahakos, D. V., & Koulouris, N. G. (2014). Impact of hemodialysis on dyspnea and lung function in end stage kidney disease patients. *BioMed Research International, 2014*, Article ID 212751. https://doi.org/10.1155/2014/212751

Restrepo, R. D., Wettstein, R., Wittnebel, L., & Tracy, M. (2011). Incentive spirometry: 2011. *Respiratory Care, 56*(10), 1600–1604. https://doi.org/10.4187/respcare.01471

Silva, V. G., Amaral, C., Monteiro, M. B., Nascimento, D. M., & Boschetti, J. R. (2011). Effects of inspiratory muscle training in hemodialysis patients. *Brazilian Journal of Nephrology (Jornal Brasileiro de Nefrologia), 33*(1), 62–68.

Smith, A. C., & Burton, J. O. (2012). Exercise in kidney disease and diabetes: Time for action. *Journal of Renal Care, 38*(1, Suppl.), 52–58. https://doi.org/10.1111/j.1755-6686.2012.00279.x

Tyson, A. F., Kendig, C. E., Mabedi, C., Cairns, B. A., & Charles, A. G. (2015). The effect of incentive spirometry on postoperative pulmonary function following laparotomy: A randomized clinical trial. *JAMA Surgery, 150*(3), 229–236. https://doi.org/10.1001/jamasurg.2014.1846

Unal, A., Tasdemir, K., Oymak, S., Duran, M., Kocyigit, I., Oguz, F., Tokgoz, B., Sipahioglu, M. H., Utas, C., & Oymak, O. (2010). The long-term effects of arteriovenous fistula creation on the development of pulmonary hypertension in hemodialysis patients. *Hemodialysis International, 14*(4), 398–402. https://doi.org/10.1111/j.1542-4758.2010.00478.x

Watanabe, F. T., Koch, V. H., Juliani, R. C., & Cunha, M. T. (2016). Six-minute walk test in children and adolescents with renal diseases: Tolerance, reproducibility and comparison with healthy subjects. *Clinics (Sao Paulo), 71*(1), 22–27. https://doi.org/10.6061/clinics/2016(01)05

Webster, A. C., Nagler, E. V., Morton, R. L., & Masson, P. (2017). Chronic kidney disease. *The Lancet, 389*(10075), 1238–1252. https://doi.org/10.1016/S0140-6736(16)32064-5

Yılmaz, S., Yildirim, Y., Yilmaz, Z., Kara, A. V., Taylan, M., Demir, M., Coskunsel, M., Kadiroglu, A. K., & Yilmaz, M. E. (2016). Pulmonary function in patients with end-stage renal disease: Effects of hemodialysis and fluid overload. *Medical Science Monitor, 22*, 2779–2784. https://doi.org/10.12659/MSM.897480

16

Development and Evaluation of a Teamwork Improvement Program for Perioperative Patient Safety

Shinae AHN[1] • Nam-Ju LEE[2]*

ABSTRACT

Background: Effective teamwork in healthcare teams improves quality of care, which positively impacts on patient safety. Teamwork is especially crucial for perioperative nurses because they provide care as a team in the operating room. Previous research on teamwork training has principally addressed the general aspects of healthcare settings and focused on interdisciplinary teamwork and has rarely considered operative settings and nursing teamwork.

Purpose: The aim of this study was to develop a teamwork improvement program for perioperative patient safety and to evaluate the effectiveness of this program.

Methods: A quasi-experimental design was applied. We developed a teamwork improvement program based on teamwork competencies that focused on the perioperative nursing practice. This research was conducted at two operating centers in a tertiary hospital in South Korea, and a total of 60 perioperative nurses participated, including 28 nurses from the cancer operating center (experimental group) and 32 nurses from the main operating center (control group). The program consisted of four sessions and was delivered to the experimental group for a period of 2 weeks. Following the intervention, the effectiveness of the intervention was measured using a self-report questionnaire, focus group interviews, and program evaluation survey. Data were analyzed using chi-square test, t test, Fisher's exact test, and content analysis.

Results: Nearly all (96.4%) of the participants were satisfied with the overall content of the teamwork improvement program. Statistically significant differences were found between the experimental and control groups with regard to teamwork knowledge, teamwork attitudes, communication self-efficacy, and teamwork skills and behaviors. Three themes were elicited from the qualitative analysis, including "recognizing the importance and content of teamwork," "improving teamwork competencies," and "contributing to safe surgery." No significant difference in the incidence of surgical nursing errors was identified between the experimental and control groups within a 4-week period.

Conclusions/Implications for Practice: The teamwork improvement program developed in this study was demonstrated as effective in improving perioperative nurses' utilization of teamwork competencies in nursing practice and positively changing teamwork. The findings of this study provide evidence that teamwork training increases nurses' teamwork competencies. The clinical application of teamwork tools using competency-based teamwork training may contribute to patient safety and safe nursing practice.

KEY WORDS:
teamwork, nursing team, program development, patient safety, operating rooms.

Introduction

Teamwork has been emphasized as essential to improving quality and safety in the healthcare delivery system. Teamwork has been defined as a dynamic interaction among healthcare providers that is aimed toward a common goal and refers to a set of interrelated knowledge, attitudes, and skills (Agency for Healthcare Research and Quality [AHRQ], 2019). Various types of healthcare providers work together to provide patient care within the complexity of healthcare systems (World Health Organization [WHO], 2011). Healthcare providers perform interdependent tasks but are rarely trained together (King et al., 2008). From this perspective, ensuring safe care is often difficult unless teamwork and effective communication exist among healthcare providers. Therefore, it is necessary to provide a strategy that strengthens teamwork to enhance patient safety.

Effective teamwork has been recognized as critical to preventing medical errors in the care process (WHO, 2011). A meta-analysis study has demonstrated that improving teamwork competency through team training in healthcare saves patient lives (Hughes et al., 2016). In addition, teamwork has been proposed in previous studies as affecting job performance positively in relation to patient safety and patient outcomes. Improving teamwork among nursing staff has been reported to

[1]PhD, RN, Assistant Professor, Department of Nursing, Wonkwang University, Jeonbuk, Republic of Korea. • [2]PhD, RN, Professor, College of Nursing, The Research Institute of Nursing Science, Seoul National University, Seoul, Republic of Korea.

reduce patients' fall rate (Kalisch et al., 2007), increase nurses' performance of missed care (Kalisch & Lee, 2010), and result in better error reporting (Hwang & Ahn, 2015). As nursing teams comprise the largest human resource in hospitals, improving teamwork competency in nurses may have financial and quality-of-care impacts across the healthcare sector (Barton et al., 2018).

Patient safety involves minimizing the incidence and impact of adverse events while maximizing recovery from these events (WHO, 2011). Patient safety competency consists of knowledge, skills, and attitudes toward patient safety (Cronenwett et al., 2007; WHO, 2011). To achieve patient safety and quality improvement goals, several international organizations have included teamwork competencies within core patient safety competencies (AHRQ, 2019; Australian Commission on Safety and Quality in Health Care, 2005; Canadian Patient Safety Institute, 2008; WHO, 2011). To ensure that nurses are competent in patient safety, education on patient safety in the nursing curriculum is required. However, because nurses receive little or no formal patient safety education in the university curriculum (Barton et al., 2018; Hwang, 2015), they may not be able to cope with patient safety issues adequately. Among patient safety competencies, nurses have demonstrated the lowest scores on teamwork competencies (Hwang, 2015). Therefore, the first step toward ensuring patient safety and quality in healthcare is to provide an education program that emphasizes teamwork competency.

Teamwork training enables healthcare providers to optimize their teamwork competencies with the teamwork knowledge, attitudes, and skills needed to become effective team members (Sherwood & Barnsteiner, 2017). The teamwork improvement program (TIP), Team Strategies and Tools to Enhance Performance and Patient Safety (TeamSTEPPS) has been applied in various healthcare settings and has proven to be effective by using an evidence-based team training method developed for improving patient safety by enhancing both communications among healthcare professionals and teamwork competencies (Cooke, 2016; Gaston et al., 2016; Parker et al., 2019).

Nurses play an important role as part of the multidisciplinary team while providing 24-hour care for patients and interaction with them. Because nurses conduct their clinical practice based on cooperation and collaboration with other nurses (Kaiser & Westers, 2018), teamwork is a critical element in effective nursing practice. Particularly, of the patient care departments in the hospital, the operating room (OR) is one of the most intricate and high-risk environments (Sonoda et al., 2018), where healthcare is provided by a temporary interprofessional team and often performed using invasive treatments under anesthesia. Teamwork between nurses in the OR is especially important because two nurses work closely as a team performing the roles of scrub nurse and circulating nurse in each operation. While participating in the operation, the perioperative nurse cannot perform tasks such as counting, timeout, supplying of aseptic surgical materials, and coping with emergency situations as an individual nurse. Therefore, perioperative nurses are required to have teamwork competencies to minimize incidents during surgery.

To provide the best surgical nursing care to patients, nursing team members must communicate effectively and coordinate properly (Sonoda et al., 2018). Thus, applying a TIP that focuses on the nursing team in the OR environment and educating nurses to understand how to apply teamwork strategies in the clinical context of their specialty settings are necessary. To successfully apply these teamwork programs in specific clinical settings, it is important to include adequate materials and resources relevant to the department in the program design (Clapper & Ng, 2013) or to develop a customized program for the target area (Vertino, 2014). The TeamSTEPPS program has been applied in several intervention studies in the OR (Dahl et al., 2017; S.-H. Lee et al., 2021) for interprofessional teams, including nursing, surgical, and anesthesia staff. However, few studies have focused on the implementation of this program within the nursing team in the OR.

Therefore, in this study, we developed a TIP for perioperative patient safety and evaluated the effectiveness and satisfaction of this program in the context of perioperative nurses.

Methods

Study Design

In this study, a quasi-experimental research design was used to evaluate the effectiveness of the developed program.

Setting and Sample

This study was conducted at one tertiary hospital in South Korea. Participants were recruited using a convenience sampling method from two operating centers (cancer operating center, main operating center), which shared a similar safety culture, unit organization, nursing staffing level, and working conditions. The inclusion criteria were (a) > 6 months of clinical experience as a perioperative staff nurse and (b) understood the purpose of the study and agreed to participate. The nurses working in the cancer operating center were assigned to the experimental group, and the nurses working in the main operating center were assigned to the control group. The groups were located at separate centers to minimize treatment diffusion.

We calculated the appropriate sample size using G*Power 3.1 (Faul et al., 2009) by specifying an effect size of 0.5, a power of .7, and a probability of alpha error of .05 for a paired t test. The required sample size was 27 in each group. A sample of 63 perioperative nurses agreed to participate, and 60 nurses actually participated.

Program Development

The process used to develop the TIP consisted of four steps (Figure 1). In the first step, the researchers identified teamwork competencies using a literature review on patient safety competencies and then combined these competencies with team-based competencies that are specifically required of perioperative nurses (Australian Commission on Safety and

Figure 1

Stages of program development and evaluation

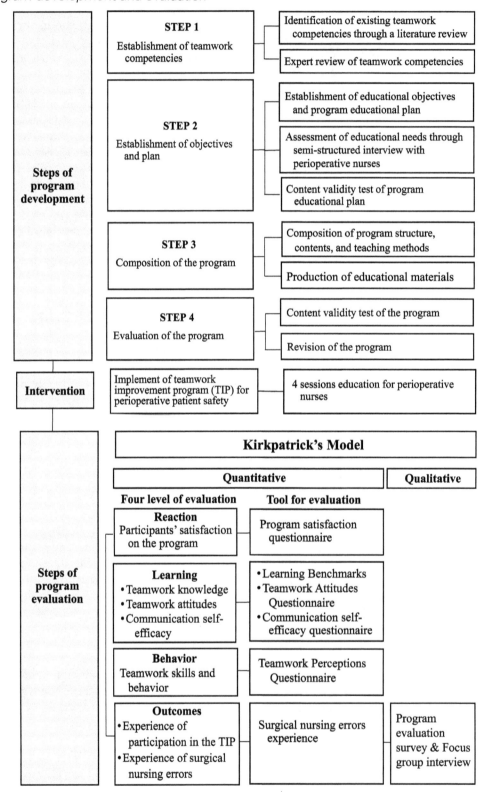

Quality in Health Care, 2005; Canadian Patient Safety Institute, 2008; Cronenwett et al., 2007; WHO, 2011). The researchers categorized the teamwork competencies based on the educational objectives and core concepts described in the TeamSTEPPS educator's guide. The list of teamwork competencies was finalized after review by a panel of experts.

Table 1

Structure of the Teamwork Improvement Program for Perioperative Patient Safety

Theme	TeamSTEPPS Modules	TeamSTEPPS Content	Applied in the TIP	TeamSTEPPS Tools	Content Added to the TIP	Tools and Teaching Strategies Added to the TIP
(Session 1) Understanding the importance of teamwork for perioperative patient safety and error prevention	Introduction	1. Faculty and participant introductions	✓		• Concept and definition of patient safety • Understanding of human factors, systems approach, and patient safety • The importance of perioperative patient safety • Understanding of surgical errors • Perioperative patient safety and teamwork	• Quiz on perioperative patient safety • Watching the news about a wrong-site surgery • Teamwork game • Speak-up video: preventing errors in your care • Speak-up video: asking your advocate to speak up • Discussion (strategies for and experience of patient participation in the OR)
		2. Overview of the master trainer course and materials				
		3. Sue Sheridan video and discussion				
		4. Barriers to team performance	✓			
		5. Patient safety movement and team training	✓			
		6. The TeamSTEPPS framework	✓			
		7. Characteristics of high performing teams	✓			
	Team structure	1. Definition of a team	✓			
		2. Teams and teamwork exercise				
		3. Partnering with patients and families	✓			
		4. Multi-team system	✓			
		5. Team structure video and discussion				
(Session 2) Understanding the concepts of communication and leadership for improving teamwork	Communication	1. Importance of communication	✓	• SBAR	• Communication failure in the OR • Root causes of sentinel event data • Importance of surgical safety checklist • Tools and resources for improving team communication in the perioperative setting • Team-guided strategies for safe perioperative clinical practice	• Review quiz • Scenario-based practice focusing on perioperative setting • Team-based method • Surgical safety checklist • Handoff tools • Discussion (experience of conflict and resolution in the OR)
		2. Communication definition, standards, and challenges	✓	• Call-out		
		3. Information exchange strategies and tools	✓	• Check-back • Handoff		
	Leadership	1. Types of and effective team leaders	✓	• Brief		
		2. Team leader strategies	✓	• Huddle		
		3. Conflict resolution	✓	• Debrief		
		4. Promoting and modeling teamwork	✓			

(continues)

TABLE 1

Structure of the Teamwork Improvement Program for Perioperative Patient Safety, Continued

Theme	TeamSTEPPS Modules	TeamSTEPPS Content	Applied in the TIP	TeamSTEPPS Tools	Content Added to the TIP	Tools and Teaching Strategies Added to the TIP
(Session 3) Understanding the concepts of situation monitoring and mutual support for improving teamwork	Situation monitoring Mutual support	1. The STEP process 2. Situation awareness 3. Shared mental models 1. Task assistance 2. Feedback 3. Advocacy and assertion 4. Conflict resolution	✓ ✓ ✓ ✓ ✓ ✓ ✓	• STEP • Cross-monitoring • The assertive statement • Two-challenge rule • CUS • DESC script	• Understanding of situation monitoring and mutual support in the perioperative setting • How to share important information to improve safety of perioperative care • Patient advocacy and self-assessment on perioperative patient safety issues	• Review quiz • Scenario-based discussion • Situation monitoring and mutual support scenario in the OR • Practical exercise for assertiveness on patient safety issues • Best practice video
(Session 4) Summary: putting it all together to improve teamwork	Summary	1. Review of teamwork skills, team effectiveness and TeamSTEPPS outcomes 2. Skills practice exercise 3. Identifying opportunities to use TeamSTEPPS 4. Practice teaching session preparation	✓ ✓	• Tools and strategies learned	• Summary of teamwork components, tools and strategies for perioperative patient safety • Teamwork training • Discussion and evaluation	• Speak-up video: preparing for surgery • Wrong-site surgery scenario that could occur in the OR • Teamwork training: scenario-based discussion and simulation

Note. The program was based on the fundamental modules of the TeamSTEPPS program, and modifications was made for application in the OR clinical environment. TeamSTEPPS = Team Strategies and Tools to Enhance Performance and Patient Safety; TIP = teamwork improvement program; OR = operating room; SBAR = situation, background, assessment, recommendation; STEP = status of the patient, team members, environment, progress toward the goal; CUS = concern, uncomfortable, safety; DESC = describe the specific situation, express your concerns about the action, suggest other alternatives, consequences should be stated.

In the second step, the educational plan for the program was constructed in accordance with the educational content of the TeamSTEPPS fundamental modules, and additional content was added to reflect the specific needs of OR environments. In addition, teamwork education needs were assessed using interviews with three perioperative nurses, and the content validity for the final educational plan was verified with four clinical experts.

In the third step, the instructional structure, methods, and materials were developed based on the results of the established educational plan. After initial development, the educational content was reviewed by an expert panel composed of a perioperative nurse with more than 15 years of clinical experience in

the OR and a nurse educator who had worked for more than 10 years in a hospital. The final program was developed after revising the content, structure, and teaching methods in accordance with the results of the validity test.

Comparisons of the structure and content between TeamSTEPPS and the developed TIP are described in Table 1. The focus in this study was on improving teamwork competencies among perioperative nurses and applying teamwork strategies to nursing practice to enhance perioperative patient safety. The content addressing patient safety concepts and teamwork was emphasized, and teaching materials (AHRQ, 2019; National Patient Safety Agency, 2011; The Joint Commission, 2016a, 2016b; WHO, 2009, 2011) included scenarios and examples closely related to daily surgical practice in OR settings. In addition, tools were integrated into the TIP that are part of the OR standard of practice, such as the surgical safety checklist, briefing, and debriefing. Moreover, handoff tools (WHO, 2009, 2011) were added to improve the communication skills of participants in actual situations.

Measures

Kirkpatrick's four levels of training evaluation model (reaction, learning, behavior, and outcomes; Kirkpatrick & Kirkpatrick, 2006) were adopted to evaluate the effectiveness of the program (Figure 1).

Program satisfaction evaluation (reaction evaluation)

Participant's satisfaction with the program was assessed using the program satisfaction questionnaire (N.-J. Lee, 2015). The program satisfaction questionnaire with modifications consisted of eight items scored using a 7-point Likert scale. The Cronbach's alpha value was .92 in this study.

Teamwork competencies (learning and behavior evaluation)

Teamwork competencies comprised teamwork knowledge, teamwork attitudes, communication self-efficacy, and teamwork skills and behavior. In the learning evaluation, teamwork knowledge, teamwork attitudes, and communication self-efficacy were measured. Teamwork skills and behavior were measured at the behavior level.

For teamwork knowledge, the Learning Benchmarks of 23 multiple-choice items was used (1 = *correct answer*, 0 = *wrong answer*), with higher total scores associated with better teamwork knowledge.

The Teamwork Attitudes Questionnaire (TAQ) was used to assess teamwork attitudes. The TAQ consists of 30 items in five subscales (team structure, leadership, situation monitoring, mutual support, and communication) scored using a 5-point Likert scale (1 = *strongly disagree* to 5 = *strongly agree*). Higher scores are associated with positive teamwork attitudes. The Cronbach's alpha values of the five subscales reported in previous research were .70, .81, .83, .70, and .74, respectively (AHRQ, 2017). The Cronbach's alpha values of the five subscales were .81, .82, .90, .60, and .67, respectively, in this study.

A 13-item questionnaire was developed in this study to measure communication self-efficacy based on the communication competencies selected in this study. This questionnaire uses a 5-point Likert scale, ranging from 1 = *strongly disagree/not at all* to 5 = *strongly agree/very much*, with higher scores associated with higher communication self-efficacy. The Cronbach's alpha value of this questionnaire was .82 in this study.

Teamwork skills and behavior were measured using the Teamwork Perceptions Questionnaire (TPQ). The TPQ consists of 35 items under the same five subscales as the TAQ that are scored using a 5-point Likert scale (1 = *strongly disagree* to 5 = *strongly agree*), with higher scores associated

with better teamwork skills and behavior. The TPQ psychometric test has been validated in the hospital setting (Keebler et al., 2014). The Korean language version of the TPQ, translated and revised by Ahn and Lee (2016), was used in this study. The Cronbach's alpha values of the five subscales were .82, .88, .76, .78, and .75, respectively, in this study.

The Learning Benchmarks, TAQ, and TPQ tools were developed by the AHRQ and the U.S. Department of Defense. Permission to use the scales was obtained from the AHRQ, and the authors of this study translated these scales from English to Korean using the committee approach. In the committee approach, all versions of a translation are reviewed by an expert team after initial translation (Tsang et al., 2017). In this study, the tools were initially translated independently by three experts, who then met together to review all of the translated versions in a reconciliation/consensus session to discuss discrepancies and reach an agreement on the translated tools. The clarity and readability of the items were tested by a group of nurses and doctoral students of nursing. After conducting a content validity test, the final questionnaire was completed for the Learning Benchmarks and TAQ.

Experience of participation in the teamwork improvement program and experience of surgical nursing errors (outcomes evaluation)

To assess the participants' experience of change after participating in the TIP, qualitative data were collected using focus group interviews (FGIs) and the program evaluation survey (PES). In addition, their experience of surgical nursing errors was investigated using pre- and postsurveys. A "surgical nursing error" refers to a nursing mistake experienced or perceived by the perioperative nursing team, which may result in unanticipated harm to a patient during an operation. In the survey, participants answered "yes" or "no" to having experienced these errors and indicated the number of error experiences encountered during the previous 4-week period.

Intervention

The program consisted of four 60-min sessions conducted twice per week over a 2-week period and participation in web-based learning. The TIP utilized a variety of educational methods, including lectures, presentations, feedback, watching videos, discussion, scenario-based discussion, and simulation. The educational materials were posted to a website so that participants could learn in advance. A research team member provided the TIP to the experimental group at a seminar room in the operating center. Based on the definition of a team (AHRQ, 2019), four or five nurses who worked together to perform the same operations with the aim of safe surgery were assigned to one team. To enhance team performance, team members participated together in team activities (e.g., teamwork games, scenario-based discussions, and a simulation) during the TIP.

Data Collection

Data were obtained between December 2016 and March 2017. After obtaining permission to collect data from a tertiary hospital, the researcher recruited nurses interested in participating by posting the recruitment poster in operating centers. This study was approved by the institutional review board at the Seoul National University (IRB No. 1608/003-010). All of the study participants read and signed the informed consent form.

The pre- and postsurveys were conducted at a 4-week interval with both control and experimental groups. In the pre-and postsurveys, we measured teamwork competencies and surgical nursing error experiences using a self-report questionnaire. After the presurvey, the experimental group underwent the TIP for 2 weeks and completed a postsurvey, including the program satisfaction questionnaire, after the 2-week intervention. In addition, the experimental group underwent a PES and FGIs.

The PES was conducted in the fourth session of the program to allow all of the participants to freely write their thoughts and feelings about the program participation experience, and we utilized the data as a basis for team discussion. We conducted two FGIs with eight nurses from the experimental group who agreed to participate in interviews 2 weeks after the intervention. The participants were divided into two groups, taking into account their duty schedule and duration of clinical career. The FGIs lasted 50–60 minutes for each group and were recorded after obtaining the consent of the participants. The key questions on the PES and FGIs were as follows: "Are there any changes in your overall thoughts about teamwork after participating in the program?" "Have you made any changes in clinical practice after participating in the program?" "Which tools or strategies that you have learned in the program would you like to try first in the OR?"

Data Analysis

SPSS 24.0 (IBM Inc., Armonk, NY, USA) was used to analyze the quantitative data in this study. The general characteristics of the experimental and control group participants were analyzed using descriptive statistics. Homogeneity tests for general and study variables were analyzed using an independent t test, χ^2 test, and Fisher's exact test. The analyses of pretest and posttest differences between the experimental and control groups were performed using a paired t test. Differences in nursing error experiences between the two groups were analyzed using a chi-square test.

The qualitative data from the PES and FGIs were analyzed using a conventional content analysis based on Hsieh and Shannon (2005). The recorded data from the interview were transcribed as text. First, the overall meaning of the text was extrapolated by repeatedly reading and rereading the data. Next, meaningful sentences and words that contained key ideas were highlighted to identify associated codes, and similar codes were sorted into subcategories. At the end of the process, the subcategories were derived into categories. To enhance rigor, an analytical discussion between two researchers was undertaken until consensus was reached to determine whether the results of the analysis reflected the participants' experiences accurately.

Results

Data on participants' recruitment and retention are summarized in Figure 2. The baseline characteristics and premeasurement scores for the intervention and control groups are shown in Table 2. No statistically significant difference in the premeasurement scores of outcome variables was identified between the two groups with regard to teamwork knowledge ($t = -1.21$, $p = .230$), teamwork attitudes ($t = -0.10$, $p = .920$), communication self-efficacy ($t = -1.00$, $p = .321$), teamwork skills and behavior ($t = -0.24$, $p = .808$), and experience of surgical nursing errors ($\chi^2 = 1.08$, $p = .406$).

Program Satisfaction

Nearly all (96.4%) of the participants were satisfied with the overall content of the TIP, and the information provided in the program was identified as helpful to their clinical practice. The participants scored each of the eight items an average of ≥ 6 points (on a 7-point scale).

Teamwork Competencies

The pretest–posttest differences for the experimental and control groups were analyzed. The pretest–posttest differences in the experimental group were significantly higher than in the control group for teamwork knowledge (mean = 0.75 ± 1.38 vs. -0.68 ± 1.35, $t = 4.07$, $p < .001$), teamwork attitudes (mean = 0.51 ± 0.31 vs. -0.00 ± 0.33, $t = 6.10$, $p < .001$), communication self-efficacy (mean = 1.12 ± 0.32 vs. 0.23 ± 0.37, $t = 9.90$, $p < .001$), and teamwork skills and behavior (mean = 0.54 ± 0.41 vs. -0.08 ± 0.39, $t = 6.04$, $p < .001$).

Experience of Participation in the Teamwork Improvement Program

Based on the results of the conventional content analysis, seven subcategories under three categories were extracted (Table 3).

Recognizing the importance and content of teamwork

Participants experienced a turning point in rethinking teamwork in their workplace after training. They realized teamwork as crucial for improving patient safety in the OR and could demonstrate teamwork through participating in team activities. Involving patients and their caregivers as team members was a new concept for participants, and they felt proud to apply it in their work. In addition, the participants realized that, to achieve a safe operation, the team should have a common goal that encompasses all members of the team, including patients and caregivers. Working in the OR, they had previously perceived that they worked alone but changed their mind after the intervention to perceive their work in the context of their team.

Figure 2

Flow diagram of participants

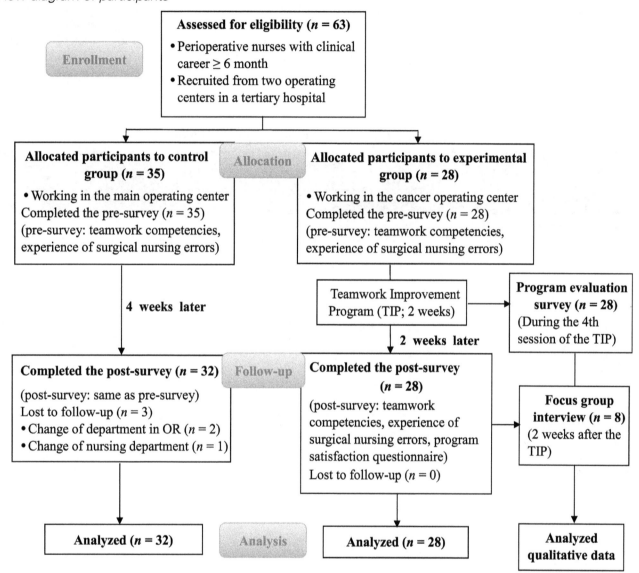

Improving teamwork competencies

Participants realized that they already had knowledge of teamwork but did not know how to apply it in their workplace. They also had a positive experience of the education, in that they were glad to learn the strategies for applying their knowledge to practice. After the training, the participants employed tools and coping strategies when patient safety was threatened, and they had a positive experience of practicing the strategies they had learned in the training program while working in OR settings.

Contributing to safe surgery

With regard to safe surgery, leading a team effectively is important, but participants were not previously aware that they could play the role of leader. They learned that there were various types of team leaders, and they became aware of the leader's role and responsibility to prevent errors

using standard OR practices, such as briefing, debriefing, and implementing the surgical safety checklist. The participants recognized that ineffective communication could impact patient safety and endeavored to use assertive strategies to ensure clear communication among team members.

Experience of Surgical Nursing Errors

In the postsurvey, 10 participants (35.7%) in the experimental group and 11 participants (34.4%) in the control group responded that they had experienced surgical nursing errors. There was not a significant difference between the two groups.

Discussion

Nurses' teamwork is an important factor in ensuring the quality of care and patient safety. To improve nursing teamwork, a competency-based education program is important to guide teaching and learning. The Quality and Safety Education for Nurses emphasizes the teamwork and collaboration competency as a core requirement of nursing education (Cronenwett et al., 2007). However, there is a lack of guidance in terms of how to teach nurses this competency. In this study, a TIP for perioperative patient safety was developed based on the teamwork competencies required for nurses, and the effectiveness of the program was assessed using Kirkpatrick's four-level evaluation model. The TIP for perioperative patient safety is the first nursing teamwork training program to be assessed as suitable for OR settings in South Korea.

Table 2

General Characteristics and Premeasurement Scores of Participants (N = 60)

Category	Total (*N* = 60)	Experimental Group (*n* = 28)	Control Group (*n* = 32)	*t*/χ²	*p*
		n (%) or *M* ± *SD*			
General characteristics					
Age (year)	28.25 ± 4.48	28.36 ± 4.72	28.16 ± 4.33	0.17	.864
Gender					
Female	58 (96.7)	28 (100.0)	30 (93.8)	1.81[a]	.494
Male	2 (3.3)	0 (0.0)	2 (6.2)		
Working hours per day	8.52 ± 0.67	8.59 ± 0.78	8.45 ± 0.56	0.77	.448
Education					
Bachelor	59 (98.3)	27 (96.4)	32 (100.0)	1.16[a]	.467
Associate degree in nursing	1 (1.7)	1 (3.6)	0 (0.0)		
Job position					
Staff nurse	42 (70.0)	21 (75.0)	21 (65.6)	0.63	.574
Senior nurse	18 (30.0)	7 (25.0)	11 (34.4)		
Clinical career (years)					
< 5	38 (63.3)	19 (67.9)	19 (59.4)	1.34	.512
5–9	12 (20.0)	6 (21.4)	6 (18.7)		
≥ 10	10 (16.7)	3 (10.7)	7 (21.9)		
Type of work					
Day	31 (51.7)	13 (46.4)	18 (56.3)	0.58	.605
Evening	29 (48.3)	15 (53.6)	14 (43.7)		
Patient safety education experience					
Yes	54 (90.0)	24 (85.7)	30 (93.8)	1.07[a]	.404
No	6 (10.0)	4 (14.3)	2 (6.2)		
Annual number of patient safety education experiences	1.48 ± 1.36	1.29 ± 0.85	1.66 ± 1.68	−1.05	.296
Teamwork education experience					
Yes	17 (28.3)	5 (17.9)	12 (37.5)	2.84	.150
No	43 (71.7)	23 (82.1)	20 (62.5)		
Annual number of teamwork education experiences	0.28 ± 0.45	0.18 ± 0.39	0.38 ± 0.49	−1.72	.090
Communication education experiences					
Yes	38 (63.3)	16 (57.1)	22 (68.8)	0.87	.425
No	22 (36.7)	12 (42.9)	10 (31.2)		
Annual number of communication education experiences	0.68 ± 0.57	0.61 ± 0.57	0.75 ± 0.57	−0.97	.335
Premeasurement scores					
Teamwork knowledge		19.82 ± 1.16	20.19 ± 1.18	−1.21	.230
Teamwork attitudes		4.13 ± 0.35	4.14 ± 0.32	−0.10	.920
Communication self-efficacy		3.31 ± 0.41	3.43 ± 0.50	−1.00	.321
Teamwork skills and behavior		3.86 ± 0.39	3.88 ± 0.36	−0.24	.808
Experience of surgical nursing errors					
Yes		7 (25.0)	12 (37.5)	1.08	.406
No		21 (75.0)	20 (62.5)		

[a] Fisher's exact test.

Table 3

Category, Subcategory, and Quotes From Content Analysis

Category	Subcategory	Quotes
Recognizing the importance and content of teamwork	Recognition of the need for teamwork improvement program	*I can now keep in mind that the most important thing for patient safety is teamwork. I had no idea about teamwork at all before, but through this teamwork training, I came to realize the importance of teamwork. (Program evaluation survey, Participant 13)* *I hope charge nurses and even nursing managers take part in this training, because they sometimes tend to blame us and take doctors' sides on patient safety issues. So, I want them to comfort us by realizing we are one team and those situations should not be ascribed to anyone. (Focus Group 2, Interviewee 1)*
	Promoting the value of team activity	*Making rings was the most impressive. Ah! During this trivial activity, we planned and experienced teamwork, so we learned that we needed teamwork. (Focus Group 2, Interviewee 2)* *I think it was meaningful to be able to apply what we learned with the last scenario to practice. Looking back at the team activities, I felt that my knowledge was integrated and organized. (Focus Group 2, Interviewee 4)*
	A new perspective about teams	*I think the largest difference after the teamwork education is about whether to include patients in our team or not. Of course, I have talked to the patient when going through the surgical safety checklist, but I had never thought it was part of teamwork with the patient. Through the teamwork education, I realized patients could be among the team members and found that providing preoperative nursing care and checking identification was a part of teamwork already. It changed my view on the patient. (Focus Group 1, Interviewee 1)* *It would be a great help to be able to work with my colleagues as a team under good conditions with pleasure. Not "my work" or "your work" but "work together"! (Program evaluation survey, Participant 23)*
Improving teamwork competencies	Joy of applying teamwork knowledge	*Some of the educational content was what I'd already learned in my undergraduate courses, but I had had no chance to apply or link it to clinical situations while working in the OR. During the training session, I realized "Oh! I should have done this, but I did not." (Focus Group 1, Interviewee 4)* *Previously, I worked with uncertainty about teamwork, but now I'm glad to be able to utilize evidence and apply more solutions in clinical situations based on my new knowledge. (Program evaluation survey, Participant 5)*
	Improvement of coping competencies in clinical situations	*Sometimes I did not know the name of the specimen exactly, but the surgeon was too scary and the operation was too speedy, so it was difficult to check the exact name one more time. However, after the teamwork training, I learned that throwing the specimen on the scrub table without saying its name could be a threat to the patient's safety. Thus, now I have become able to use teamwork strategies such as "call out" when I feel something is wrong. (Focus Group 2, Interviewee 3)*

TABLE 3

Category, Subcategory, and Quotes From Content Analysis, Continued

Category	Subcategory	Quotes
Contributing to safe surgery	Responsibility and leadership for patient safety	*I came to think it is important to more actively participate during surgery. After training, I realized my role and responsibility for patient safety. Therefore, I came to be more actively involved in the briefing and debriefing process.* (Focus group 1, Interviewee 2) *I had been thinking that I was not a powerful person in my team. But after training, it seems that I have a sense of awareness of the team and our responsibility because we can become situational leaders by being educated.* (Program evaluation survey, Participant 20)
	Assertive communication on safety issues	*No matter how scary it is to start to speak because he is a stubborn doctor or she is a senior nurse, the only way of providing some information is verbal communication. It's very, very difficult to use "Call out" or the "Two-Challenge Rule," but it is important to communicate with such a person.* (Focus Group 1, Interviewee 2) *I think patient safety issues are likely to happen in emergency situations. So, I want to try CUS (concern, uncomfortable, safety) when I'm confronted with safety issues in the OR because this communication tool is easy to apply and effective for preventing errors.* (Program evaluation survey, Participant 16)

The findings of this study provide evidence that teamwork training increases nurses' teamwork competencies in terms of teamwork knowledge, attitudes, skills and behavior, and communication self-efficacy, which is consistent with previous findings (Cooke, 2016; Gaston et al., 2016; Parker et al., 2019; Thomas & Galla, 2013). After participating in a teamwork program, the improvements in teamwork competency were found to affect various aspects of patient safety, including patient safety culture (Gaston et al., 2016; Staines et al., 2019; Thomas & Galla, 2013) and patient outcomes (Kalisch et al., 2007). In addition, increased teamwork competencies may impact nurses' job satisfaction and retention, which in turn may positively impact the healthcare work environment for nurses. Kalisch et al. (2010) found that nurses who scored higher on teamwork were more likely to be satisfied with their occupation. Moreover, teamwork interventions that include a 4-hour TeamSTEPPS training course and a simulation session were shown to increase the job satisfaction and slightly decrease the turnover rate among nurses (Baik & Zierler, 2019). Therefore, ongoing teamwork training is needed to improve patient safety, provide high-quality patient care, and ensure adequate nursing staffing.

Compared with previous studies that have applied the TeamSTEPPS program in OR settings (Dahl et al., 2017; S.-H. Lee et al., 2021), the TIP used in this study focused on knowledge of nursing teamwork in the perioperative setting, patient safety concepts, and the relationship between teamwork and patient safety in the healthcare system. Scenarios and examples were added in the teaching materials to supplement the concept-oriented materials of TeamSTEPPS and to help participants better understand the content. The qualitative data in this study indicate that participants showed improvement in recognizing the importance and content of teamwork. It is important that participants' attitudes and perceptions of teamwork improved. Teamwork depends on team members' willingness to cooperate and communicate together with the shared goal of achieving optimal outcomes for patients (King et al., 2008).

To develop teamwork competencies, nurses should not only be equipped with relevant knowledge, attitudes, and skills but also be supported to use the tools they have learned in clinical practice (Barton et al., 2018). The TIP developed in this study includes various tools that nurses may apply in actual work situations. It is particularly meaningful that participants perceived that their coping skills improved and that they applied communication tools based on teamwork knowledge, demonstrating positive changes in perioperative nurses' teamwork skills and behavior. This is consistent with previous findings that 89% of healthcare professionals used a tool in clinical practice after team training (Gaston et al., 2016). In terms of patient safety competencies, teamwork competencies have a critical impact on the safety climate (Hwang, 2015). Therefore, these outcomes may contribute to a positive safety climate and culture.

Showing the *Speak-up* video during the intervention and having the participants watch it repeatedly on the website/mobile applications is thought to be effective in improving communication self-efficacy and leadership. The qualitative data analysis in this study showed that the participants were willing to use assertiveness strategies and team-guided strategies such as the two-challenge rule, call-out, CUS (concern, uncomfortable, safety), briefing, and debriefing, all of which were emphasized in teamwork training. Effective communication and leadership skills are required to improve patient safety and teamwork in healthcare. Thus, teaching health professionals how to speak up and express themselves when they have safety concerns is a key factor in achieving safe patient care (WHO, 2011). In addition, assertive communication education is needed on an ongoing basis to prevent potential errors in the OR. Therefore, it is necessary to create an environment in which team members feel safe to encourage them to communicate effectively and speak up with each other.

To improve quality and safety competencies, it is necessary to use various teaching strategies that include not only didactic or web-based modules but also case studies and simulations (Cronenwett et al., 2007). This study incorporated various teaching methods such as teamwork games, videos, scenario-based small group discussions, and lectures to engage participants. Simulation using the TeamSTEPPS may be an effective way to improve the teamwork and collaboration competency proposed by Quality and Safety Education for Nurses (Sherwood & Barnsteiner, 2017). In this study, simulation training was performed using the OR scenarios in which participants could apply all of the teamwork competencies learned in the last lesson of the developed program. In the simulation, nurses not only integrated teamwork knowledge into practice but also took into account the attributes and performance of other team members participating in the scenario and made situational judgments (Barton et al., 2018). Therefore, using a scenario that reflects the clinical situation in teamwork training strengthens the learning effect and is effective in linking learned teamwork knowledge to teamwork skills and behavior.

This study has several limitations. First, this research was conducted at a tertiary hospital in a metropolitan city. Thus, the results may not be generalizable to other nurses. In future research, the sample size may be increased, and perioperative nurses working at different organizational levels and in different cultures may be recruited. Second, this research measured short-term outcomes using a self-reported questionnaire. Thus, the insignificant pretest–posttest difference in surgical nursing error experience may be due to the short time between intervention and postmeasurement or reflect a subjective measurement bias. Therefore, a long-term outcome measure using objective data will be necessary to examine the association between teamwork competencies and clinical errors.

Conclusions

Effective teamwork in nursing teams is an essential factor in the OR that may be learned using a systematic competency-based teamwork program. The TIP developed in this study was effective in improving the teamwork competencies of the perioperative nurses. The clinical application of teamwork strategies may be expected to contribute to patient safety by promoting effective communication, leadership, situation monitoring, and mutual support with other health professionals based on teamwork knowledge. When providing teamwork training, educational materials that reflect healthcare professionals' clinical settings should be used to strengthen the connection between patient safety concepts and teamwork. To promote a safe nursing practice, hospital executives and nurse managers should create an environment that supports the implementation of learned teamwork strategies. Finally, in the future, applying and evaluating the effectiveness of the TIP with not only nursing staff but also other healthcare professionals who work together in the OR will be necessary.

Acknowledgment

This research was supported by Basic Science Research Program through the National Research Foundation of Korea funded by the Ministry of Education (No. 2014R1A1A2055166).

Author Contributions

Study conception and design: SA, NJL
Data collection: SA
Data analysis and interpretation: SA, NJL
Drafting of the article: SA, NJL
Critical revision of the article: SA, NJL

References

Agency for Healthcare Research and Quality. (2017). *TeamSTEPPS® Teamwork Attitudes Questionnaire manual.* https://www.ahrq.gov/teamstepps/instructor/reference/teamattitudesmanual.html

Agency for Healthcare Research and Quality. (2019). *TeamSTEPPS 2.0.* https://www.ahrq.gov/teamstepps/instructor/index.html

Ahn, S. A., & Lee, N.-J. (2016). The effect of operating room nursing and medical staff teamwork and perception of patient safety culture on the performance of surgical patient safety protocol. *Journal of Korean Critical Care Nursing, 9*(1), 27–39. (Original work published in Korean)

Australian Commission on Safety and Quality in Health Care. (2005). *National patient safety education framework.* https://www.safetyandquality.gov.au/publications-and-resources/resource-library/national-patient-safety-education-framework

Baik, D., & Zierler, B. (2019). RN job satisfaction and retention after an interprofessional team intervention. *Western Journal of Nursing Research, 41*(4), 615–630. https://doi.org/10.1177/0193945918770815

Barton, G., Bruce, A., & Schreiber, R. (2018). Teaching nurses teamwork: Integrative review of competency-based team training in nursing education. *Nurse Education in Practice, 32,* 129–137. https://doi.org/10.1016/j.nepr.2017.11.019

Canadian Patient Safety Institute. (2008). *The safety competencies.* http://www.patientsafetyinstitute.ca/en/toolsResources/safetyCompetencies/Pages/default.aspx

Clapper, T. C., & Ng, G. M. (2013). Why your TeamSTEPPS™ program may not be working. *Clinical Simulation in Nursing, 9*(8), e287–e292. https://doi.org/10.1016/j.ecns.2012.03.007

Cooke, M. (2016). TeamSTEPPS for health care risk managers: Improving teamwork and communication. *Journal of Healthcare Risk Management, 36*(1), 35–45. https://doi.org/10.1002/jhrm.21233

Cronenwett, L., Sherwood, G., Barnsteiner, J., Disch, J., Johnson, J., Mitchell, P., Sullivan, D. T., & Warren, J. (2007). Quality and safety education for nurses. *Nursing Outlook, 55*(3), 122–131. https://doi.org/10.1016/j.outlook.2007.02.006

Dahl, A. B., Abdallah, A. B., Maniar, H., Avidan, M. S., Bollini, M. L., Patterson, G. A., Steingerg, A., Scaggs, K., Dribin, B. V., & Ridley, C. H. (2017). Building a collaborative culture in cardiothoracic operating rooms: Pre- and postintervention study protocol for evaluation of the implementation of TeamSTEPPS training and the impact on perceived psychological safety. *BMJ Open, 7*(9), Article e017389. https://doi.org/10.1136/bmjopen-2017-017389

Faul, F., Erdfelder, E., Buchner, A., & Lang, A. G. (2009). Statistical power analyses using G*Power 3.1: Tests for correlation and regression analyses. *Behavior Research Methods, 41*(4), 1149–1160. https://doi.org/10.3758/BRM.41.4.1149

Gaston, T., Short, N., Ralyea, C., & Casterline, G. (2016). Promoting patient safety: Results of a TeamSTEPPS® initiative. *The Journal of Nursing Administration, 46*(4), 201–207. https://doi.org/10.1097/NNA.0000000000000333

Hsieh, H.-F., & Shannon, S. E. (2005). Three approaches to qualitative content analysis. *Qualitative Health Research, 15*(9), 1277–1288. https://doi.org/10.1177/1049732305276687

Hughes, A. M., Gregory, M. E., Joseph, D. L., Sonesh, S. C., Marlow, S. L., Lacerenza, C. N., Benishek, L. E., King, H. B., & Salas, E. (2016). Saving lives: A meta-analysis of team training in healthcare. *Journal of Applied Psychology, 101*(9), 1266–1304. https://doi.org/10.1037/apl0000120

Hwang, J.-I. (2015). What are hospital nurses' strengths and weaknesses in patient safety competence? Findings from three Korean hospitals. *International Journal for Quality in Health Care, 27*(3), 232–238. https://doi.org/10.1093/intqhc/mzv027

Hwang, J.-I., & Ahn, J. (2015). Teamwork and clinical error reporting among nurses in Korean hospitals. *Asian Nursing Research, 9*(1), 14–20. https://doi.org/10.1016/j.anr.2014.09.002

Kaiser, J. A., & Westers, J. B. (2018). Nursing teamwork in a health system: A multisite study. *Journal of Nursing Management, 26*(5), 555–562. https://doi.org/10.1111/jonm.12582

Kalisch, B. J., Curley, M., & Stefanov, S. (2007). An intervention to enhance nursing staff teamwork and engagement. *Journal of Nursing Administration, 37*(2), 77–84. https://doi.org/10.1097/00005110-200702000-00010

Kalisch, B. J., Lee, H., & Rochman, M. (2010). Nursing staff teamwork and job satisfaction. *Journal of Nursing Management, 18*(8), 938–947. https://doi.org/10.1111/j.1365-2834.2010.01153.x

Kalisch, B. J., & Lee, K. H. (2010). The impact of teamwork on missed nursing care. *Nursing Outlook, 58*(5), 233–241. https://doi.org/10.1016/j.outlook.2010.06.004

Keebler, J. R., Dietz, A. S., Lazzara, E. H., Benishek, L. E., Almeida, S. A.,

Toor, P. A., King, H. B., & Salas, E. (2014). Validation of a teamwork perceptions measure to increase patient safety. *BMJ Quality and Safety, 23*(9), 718–726. https://doi.org/10.1136/bmjqs-2013-001942

King, H. B., Battles, J., Baker, D. P., Alonso, A., Salas, E., Webster, J., Toomey, L., & Salisbury, M. (2008). TeamSTEPPS™: Team strategies and tools to enhance performance and patient safety. In K. Henriksen, J. B. Battles, M. A. Keyes, & M. L. Grady (Eds.), *Advances in patient safety: New directions and alternative approaches (Vol. 3: performance and tools).* Agency for Healthcare Research and Quality.

Kirkpatrick, D. L., & Kirkpatrick, J. D. (2006). *Evaluating training programs.* Berrett-Koehler.

Lee, N.-J. (2015, May). *Undergraduate nursing students' perceptions of patient safety competencies.* Oral session presented at 2015 QSEN National Forum Conference, San Diego, CA.

Lee, S.-H., Khanuja, H. S., Blanding, R. J., Sedgwich, J., Pressimone, K., Ficke, J. R., & Jones, L. C. (2021). Sustaining teamwork behaviors through reinforcement of TeamSTEPPS principles. *Journal of Patient Safety, 17*(7), e582-e586. https://doi.org/10.1097/PTS.0000000000000414

National Patient Safety Agency. (2011). *'How to guide': Five steps for safe surgery.* https://www.patientsafetysolutions.com/docs/January_11_2011_NPSA_UK_How_to_Guide_Five_Steps_to_Safer_Surgery.htm

Parker, A. L., Forsythe, L. L., & Kohlmorgen, I. K. (2019). TeamSTEPPS®: An evidence-based approach to reduce clinical errors threatening safety in outpatient settings: An integrative review. *Journal of Healthcare Risk Management, 38*(4), 19–31. https://doi.org/10.1002/jhrm.21352

Sherwood, G., & Barnsteiner, J. (2017). *Quality and safety in nursing: A competency approach to improving outcomes* (2nd ed.). Wiley-Blackwell.

Sonoda, Y., Onozuka, D., & Hagihara, A. (2018). Factors related to teamwork performance and stress of operating room nurses. *Journal of Nursing Management, 26*(1), 66–73. https://doi.org/10.1111/jonm.12522

Staines, A., Lécureux, E., Rubin, P., Baralon, C., & Farin, A. (2019). Impact of TeamSTEPPS on patient safety culture in a Swiss maternity ward. *International Journal for Quality in Health Care, 32,* 618–624. https://doi.org/10.1093/intqhc/mzz062

The Joint Commission. (2016a). *Speak up campaigns.* https://www.jointcommission.org/speakup.aspx

The Joint Commission. (2016b). *Sentinel event data root causes by event type.* https://www.jointcommission.org/sentinel_event.aspx

Thomas, L., & Galla, C. (2013). Building a culture of safety through team training and engagement. *BMJ Quality and Safety, 22*(5), 425–434. https://doi.org/10.1136/bmjqs-2012-001011

Tsang, S., Royse, C. F., & Terkawi, A. S. (2017). Guidelines for developing, translating, and validating a questionnaire in perioperative and pain medicine. *Saudi Journal of Anaesthesia, 11*(5), 80–89. https://doi.org/10.4103/sja.SJA_203_17

Vertino, K. A. (2014). Evaluation of a TeamSTEPPS© initiative on staff attitudes toward teamwork. *The Journal of Nursing Administration, 44*(2), 97–102. https://doi.org/10.1097/NNA.0000000000000032

World Health Organization. (2009). *WHO guidelines for safe surgery: Safe surgery saves lives.* Author. https://www.who.int/publications/i/item/9789241598552

World Health Organization. (2011). *Patient safety curriculum guide: Multi-professional edition.* Author. https://www.who.int/publications/i/item/9789241501958

17

Development of Fertility Preparedness Scale for Women Receiving Fertility Treatment

Sevcan FATA[1]* • Merlinda ALUŞ TOKAT[2]

ABSTRACT

Background: Stress has a negative impact on fertility by suppressing the secretion of fertility hormones. Although it is known that stress reduces the probability of conception and affects fertility negatively, scales that are now widely used to evaluate fertility preparedness include negative items. Positive statements are crucial to relieving stress in women. Using positive items in assessments of fertility preparedness in women may help reduce related stress.

Purpose: This study was designed to develop the Fertility Preparedness Scale for women receiving fertility treatments.

Methods: A methodological study was conducted in four fertility clinics between December 2015 and March 2016. Two hundred thirty women who had been diagnosed with primary or secondary infertility were enrolled as participants. A personal information form and the Fertility Preparedness Scale were used to collect data.

Results: The Cronbach's alpha was .84 for the total scale and .76–.79 for the subscales. Factor analysis extracted three subscales that explained 52.93% of the total variance. The confirmatory factor analysis found a goodness of fit index of .80, a comparative fit index of .95, and a nonnormed fit index of .94.

Conclusions/Implications for Practice: This scale is valid and reliable for measuring the fertility preparedness of women who receive fertility treatment.

KEY WORDS
fertility, fertility preparedness, reliability, scale, validity.

Introduction

Infertility is a significant source of stress for most couples. Although some studies have found stress to play an important role in reducing the chances of conception by suppressing the secretion of fertility hormones (Behboodi-Moghadam, Salsali, Eftekhar-Ardabily, Vaismoradi, & Ramezanzadeh, 2013; Matthiesen, Frederiksen, Ingerslev, & Zachariae, 2011; Yusuf, 2016), others have found that stress has no effect on fertility outcomes (Anderheim, Holter, Bergh, & Möller, 2005; Cesta et al., 2018). Stress disrupts endocrine signaling in the hypothalamic–pituitary–gonadal axis. The pituitary gonadotropes are suppressed through receptors in the hypothalamus, and follicle development is disrupted in the ovaries. Consequently, the release of estrogen and progesterone is reduced (Whirledge & Cidlowski, 2010). In addition, it is known that, among women who are stressed, the number of healthy follicles, implantation rates, and pregnancy outcomes are affected more negatively (An, Sun, Li, Zhang, & Ji, 2013; Gourounti, Anagnostopoulos, & Vaslamatzis, 2011; Younis et al., 2012). Globally, women with fertility problems in many assisted reproduction centers are treated using only interventional procedures. During psychological assessments, the stress levels of these women are mostly evaluated using questions with negative meanings such as "Do you feel drained or worn out because of fertility problems?" and "Do you feel sad and depressed about your fertility problems?" (Boivin, Takefman, & Braverman, 2011). The process of answering the negative items on these scales may elevate perceive stress. However, during these psychological assessments, preparedness associated with fertility is not assessed. Women begin their fertility treatment without assessing whether they are psychologically prepared. Preparedness as a concept has been studied in terms of patients' ability to perform self-care to change lifestyles. Under this concept, preparedness is tied as much to learning as to appraising the situation and one's own abilities, considering available options, and rehearsing or trying out new solutions (Dalton & Gottlieb, 2003). It consists of several components, including an awareness phase, an appraisal phase, and a planning phase. The first phase is becoming aware of what needs to change. The second phase involves appraising the costs and benefits of changing and trying to envisage how life would be if they do change. The last phase is planning for action (Dalton, 1998).

Many healthcare providers explain the success or failure of a patient's willingness to change or to comply with a medical regimen as lack of preparedness. Higher preparedness is associated with better treatment results (Dalton & Gottlieb, 2003). Therefore, assessing women's preparedness is a very important step in fertility treatment. In the literature, no scale for measuring fertility preparedness has been published. Thus, the development of a related scale is needed to evaluate

[1]PhD, Research Assistant Doctor, Gynecology & Obstetrics Nursing Department, Nursing Faculty, Dokuz Eylul University, Izmir, Turkey • [2]PhD, Associate Professor, Gynecology & Obstetrics Nursing Department, Nursing Faculty, Dokuz Eylul University, Izmir, Turkey.

women's preparedness positively. At the same time, it is important to assess the positive aspects of change in the cost and benefits phase. Focusing on positive aspects accelerates preparedness (Dalton, 1998). If all of the items of the scale are positive items, it can contribute positively to the treatment process while the women are reading these scale items. For this reason, the aim of this study was to develop the "Fertility Preparedness Scale for Women Receiving Fertility Treatment," to evaluate fertility preparedness using only positive items.

Methods

Participants and Settings

This was a methodological study, conducted at four fertility clinics in Turkey between December 2015 and March 2016. The participants were 230 women who were (a) able to speak, read, and write Turkish; (b) diagnosed with primary or secondary infertility; and (c) without psychiatric illness. In Turkey, there is a wide variation in educational status among women. To ensure that the scale could be used efficaciously with women of all educational backgrounds, participants were selected according to their education status using a stratified sampling method with an optimum delivery method.

Steps of Developing the Scale

Item pool

An item pool (30 items) was prepared by reviewing the literature and the opinions of researchers and fertility experts (Buyukozturk, 2011). To assess the appropriateness of item contents, 10 nurses and doctors who were infertility experts in either a clinical or an academic setting reviewed the items. They rated each item on a scale of 1 = *not suitable* to 4 = *quite suitable* for the evaluation of fertility preparedness. To examine the suitability of items of the scale and the ability of the scale to measure preparedness, the Item Content Validity Index (ICV-I) and Scale Content Validity Index were calculated, respectively. According to the literature, the ICV-I score should exceed .78 (Polit & Beck, 2006). The ICV-I in our results varied between .80 and 1.00. When all of the experts gave 4 points for any item, the ICV-I of that item was 1. To develop the scale from items that are reasonably suitable, those items with ICV-I < 1 were removed. The Scale Content Validity Index was found to be .96 (minimum recommended score is .90; Polit & Beck, 2006). As a result of this analysis process, the 25-item Fertility Preparedness Scale (FPS) was developed.

The 23-item Fertility Preparedness Scale

To confirm the ease of comprehension of items, a pilot study was performed with 30 women who met the previously mentioned inclusion criteria. The items were read to these participants, and they were asked to assess the comprehensibility of each. The two items that were not understood were removed because it

was decided that the remaining items were sufficient to measure preparedness. In addition, minor changes were made to some items based on the participants' suggestions. After these changes, the final 23-item FPS was composed.

Data Collection

After informed consent procedures, the personal information form and 23-item FPS were completed by women who applied to fertility clinics. The data collection process took a maximum of 10 minutes to complete per participant. The personal information form contained 15 questions related to sociodemographic characteristics and fertility history. The 23-item FPS was scored using a 5-point Likert scale, with minimum and maximum scores of 23 and 115, respectively. The median of the scale score is 56 points, which was considered the cutoff value. A scale score of below 56 indicates that a participant is not sufficiently prepared for fertility, and a scale score of 56 or higher indicates sufficient fertility preparedness.

In this study, three bilingual experts translated the scale independently from Turkish into English. Back-translation from English into Turkish using blind back-translation procedures was completed by a lay person who had not seen the original Turkish version of the scale and who knew both languages, but whose native language was English.

Ethical Considerations

Ethical approval was obtained from the Dokuz Eylul University Ethics Committee for Noninterventional Studies (2015/22-16). Moreover, permission from each fertility clinic and written consent from participants were obtained.

Data Analysis

Sociodemographic characteristics and fertility history were analyzed using descriptive statistics. For FPS, validity and reliability analyses were performed. SPSS Version 15.0 (SPSS, Inc., Chicago, IL, USA) and linear structural relations were used for analysis.

Validity analysis

The factor structure of the instrument was tested using exploratory factor analysis (EFA) and confirmatory factor analysis (CFA). EFA is used to identify the factor structure for a set of variables based on data instead of theory. In contrast, CFA is generally based on a strong theoretical and empirical foundation that allows an investigator to specify a hypothesized factor structure in advance and then test it. Thus, CFA may be used to determine how well a proposed model fits the data (Tabachnick & Fidell, 2007).

EFA was performed as a part of determining construct validity. To measure sampling adequacy for EFA, the Kaiser–Meyer–Olkin (KMO) procedure was used, and normal distribution was determined using Bartlett's test of sphericity. Moreover, principal component analysis with varimax rotation was used to develop the subscales.

CFA was the second part of establishing construct validity. CFA allowed the researcher to test the hypothesis of a relationship between the observed variables and the subscales developed. A structural equation model was performed, and chi-square degrees-of-freedom statistics (χ^2/df), root mean square error approximation (RMSEA), goodness of fit index (GFI), comparative fit index (CFI), normed fit index (NFI), and nonnormed fit index (NNFI) were calculated.

Reliability analysis

Cronbach's alpha, split-half reliability, item–total correlation, and Hotelling's T^2 test were used to determine reliability. Internal consistency was examined using two approaches: Cronbach's alpha (coefficient alpha) and split-half reliability (Spearman–Brown test). The item–total correlations were used to explain the relationships among each item and the scale. Furthermore, the relationships among each item of the subscale and the overall subscale were evaluated in the same manner. In scale development, it is important to observe whether item means are equal or not, which was analyzed using Hotelling's T^2 test.

Results

Sample Characteristics

The mean age of participants was 32.1 (SD = 5.55) years, and 36.5% were employed. Regarding educational level, 33.5% had completed primary school, 33% had completed high school, and 33.5% had completed postgraduate studies. The average duration of fertility treatment was 2.22 (SD = 1.08) years, and 92.6% had primary infertility. Among the participants, 36.5% reported female infertility, 87.8% had experienced ovulation induction, 55.7% had received intrauterine insemination, and 49.6% had undergone in vitro fertilization.

Validity

In the EFA, the KMO coefficient was .898 and the result of Bartlett's sphericity test was χ^2 = 2.790E3, p < .001. In the principal component analysis, all item eigenvalues were greater than 1. In addition, three subscales were exposed to explanatory analysis: "hope and awareness," "positive feelings and thoughts," and "prepared body and brain." The subscales were composed of the components of preparedness concept (see Figure 1). These three subscales explained 52.93% of the total variance, which shows the power of the factor structure of the scale (see Table 1). Regarding the relationship between each item and the overall subscale, factor loading was calculated and only one item factor loading (Item 18) was found to be below the suggested levels, with a score of .24. The factor loadings for all other items were between .41 and .82.

In the CFA, the calculated values were as follows: χ^2/df = 2.85, RMSEA = .08, GFI = .80, CFI = .95, NFI = .92 and NNFI = .94. Correlations between subscales were between .67 and .75, and p value was < .001 (see Figure 1).

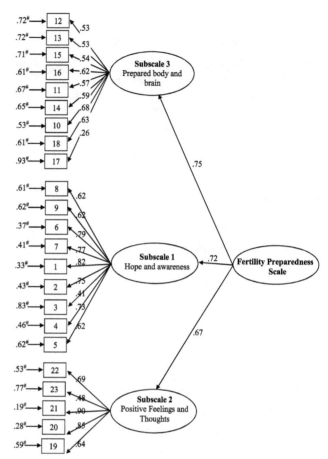

Figure 1. Confirmatory factor analysis of Fertility Preparedness Scale. *Error variance: the part of the total variance caused by irrelevant factors that were not experimentally controlled.

The relationship between the scale and the items (factor load) tested using EFA is shown in the table. The factor correlation and item correlation tested using CFA are given in the figure.

Reliability

The item–total score correlation coefficients ranged between .45 and .71. The Pearson correlation coefficients between subscale scores and scale total scores were between .80 and .83.

The total Cronbach's alpha was .84. The Cronbach's alpha coefficients of the subscales ranged from .76 to .79 (see Table 1). According to the Spearman–Brown analysis, the split-half correlation coefficient was .811. Item scores were different from each other (Hotelling's T^2 = 299.445, p < .001).

Discussion

Validity

A KMO value of between .80 and .90 is considered "very good." The KMO value of this scale was found to be .898,

TABLE 1.
Reliability and Validity Analysis of Fertility Preparedness Scale (N = 230)

Subscale	Percentage Variance	Cronbach's Alpha
Subscale 1: hope and awareness	20.91	.77
Subscale 2: positive feelings and thoughts	15.83	.79
Subscale 3: prepared body and brain	16.19	.76
Fertility Preparedness Scale	52.93	.84

Item	Factor Loading	Mean	SD	Item–Total Correlation
Subscale 1: hope and awareness				
8. Treatment will be beneficial to help me conceive.	.72	4.42	0.79	.67
9. I think positively about new medical options.	.76	4.39	0.77	.62
6. I think positively about traditional practices.	.47	3.76	1.14	.45
7. I am aware that balanced and regular nutrition increases my chance of pregnancy.	.78	4.33	0.83	.65
1. I am aware that regular exercise increases my chance of pregnancy.	.68	4.13	0.93	.60
2. Positive thoughts can be beneficial to my reproductive organs.	.71	4.22	0.86	.70
3. I look forward to future with the hope.	.62	4.33	0.89	.65
4. When I relaxed, more oxygen and blood go to my reproductive organs.	.58	4.00	0.96	.65
5. When I relaxed, hormones are regularly released.	.55	4.00	0.97	.65
Subscale 2: positive feelings and thoughts				
22. I can positively control my feelings.	.59	3.89	0.94	.65
23. I'm just focusing on positive thinking about becoming pregnant.	.81	4.04	0.95	.64
21. I try to increase my positive thoughts about pregnancy.	.82	3.98	1.01	.71
20. I only use positive words about pregnancy.	.58	4.02	0.93	.65
19. I just get positive messages about becoming pregnant.	.39	3.96	1.12	.56
Subscale 3: prepared body and brain				
12. My reproductive hormones are healthy and balanced.	.59	3.93	0.94	.68
13. I can feel comfortable while waiting for my test results.	.64	3.33	1.23	.59
15. My body works perfectly for becoming pregnant.	.73	3.71	1.03	.53
16. My uterus is now ready for pregnancy.	.63	3.95	0.92	.55
11. Listening to relaxing music will make it easier to conceive.	.56	3.51	1.10	.60
14. I do everything I can to feel relaxed during treatments.	.53	4.16	0.93	.54
10. I can feel comfortable while waiting control day.	.52	3.67	1.18	.66
18. I trust my body and mind.	.24	3.85	1.00	.67
17. I can positively impact my hormones.	.41	3.84	0.98	.62

which means that the sample size was suitable for the factor analysis. In the factor analysis, normality and linearity properties are also important, along with sample size. Whether the data follow a multivariate normal distribution is typically tested using Bartlett's sphericity test (Tavsancil, 2010). In this study, the result of this test was significant at an advanced level (χ^2 = 2.790E3, $p < .001$), showing that the correlation matrix is suitable for the factor analysis.

In the principal component analysis, items with an eigenvalue greater than 1 are significant for evaluating the main component of the scale (Akgul, 2005). The fact that eigenvalues of all of the items exceeded 1 in the FPS indicates that

each item is suitable for measuring preparedness. In addition, the higher variance rates (52.93%) indicate the suitability of the subscales for explaining preparedness. Variance rates between 40% and 60% are accepted as sufficient (Sencan, 2005). To test whether an item is related to the subscale, it is necessary to check its factor loading (Sencan, 2005). Factor loadings ranging from .30 to .40 may be considered as the lower cutoff points to create the factor pattern (Tavsancil, 2010). Buyukozturk defined factor load values of greater than .60 as high, between .30 and .59 as medium, and .29 or below as low. At the same time, he indicated that the factor load values should be evaluated together with variance and that items with low factor loads may be used (Buyukozturk, 2011). All items except one were within this value range, indicating that the quality of these items makes them suitable for inclusion in the subscales. The item with a factor loading of .24 was not excluded because the researchers decided that it was the basic item of the scale.

In the CFA, results were found to fit well with the EFA results. It is suggested in the literature that χ^2/df should be between 3/1 and 5/1 and that CFI, NFI, and NNFI values should be more than > .90. It has been generally reported that the RMSEA should be between 0 and 1, with lower scores showing a well-fitting model. The upper limit should be greater than .08. A GFI ranging between 0 and 1 or higher indicates a well-fitting model. The findings show that the model has good compliance (Kalayci, 2010; Ozdamar, 2009). It was found that the scale is suitable for measuring fertility preparedness. The CFA confirmed that the relationships among subscales were significant and positive, indicating that the subscales were compatible with each other in measuring fertility preparedness.

Reliability

The correlation coefficients of the scale items were high and statistically significant. A high item–total correlation shows that items exemplify similar behaviors and that the internal consistency of the test is high (Buyukozturk, 2011). In the literature, Pearson's correlation coefficient has been classified as follows: .26–.49, weak; .50–.69, moderate; .70–.89, high; and .90–1.00, very high (Sencan, 2005). Items with a high item–total correlation distinguish individuals very well. Item–total score correlations under .25 indicate no correlation between items and the scale and that these items cannot be used in distinguishing individuals (Akgul, 2005). In our results, the item–total score correlation coefficients ranged between .45 and .71, showing that every item evaluates fertility preparedness. Pearson correlation coefficients between subscale and total scale scores (.80–.83) showed that subscales are able to distinguish individuals in terms of preparedness.

On the basis of the literature, Cronbach's alpha coefficients between $.60 \leq \alpha \leq .80$ and $.80 \leq \alpha \leq 1.00$ are evaluated as "quite reliable" and "highly reliable," respectively (Simsek, 2007). This study shows that the FPS is highly reliable. It was detected that Subscales 1 and 2 were "quite reliable" and that Subscale 3 was "highly reliable." These findings show that items of the scale are homogenous and that they measure the same feature.

The split-half coefficient should be at least .70 (Sencan, 2005). In this study, it was determined to be above .70 and was found that, when the scale was randomly divided into two halves, it was still reliable in measuring fertility preparedness.

In methodological studies, it is important to assess whether the mean scores of items are similar (Simsek, 2007). It was detected through Hotelling's T^2 test that the items of the FPS are perceived by women in the same way.

Infertility is seen as an important problem in Turkish culture. Part of being a woman is giving birth to children. So, women want to have children for their spouse and family rather than for their own purposes. It is thought that assessing psychological preparedness before fertility treatment positively affects the treatment process. As the scale contains only 23 items, it may be easily applied in practice and also easily answered by women. Its other positive aspect is its providing positive messages to women during fertility treatment. When women read positive items, they may take a more positive perspective on fertility treatment (Gilbert, 2013). Because the treatment process is expensive and stressful, if a woman starts well prepared in this process, financial loss may be prevented and the treatment success may be improved. It would be useful to measure the preparedness of women by applying this scale in clinics before treatment.

Conclusions and Recommendations

In conclusion, the FPS is valid and reliable for measuring the fertility preparedness of women who receive fertility treatment. It may be used before or during fertility treatment. The scale is clinically feasible, short, and cost free, which are crucial factors in daily practice for both healthcare professionals and patients. We expect that future applications of this scale will enable health professionals to assess preparedness and plan necessary initiatives.

Author Contributions

Study conception and design: All authors
Data collection: SF
Data analysis and interpretation: All authors
Drafting of the article: All authors
Critical revision of the article: All authors

References

Akgul, A. (2005). *Statistical analysis SPSS practices techniques in medical research* (3rd ed., p. 384). Ankara, Turkey: Emek Ofset. (Original work published in Turkish)

An, Y., Sun, Z., Li, L., Zhang, Y., & Ji, H. (2013). Relationship between psychological stress and reproductive outcome in women undergoing in vitro fertilization treatment: Psychological and neurohormonal assessment. *Journal of Assisted Reproduction & Genetics, 30*(1), 35–41. https://doi.org/10.1007/s10815-012-9904-x

Anderheim, L., Holter, H., Bergh, C., & Möller, A. (2005). Does psychological stress affect the outcome of *in vitro* fertilization? *Human Reproduction, 20*(10), 2969–2975. https://doi.org/10.1093/humrep/dei219

Behboodi-Moghadam, Z., Salsali, M., Eftekhar-Ardabily, H., Vaismoradi, M., & Ramezanzadeh, F. (2013). Experiences of infertility through the lens of Iranian infertile women: A qualitative study. *Japan Journal of Nursing Science, 10,* 41–46. https://doi.org/10.1111/j.1742-7924.2012.00208.x

Boivin, J., Takefman, J., & Braverman, A. (2011). The fertility quality of life (FertiQol) tool: Development and general psychometric properties. *Fertility & Sterility, 96*(2), 409–415.e3.

Buyukozturk, S. (2011). *Data analysis handbook for social sciences: Statistics, research design, SPSS practices and interpretation* (14th ed.). Ankara, Turkey: Pegem Academy. (Original work published in Turkish)

Cesta, C. E., Johansson, A. L. V., Hreinsson, J., Rodriguez-Wallberg, K. A., Olofsson, J. I., Holte, J., … Nyman Iliadou, A. (2018). A prospective investigation of perceived stress, infertility-related stress, and cortisol levels in women undergoing in vitro fertilization: Influence on embryo quality and clinical pregnancy rate. *Acta Obstetricia et Gynecologica Scandinavica, 97*(3), 258–268. https://doi.org/10.1111/aogs.13280

Dalton, C. (1998). *Readiness to engage in health work: A concept analysis* (Unpublished master's thesis). School of Nursing, McGill University, Montreal, Canada.

Dalton, C. C., & Gottlieb, L. N. (2003). The concept of readiness to change. *Journal of Advanced Nursing, 42*(2), 108–117. https://doi.org/10.1046/j.1365-2648.2003.02593.x

Gilbert, S. (2013). *Fertility support program.* Scottsdale, AZ: Hypnobirthing Institute.

Gourounti, K., Anagnostopoulos, F., & Vaslamatzis, G. (2011). The relation of psychological stress to pregnancy outcome among women undergoing in-vitro fertilization and intracytoplasmic sperm injection. *Women & Health, 51*(4), 321–339. https://doi.org/10.1080/03630242.2011.574791

Kalayci, S. (2010). *SPSS applied multivariate statistical techniques* (5th ed., pp. 321–331). Ankara, Turkey: Asil Publication Distribution. (Original work published in Turkish)

Matthiesen, S. M., Frederiksen, Y., Ingerslev, H. J., & Zachariae, R. (2011). Stress, distress and outcome of Assisted Reproductive Technology (ART): A meta-analysis. *Human Reproduction, 26*(10), 2763–2776. https://doi.org/10.1093/humrep/der246

Ozdamar, K. (2009). *Statistical data analysis with packet programs* (7th ed., pp. 274–275). Eskisehir, Turkey: Kaan Bookstore. (Original work published in Turkish)

Polit, D. F., & Beck, C. T. (2006). The content validity index: Are you sure you know what's being reported? Critique and recommendations. *Research in Nursing & Health, 29*(5), 489–497. https://doi.org/10.1002/nur.20147

Sencan, H. (2005). *Reliability and validity in social and behavioral measurements* (1st ed.). Ankara, Turkey: Seckin. (Original work published in Turkish)

Simsek, O. F. (2007). *Introduction to structural equation modeling, basic principles and LISREL applications* (pp. 12–18). Ankara, Turkey: Cem Web Ofset. (Original work published in Turkish)

Tabachnick, B. G., & Fidell, L. S. (2007). *Using multivariate statistics* (5th ed.). New York, NY: Allyn & Bacon.

Tavsancil, E. (2010). *Attitude measurement and data analysis with SPSS* (4th ed.). Ankara, Turkey: Nobel Publication Distribution. (Original work published in Turkish)

Whirledge, S., & Cidlowski, J. A. (2010). Glucocorticoids, stress, and fertility. *Minerva Endocrinology, 35*(2), 109–125.

Younis, A., Clower, C., Nelsen, D., Butler, W., Carvalho, A., Hok, E., & Garelnabi, M. (2012). The relationship between pregnancy and oxidative stress markers on patients undergoing ovarian stimulations. *Journal of Assisted Reproduction and Genetics, 29*(10), 1083–1089. https://doi.org/10.1007/s10815-012-9831-x

Yusuf, L. (2016). Depression, anxiety and stress among female patients of infertility: A case control study. *Pakistan Journal of Medical Science, 32*(6), 1340–1343. https://doi.org/10.12669/pjms.326.10828

18

Factors Associated With Adherence to Fluid Restriction in Patients Undergoing Hemodialysis in Indonesia

Melyza PERDANA[1] • Miaofen YEN[2]*

ABSTRACT

Background: The factors related to fluid intake adherence among patients undergoing hemodialysis have been explored in many studies. However, most of these were conducted in Western countries and have produced inconsistent results. A study of this issue in Indonesia, a tropical country with strong herbal medicine traditions, may show different results. In addition to demographic characteristics, self-efficacy is a standard measurement used in chronic care management activities such as hemodialysis treatment. Understanding the reasons behind patient nonadherence in Indonesia may help nurses better manage the fluid intake of patients.

Purpose: This study was designed to determine the factors that predict patient adherence to fluid intake restrictions.

Methods: A cross-sectional study was conducted on 153 patients undergoing hemodialysis at two hospitals. Intradialytic weight gain over a 1-month period was recorded to assess the participants' adherence to fluid intake restrictions. Intradialytic weight gains of more than 2 kg was considered to be nonadherent. A daily urine output and level of thirst were also recorded. The participants completed an adapted self-efficacy questionnaire, Swedish Fluid Intake Appraisal Inventory, and the data were analyzed together with demographic characteristic and clinical parameters using hierarchical multiple regression.

Results: The results revealed that most of the respondents did not adequately adhere to fluid intake restrictions (59.5%). Intradialytic weight gain was shown to strongly correlate with self-efficacy ($p < .05$, $\beta = -.201$), gender ($p < .05$, $\beta = -.179$), educational background ($p = .05$, $\beta = .159$), and urine output ($p < .05$, $\beta = -.168$). Demographic characteristic explained 10.6% and self-efficacy explained 3.9% of the variance in fluid adherence.

Conclusions/Implications for Practice: Female participants with higher self-efficacy scores reported the lowest average level of intradialytic weight gain, indicating better adherence to fluid intake restrictions. Several demographic factors as well as self-efficacy were identified as potential predictors of fluid intake restriction adherence. Therefore, measuring self-efficacy periodically is a good initial step toward detecting those patients who are at higher risk of noncompliance with fluid intake restrictions.

KEY WORDS:
adherence, fluid restriction, hemodialysis, interdialytic weight gain (IDWG), self-efficacy.

Introduction

Chronic kidney disease (CKD) is a major health problem worldwide and is considered a key factor in poor health outcomes for most noncommunicable diseases, including cardiovascular disease, hypertension, and diabetes (Luyckx et al., 2018). CKD affects up to 13% of the world's population, and its mortality rate is continuing to increase, especially in developing countries (GBD Chronic Kidney Disease Collaboration, 2020; Hill et al., 2016). The number of patients requiring renal replacement therapy, particularly hemodialysis (HD), also continue to increase over time. In Indonesia, HD is the most widely used treatment among patients with CKD (rate of usage among Indonesian patients with CKD is approximately 98%; Indonesian Renal Registry, 2018). Many previous studies have confirmed the high financial and physical burdens imposed by CKD. Because of the high costs associated with HD treatment, CKD has a significant and negative financial impact on the public healthcare system. Indonesian National Health Insurance ranks CKD as one of the top four diseases in terms of share of national healthcare expenditures (Social Insurance Administration Organization of Indonesia, 2020). Moreover, the decrease in patient income associated with repeated hospitalizations and physical limitations also increases health expenditures (Kerr et al., 2012; Kustimah et al., 2019).

Patients receiving HD are expected to adhere to recommended therapeutic regimens such as fluid restrictions, dietary guidelines, prescribed medications, and routine dialysis sessions to maintain their health, prevent complications, and improve quality of life (Lin et al., 2017; Naderifar et al., 2019). Previous studies have identified fluid restriction as the hardest regimen to follow (Mollaoğlu & Kayataş, 2015;

[1]MS, Lecturer, Department of Medical Surgical Nursing, Universitas Gadjah Mada, Yogyakarta, Indonesia • [2]PhD, RN, Professor, Department of Nursing, National Cheng Kung University, Tainan City, Taiwan, ROC.

Ozen et al., 2019). Unrestricted fluid intake results in fluid accumulation, leading to more complications such as faster declining in estimated Glomerulo Filtration Rate, hypertension, and heart failure (Hung et al., 2015). Therefore, knowing the factors that contribute to adhering to fluid intake restrictions will be useful to help patients avoid more severe conditions.

Many studies have been conducted to identify the factors that contribute to fluid adherence behavior. Although sociodemographic characteristics such as age, gender, educational level, years on dialysis, social support, and perception of self-efficacy have been found to affect adherence to fluid intake restrictions, the degrees of effect vary across countries (Beerendrakumar et al., 2018; Chan et al., 2012; Khalil et al., 2013; Lee et al., 2014). Self-efficacy is a critical aspect in chronic disease management (Grady & Gough, 2014). Measuring self-efficacy is helpful in predicting patient adherence behavior with regard to some medication regimens such as fluid intake (Wu et al., 2016). Self-efficacy describes the expectation of an individual regarding their capacity in terms of a behavior or action to achieve a particular outcome (Bandura, 1977). Self-efficacy is not a personal characteristic but rather a judgment of self-confidence regarding the ability to accomplish some future task. Self-efficacy may be strengthened by nurses to enhance patients' self-management efficacy in long-term treatments such as HD (Lindberg & Fernandes, 2010; Winters et al., 2012). Assessing self-efficacy, specifically with regard to fluid intake restrictions, will be very helpful for nurses as an initial step to assist patients to improve their fluid intake adherence.

Furthermore, sociocultural context should be highlighted to improve scholarly understanding of patient fluid adherence behaviors (Guerra-Guerrerro et al., 2014). Traditional Indonesian beliefs regarding medications must be assessed as a factor that affects fluid intake issues. Many patients in Indonesia with end-stage renal disease undergoing HD still use *jamu*, a traditional medicinal herbal beverage, as an alternative or complementary therapy (Kustimah et al., 2019). In addition to its accessibility and affordability, many Indonesian people perceive *jamu* as more natural and less harmful than modern, chemical-based drugs (Torri, 2013). Thus, approximately 44.3% Indonesian people still adhere to a combined Western medical and *jamu* treatment approach (The Indonesia Agency of Health Research and Development, 2018). However, natural herbs such as *jamu* pose a significant health risk to patients with failing renal function.

To date, no studies addressing the factors related to adherence to fluid intake limitations in Indonesian HD patients have been published. Prior studies have focused only on adherence to attendance in HD treatment (Agustina et al., 2019). Understanding the factors affecting adherence to fluid intake restrictions will help nurses improve health outcomes in patients undergoing HD. Therefore, this study was designed to determine the factors that significantly predict patient adherence to fluid intake restrictions.

Methods

Design

This was designed as a descriptive, cross-sectional study. Interdialytic weight gain (IDWG) over a 1-month period was recorded to determine adherence to fluid intake restrictions. Data on self-efficacy were collected using the Indonesian Fluid Intake Appraisal Inventory (I-FIAI).

Participants

One hundred fifty-three patients participated in this study, which was conducted during 2014. All of the participants were HD patients who regularly attended one of two HD units located in government hospitals in Yogyakarta. Participation was voluntary, and the participants were informed that all collected information would be anonymized and kept confidential.

Inclusion criteria were as follows: patients diagnosed with CKD Stage V, received HD for at least 6 months, more than 18 years old, and able to understand Bahasa. Otherwise qualified patients with a psychological disorder were excluded. Prior to enrollment, potential participants were given information about the research procedure. Patients were enrolled in the study only after they had provided written informed consent to the researcher.

Ethical Considerations

Ethical approval was obtained by the institutional research board of Universitas Gadjah Mada under Ethical Approval No. KE/FK/151/EC. Written informed consent was given by all participants following appropriate guidance. The written informed consent was sealed and coded to respect the participants' privacy. Participants could withdraw from the study at any time.

Measures

Participants were approached during their dialysis sessions by the researcher and coresearchers. After consenting to participate, participants completed the questionnaire (demographic data sheet and I-FIAI). The urine output sheet was brought by the patients to record their daily urine output. The researcher recorded their IDWG for 1 month using a special form by inputting participants' pre- and postdialysis weights. Every sheet of the form contained the participant's randomly assigned number, which corresponded to the demographic data form and questionnaire.

The following measures were included in the study questionnaire:

1. Demographic and clinical details

Age, gender, educational background, employment status, length of time on dialysis, dialysis hours per week, and *jamu* (Indonesian herbs) consumption were all recorded. A visual analog scale was used to measure level of thirst. A special daily urine output record was completed by each patient.

2. Self-efficacy measure

A modified Swedish Fluid Intake Appraisal Inventory (S-FIAI) was used to measure self-efficacy in fluid intake restriction. The S-FIAI consists of 33 items and is framed on four situation-specific factors, including physiological, affective, social, and environmental (Lindberg et al., 2007). Compared to other scales designed to measure fluid adherence, the S-FIAI is currently the only one that focuses specifically on fluid adherence. This scale is a validated instrument with internal consistency (Cronbach's α = .96 in the Swedish version) and has been translated and used in other languages such as Dutch (Cronbach's α = .982) and Portuguese (Cronbach's α = .95; Lindberg & Fernandes, 2010; Lindberg et al., 2007; Winters et al., 2012). Items are scored on an 11-point scale, ranging from 0 (*not at all confident*) to 10 (*totally confident*), based on the general question: "How do you assess your ability to limit your fluid intake on these following occasions?" The maximum possible raw score for this instrument is 330, with the sum of all item scores interpreted as the respondent's level of self-efficacy (Lindberg et al., 2007) and higher inventory total scores associated with greater self-confidence in being able to restrict fluid consumption.

In this study, the S-FIAI was translated and modified into an Indonesian language version (I-FIAI). The translation was done by two native Indonesian speakers who are fluent in both Indonesian and Swedish. The process also involved the original author confirming the original concepts of the instrument. After translation, the I-FIAI was validated by a panel of experts (including two nephrology nurses, four nursing faculty, and two nephrologists) to ensure content validity. The content validity index for the I-FIAI had five items that initially scored less than .85 and were subsequently modified. The mean content validity index values of .937 for the I-FIAI and .919 for the S-FIAI demonstrated the excellent content validity of this instrument. The internal consistency reliability for the I-FIAI, as tested using Cronbach's alpha coefficient, was .952. Thus, the I-FIAI should be considered valid and reliable.

3. Measure of adherence

IDWG was recorded at every HD session as an objective measurement of fluid intake adherence. IDWG average values were obtained during HD sessions over a 1-month period. IDWG is a valid and reliable objective measure of fluid adherence and is used in both clinical and research settings. Patients were weighed before and after each dialysis session. IDWG was calculated by subtracting the individual's predialysis weight in the current HD session from the postdialysis weight taken in the immediately preceding session (Hecking et al., 2018), with higher IDWG values indicating poorer adherence to fluid intake restrictions (Lindberg et al., 2007). In this study, the threshold for

nonadherence was defined as having a 1-month mean IDWG value of > 2 kg (Association of Indonesian Nephrologists, 2011).

4. Level of thirst

Level of thirst was measured using a visual analog scale ranging from 0 to 10, with 0 indicating that the patient had perceived no thirst sensation over the previous 2 months and 10 indicating extreme thirst perception over the previous 2 months (Wirth & Folstein, 1982). Level of thirst was recorded at the same time the participants completed the self-efficacy questionnaire.

5. Urine output

Mean urine output was measured by summarizing the daily urine output (ml/day) recorded by patients over a 30-day period. A urine output of less than 100 ml/24 hours was considered as anuria (Kabbani, 2014).

Analysis

Analyses were performed using SPSS Windows Version 17 (SPSS, Inc., Chicago, IL, USA). Data were presented as means and standard deviations for the continuous data and as percentages for the categorical data. Each demographic characteristic, clinical indicator, and self-efficacy score were compared between adherent and nonadherent patients using an independent t test. Hierarchical multivariate linear regression analysis was used to determine the factors that influenced adherence to fluid intake, and any variables with a p value of $\leq$ .05 in the single comparisons were included in the regression analysis as candidates (i.e., gender, educational background, daily urine output, and self-efficacy). Statistical significance was defined at p < .05. In this final analysis, the dependent variable (patient adherence) was a continuous variable that was generated by IDWG and measured in kilograms.

Results

Sample Characteristics

A total of 153 patients from the HD units in two government hospitals in Yogyakarta were enrolled as participants in this study. As shown in Table 1, the mean age of the participants was 50.18 years (*SD* = 12.33), the male-to-female ratio was nearly equal (49.7:50.3), nearly half (46.4%) had completed compulsory education (secondary school) in Indonesia, and more than half were currently unemployed (64.7%). Almost all of the participants (92.8%) followed a twice-weekly HD schedule, with an average duration of HD treatment in the study sample of 36 months. Slightly more than half were anuric (52.3%), with nonadherent patients showing a significantly lower level of daily urine output (209.99 ml). Surprisingly, only 29 participants (19%) reported consuming *jamu* on a daily basis, whereas seven patients (4.5%) reported still consuming *jamu* sometimes. The mean level of

Table 1

Demographic and Clinical Data of Participants (N = 153)

Characteristic	Total (n = 153)		Adherent (n = 62)		Nonadherent (n = 91)		t/χ^2	p
	n	%	n	%	n	%		
Age (years), M and SD	50.18	12.33	51.82	11.47	48.95	12.63	t = 1.42	.15
Gender							10.75	.03*
Male	76	49.7	24	38.7	52	57.1		
Female	77	50.3	38	61.3	39	42.9		
Education							5.01	.03*
Primary school	52	33.99	29	26.8	23	25.3		
Secondary school	71	46.41	24	38.7	47	51.6		
Higher education	30	19.60	9	14.5	21	23.1		
Employment							3.44	.17
Unemployed	99	64.7	44	70.9	55	60.5		
Employed	54	35.3	18	29.1	36	39.5		
Frequency of HD/week							1.62	.44
2×/week	142	92.8	59	95.2	83	91.2		
Other	11	7.2	3	4.8	8	8.8		
Herbs consumption							0.53	.48
Yes	29	19.0	7	11.3	22	24.2		
No	117	76.5	54	87.1	63	69.2		
Sometimes	7	4.5	1	1.6	6	6.6		
Urine output (ml), M and SD	231.35	296.95	262.69	294.82	209.99	298.11	3.93	.04*
< 100	80	52.3	27	43.5	53	58.2		
≥ 100	73	47.7	35	56.5	38	41.8		
	Mean	SD	Mean	SD	Mean	SD	t	p
IDWG (kg)	2.49	1.09	1.49	0.66	3.1	0.76	−14.21	< .001
Duration of HD (month)	36.00	34.84	31.85	32.64	38.54	36.29	−1.16	.24
Thirst level (0–10)	5.64	1.82	5.42	1.68	5.69	1.98	−0.89	.37
Hemoglobin (g/dl)	8.83	1.32	8.35	1.29	8.41	1.36	−0.25	.80

Note. IDWG = interdialytic weight gain; HD = hemodialysis.
*$p < .05$.

thirst was 5.64 on a scale of 1–10. The average hemoglobin level was 8.83 g/dl. Interestingly, regarding adherence to fluid intake level, the mean IDWG of all participants was 2.49 kg with more than half of the participants assessed as noncompliant with fluid intake restrictions (59.5%). The level of nonadherence to fluid intake restrictions, as determined using IDWG, is lower in Indonesia than other countries (Efe & Kocaöz, 2015).

Self-Efficacy

Using the I-FIAI instrument, total instrument scores for the participants ranged from 112 to 330, with a mean score of 228.73 (SD = 45.67; Table 2). Nonadherent participants earned self-efficacy scores (221.81 ± 44.24) that were significantly lower than their adherent peers (236.50 ± 50.09). Furthermore, with regard to the four specific factors related to self-efficacy, only the physiological factor was found to be significantly different between adherent and nonadherent participants (p = .02), with the latter scoring higher (71.27 ± 13.09).

Finally, to examine the strongest predictor of adherence to fluid intake restrictions after controlling for other significant factors, a two-step multiple hierarchical linear regression analysis was performed. Based on the results presented in Table 3, adding self-efficacy to the second model showed a statistical significance of the overall model, $F(5, 147) = 4.055$, $p < .05$. Demographic variables (gender, educational background, and urine output) explained 10.6% of the variance in fluid adherence. The main variable, self-efficacy, in Step 2 explained an additional 3.9% of variance in fluid nonadherence after controlling for other predictors ($\beta = -.201$, $p < .05$).

Discussion

The aim of the current research was to determine factors contributing to nonadherence to fluid intake restrictions, as

Table 2
Self-Efficacy Score Among Participants (N = 153)

Variable/Subvariable	Achievable Range	Total (*n* = 153)		Adherent (*n* = 62)		Nonadherent (*n* = 91)		*t*	*p*
		Mean	SD	Mean	SD	Mean	SD		
Total I-FIAI score	112–330	228.73	45.67	236.50	50.09	221.81	44.24	1.91	.05*[a]
Physiological	36–100	69.01	15.21	65.67	17.45	71.27	13.09	2.27	.02*[a]
Affective	15–50	38.84	8.32	37.89	9.60	39.49	7.32	−1.17	.24 [b]
Social	14–110	75.14	18.70	74.01	21.39	75.91	16.71	−0.61	.54 [b]
Environmental	15–70	44.77	12.22	43.09	13.77	45.91	10.98	1.40	.16 [b]

Note. I-FIAI = Indonesian Fluid Intake Appraisal Inventory.
[a] Independent *t* test; [b] Mann–Whitney test.
*$p < .05$.

represented by IDWG, in patients undergoing HD. The results showed that most of the participants in this study were noncompliant. In general, female patients with better self-efficacy had less intradialytic weight gain, indicating better adherence to fluid intake restrictions.

As predicted, self-efficacy was found to be the most important predictor of fluid adherence. Patients with higher self-efficacy had lower IDWG. These results are consistent with previous studies of self-efficacy and health-related behaviors, in which self-efficacy was found to be the most important predictor of behavior (Agustina et al., 2019; Brady et al., 1997). Although self-efficacy is a major and complex factor that deserves to be focused on when a particular behavior is believed to be important, doing so is very challenging (Krespi-Boothby & Salmon, 2013). To strictly comply with fluid intake restrictions, patients undergoing HD must compensate not only for external factors but also for personal perceptions, including self-efficacy (Lin et al., 2017). Patients on HD regularly struggle to control the temptation

Table 3
Multiple Hierarchical Linear Regression of IDWG on Gender, Educational Background, Average Daily Urine Output, and Self-Efficacy

Predictor	Model I			Model II		
	β	*p*	*t*	β	*p*	*t*
Gender	−.18	.03	−2.24	−.18	.02	−2.32
Education	.16	.05	1.98	.13	.11	1.60
Urine output	−.17	.03	−2.15	−.14	.07	−1.86
Self-efficacy				−.20	.01	−2.59
R^2	.11			.15		
Adjusted R^2	.09			.12		
R^2 change				.04		
F	4.05*			4.06*		

Note. IDWG = interdialytic weight gain.
*$p < .05$.

to drink fluids and must learn to live with fluid intake limitations for the rest of their lives. Therefore, identifying potential factors associated with self-efficacy and developing interventions to enhance self-efficacy should offer a better solution for the long term.

Compared to the patients in studies conducted in European countries, patients undergoing HD in Indonesia exhibited better self-efficacy (Lindberg & Fernandes, 2010; Lindberg et al., 2007; Winters et al., 2012). Indonesian people hold a strong traditional belief called *nrimo*, which encourages them to accept their fate (Murtisari, 2013). This belief helps Indonesian people face all "God-ordained" situations with a good attitude. These situations include strict regimens prescribed by health providers. Furthermore, in terms of the situation-specific factors, self-efficacy in the physiological factor dimension was better in the nonadherent participants than their adherent peers. The physiological items represent situations with treatment-related symptoms, swallowing foods, and physical sensations such as thirst, salty taste, and breathlessness (Lindberg et al., 2007). The nonadherent participants were more confident in their ability to avoid drinking in the face of thirst, dry mouth, or in the aftermath of consuming salty food. They interpreted the thirst sensation as a sign for them to limit fluid intake. Physiological indicators have previously been highlighted as important in modifying self-efficacy. Furthermore, according to Bandura, some people consider their physical and emotional states as factors that may bolster their performance on certain behaviors (Bandura, 1994).

In addition to self-efficacy, gender has been suggested as a significant predictor in fluid intake adherence. In this study, average IDWG scores were higher in male participants than female participants. This finding is similar to those of several prior studies (Beerendrakumar et al., 2018; Ozen et al., 2019). The male participants in this study showed poorer adherence to fluid intake restrictions, possibly because men are generally less aware of their health status than women. Frequently, Indonesian male patients ignore medical advice and have a relatively low rate of participation in health checkups (Intarti & Khoriah, 2018). Moreover, men are generally more physically active and thus require more caloric and water intake than women (Riskesdas, 2019). These hegemonic masculinities may have influenced the negative results found in this study for the male participant in terms of excessive consumption of both water and liquids (Peak & Gast, 2014).

An interesting result was found for the educational background factor, with more highly educated part exhibiting higher IDWG scores. This result is the opposite of previous studies (Khalil et al., 2013; Mollaoğlu & Kayataş, 2015; Ozen et al., 2019) that found more years of education decreased the IDWG score. In behavioral change theory, educational level often acts as a mediator rather than an influencing factor in adherence to medical treatment (Margolis, 2013). However, when assessed together with other significant factors such as self-efficacy using multivariate analysis, educational background was no longer a significant predictor. The results of further analysis suggested that an intercorrelation exists between educational background, self-efficacy, and fluid adherence. Besides being associated with IDWG, an independent t test showed that patients with higher education had lower self-efficacy. The strong association between educational background and self-efficacy likely affected the relationship between educational background and fluid adherence in this study.

The analysis in this study found an association between lower daily urine output and higher IDWG, which is consistent with previous studies (Dantas et al., 2013; Lee et al., 2014). Urine output as one factor of fluid adherence implies that patients with anuria have more difficulties complying with fluid restrictions and are thus more prone to nonadherence. Moreover, a previous study suggested that urine output is a clinical indicator of residual renal function and also plays an important role in IDWG, with more urine output associated with both lower IDWG scores and a better survival rate (Hecking et al., 2019). Therefore, conducting an initial assessment of residual urine output may be helpful to identifying patients at significant risk of nonadherence.

Contrary to expectations, *jamu* consumption as a cultural issue was found to be nonsignificantly associated with IDWG. Nearly one quarter of the participants in this study consumed *jamu* on a daily basis, which is in line with a previous study that also found only a few patients with CKD drank herbal drinks (Indrayanti et al., 2019). Even though most Indonesians are satisfied with the effects of *jamu* (Elfahmi et al., 2014), this study found that three quarters of participants avoided consuming this beverage. Most patients undergoing HD avoid herbal drinks as a daily beverage because of concerns over potentially negative effects such as excessive fluid volumes and shortness of breath (Kustimah et al., 2019).

In summary, the results of this study suggest that, in addition to demographic factors, self-efficacy is a potential predictor of fluid intake restriction adherence in patients receiving HD. Therefore, measuring self-efficacy is a good initial step toward detecting which patients are at risk of poor fluid intake restriction adherence. Evaluating self-efficacy on a regular basis is highly recommended for nurses in the field of nephrology, as self-efficacy may change over time. Furthermore, further studies should be conducted to identify which interventions targeting the promotion of self-efficacy are the best options for improving patient adherence to fluid intake restrictions, particularly ones that help enhance physiological-specific self-efficacy, as most participants in this study were not sufficiently confident to limit their fluid consumption because of physiological changes in their body.

Conclusions

The findings of this study support self-efficacy and gender as the strongest predictors of fluid intake restriction adherence in patients receiving HD in Indonesia. Patients who are female and have higher self-efficacy scores tend to comply better with these restrictions. The findings of this study may be used by nurses as a reference for placing greater attention on male patients to promote appropriate control of their fluid intake. Moreover, self-efficacy seems to be a promising concept that may be improved to further increase adherence to fluid intake restrictions. Measuring self-efficacy on a periodic basis may be a good initial step in detecting those patients who are most at risk of noncompliance with fluid intake restriction.

Author Contributions

Study conception and design: MP, MY
Data collection: MP
Data analysis and interpretation: MP, MY
Drafting of the article: MP, MY
Critical revision of the article: MY

References

Agustina, F., Yetti, K., & Sukmarini, L. (2019). Contributing factors to hemodialysis adherence in Aceh, Indonesia. *Enfemeria Clinica, 29*(2, Suppl.), 238–242. https://doi.org/10.1016/j.enfcli.2019.04.028

Association of Indonesian Nephrologists. (2011). *Nutritional consensus on patients with chronic kidney disease.* PERNEFRI. (Original work published in Indonesian)

Bandura, A. (1977). Self-efficacy: Toward a unifying theory of behavioral change. *Psychological Review, 84*, 191–215. https://doi.org/10.1037/0033-295X.84.2.191

Bandura, A. (1994). Self-efficacy. In V. S. Ramachaudran (Ed.), *Encyclopedia of human behaviour* (Vol. *4*, pp. 71–81). Academic Press.

Beerendrakumar, N., Ramamoorthy, L., & Haridasa, S. (2018). Dietary and fluid regime adherence in chronic kidney disease patients. *Journal of Caring Sciences, 7*(1), 17–20. https://doi.org/10.15171/jcs.2018.003

Brady, B. A., Tucker, C. M., Alfino, P. A., Tarrant, D. G., & Finlayson, G. C. (1997). An investigation of factors associated with fluid adherence among hemodialysis patients: A self-efficacy theory based approach. *Annals of Behavioural Medicine, 19*, 339–343. https://doi.org/10.1007/BF02895151

Chan, Y. M., Zalilah, M. S., & Hii, S. Z. (2012). Determinants of compliance behaviours among patients undergoing hemodialysis in Malaysia. *PLOS ONE, 7*(8), Article e41362. https://doi.org/10.1371/journal.pone.0041362

Dantas, L. G., Cruz, C., Rocha, M., Moura, J. A. Jr., Paschoalin, E., Paschoalin, S., & Marcilio de Souza, M. (2013). Prevalence and predictors of nonadherence to hemodialysis. *Nephron Clinical Practice, 124*(1-2), 67–71. https://doi.org/10.1159/000355866

Efe, D., & Kocaöz, S. (2015). Adherence to diet and fluid restriction of individuals on hemodialysis treatment and affecting factors in Turkey. *Japan Journal of Nursing Science, 12*, 113–123. https://doi.org/10.1111/jjns.12055

Elfahmi, Woerdenbag, H. J., & Kayser, O. (2014). Jamu: Indonesian traditional herbal medicine towards rational phytopharmacological use. *Journal of Herbal Medicine, 4*(2), 51–73. https://doi.org/10.1016/j.hermed.2014.01.002

GBD Chronic Kidney Disease Collaboration. (2020). Global, regional, and national burden of chronic kidney disease, 1990–2017: A systematic analysis for the Global Burden of Disease Study 2017. *The Lancet, 395*(10225), 709–733. https://doi.org/10.1016/S0140-6736(20)30045-3

Grady, P. A., & Gough, L. C. (2014). Self-management: A comprehensive approach to management of chronic conditions. *American Journal of Public Health, 108*, 430–436. https://doi.org/10.2105/AJPH.2014.302041r

Guerra-Guerrerro, V., Plazas Mdel, P., Cameron, B. L., Santos Salas, A. V., & González, C. G. (2014). Understanding the life experience of people on hemodialysis: Adherence to treatment and quality of life. *Nephrology Nursing Journal, 41*(3), 289–298.

Hecking, M., McCullough, K. P., Port, F. K., Bieber, B., Morgenstern, H., Yamamoto, H., Suri, R. S., Jadoul, M., Gesualdo, L., Perl, J., & Robinson, B. M. (2019). Self-reported urine volume in hemodialysis patients: Predictors and mortality outcomes in the international Dialysis Outcomes and Practice Patterns Study (DOPPS). *American Journal of Kidney Disease, 74*(3), 425–428. https://doi.org/10.1053/j.ajkd.2019.02.012

Hecking, M., Moissl, U., Genser, B., Rayner, H., Dasgupta, I., Stuard, S., Stopper, A., Chazot, C., Maddux, F. W., Canaud, B., Port, F. K., Zoccali, C., & Wabel, P. (2018). Greater fluid overload and lower interdialytic weight gain are independently associated with mortality in a large international hemodialysis population. *Nephrology Dialysis Transplantation, 33*(10), 1832–1842. https://doi.org/10.1093/ndt/gfy083

Hill, N. R., Fatoba, S. T., Oke, J. L., Hirst, J. A., O'Callaghan, C. A., Lasserson, D. S., & Hobbs, F. D. (2016). Global prevalence of chronic kidney disease—A systematic review and meta-analysis. *PLOS ONE, 11*(7), Article e0158765. https://doi.org/10.1371/journal.pone.0158765

Hung, S.-C., Lai, Y.-S., Kuo, K.-L., & Trang, D.-C. (2015). Volume overload and adverse outcomes in chronic kidney disease: Clinical observational and animal studies. *Journal of the American Heart Association, 4*(5), Article e001918. https://doi.org/10.1161/JAHA.115.001918

Indonesian Renal Registry. (2018). *11th Report of Indonesian renal registry 2018.* https://www.indonesianrenalregistry.org/data/IRR%202018.pdf (Original work published in Indonesian)

Indrayanti, S., Ramadaniati, H., Anggriani, Y., Sarnianto, P., & Andayani, N. (2019). Risk factors for chronic kidney disease: A case–control study in a district hospital in Indonesia. *Journal of Pharmaceutical Sciences and Research, 1*(7), 2549–2554.

Intarti, W. D., & Khoriah, S. N. (2018). Factors associated with participation in elderly community services. *Journal of Health Studies, 2*(1), 110–122. http://doaj.org/toc/2549-3353 (Original work published in Indonesian)

Kabbani, A. R. (2014). Oliguria/anuria. In A. Merseburger, M. Kuczyk, & J. Moul (Eds.), *Urology at a glance.* Springer. https://doi.org/10.1007/978-3-642-54859-8_25

Kerr, M., Bray, B., Medvalf, J., O'Donoghue, D. J., & Matthews, B. (2012). Estimating the financial cost of chronic kidney disease to the NHS in England. *Nephrology Dialysis Transplantation, 27*(3, Suppl.), iii73–iii80. https://doi.org/10.1093/ndt/gfs269

Khalil, A. A., Darawad, M., Al Gamal, E., Hamdan-Mansour, A. M., & Abed, M. A. (2013). Predictors of dietary and fluid nonadherence in Jordanian patients with end-stage renal disease receiving haemodialysis: A cross-sectional study. *Journal of Clinical Nursing, 22*(1–2), 127–136. https://doi.org/10.1111/j.1365-2702.2012.04117.x

Krespi-Boothby, M. R., & Salmon, P. (2013). Self-efficacy and hemodialysis treatment: A qualitative and quantitative approach. *Turkish Journal of Psychiatry, 24*(2), 84–93.

Kustimah, K., Siswadi, A. G. P., Djunaidi, A., & Iskandarsyah, A. (2019). Factors affecting non-adherence to treatment in end stage renal disease (ESRD) patients undergoing hemodialysis in Indonesia. *The Open Psychology Journal, 12*, 141–146. https://doi.org/10.2174/1874350101912010141

Lee, M. J., Doh, F. M., Kim, C. H., Koo, H. M., Oh, H. J., Park, J. T., Han, S. H., Yoo, T.-H., Kim, Y.-L., Kim, Y. S., Yang, C. W., Kim, N.-H., & Kang, S.-W. (2014). Interdialytic weight gain and cardiovascular outcome in incident haemodialysis patients. *American Journal of Nephrology, 39*, 427–435. https://doi.org/10.1159/000362743

Lin, M.-Y., Liu, M. F., Hsu, L.-F., & Tsai, P.-S. (2017). Effects of self-management on chronic kidney disease: A meta-analysis. *International Journal of Nursing Studies, 74*, 128–137. https://doi.org/10.1016/j.ijnurstu.2017.06.008

Lindberg, M., & Fernandes, M. A. M. (2010). Self-efficacy in relation to limited fluid intake amongst Portuguese haemodialysis patients. *Journal of Renal Care, 36*(3), 133–138. https://doi.org/10.1111/j.1755-6686.2010.00182.x

Lindberg, M., Wikström, B., & Lindberg, P. (2007). Fluid Intake Appraisal Inventory: Development and psychometric evaluation of a situation-specific measure for haemodialysis patients' self-efficacy to low fluid intake. *Journal of Psychosomatic Research, 63*(2), 167–173. https://doi.org/10.1016/j.jpsychores.2007.03.013

Luyckx, V. A., Tonelli, M., & Stanifier, J. W. (2018). The global burden of kidney disease and the sustainable development goals. *Bulletin of the World Health Organisation, 96*(6), 414–422D. https://doi.org/10.2471/BLT.17.206441

Margolis, R. (2013). Educational differences in healthy behavior changes and adherence among middle-aged Americans. *Journal of Health and Social Behaviour, 54*(3), 353–368. https://doi.org/10.1177/0022146513489312

Ministry of Health, Indonesia. (2019). *National report: Riskesdas 2018.* Health Research and Development Agency.

Mollaoğlu, M., & Kayataş, M. (2015). Disability is associated with nonadherence to diet and fluid restrictions in end-stage renal disease patients undergoing maintenance hemodialysis. *International Urology & Nephrology, 47*(11), 1863–1870. https://doi.org/10.1007/s11255-015-1102-1

Murtisari, T. M. (2013). Some traditional Javanese values in NSM: From God to social interaction. *International Journal of Indonesian Studies, 1*, 110–125. https://arts.monash.edu/__data/assets/pdf_file/0010/1793611/6-Elisabeth.pdf

Naderifar, M., Tafreshi, M. Z., Ilkhani, M., Akbarizadeh, M. R., & Ghaljaei, F. (2019). Correlation between quality of life and adherence to treatment in hemodialysis patients. *Journal of Renal Injury Prevention, 8*(1), 22–27. https://doi.org/10.15171/jrip.2019.05

Ozen, N., Cinar, F. I., Askin, D., Mut, D., & Turker, T. (2019). Nonadherence in hemodialysis patients and related factors: A multicentre study. *The Journal of Nursing Research, 27*(4), Article e36. https://doi.org/10.1097/jnr.0000000000000309

Peak, T., & Gast, J. A. (2014). Aging men's health-related behaviors. *SAGE Open, 4*(4), 1–10. https://doi.org/10.1177/2158244014558044

Social Insurance Administration Organization of Indonesia. (2020). *Annual program and financial report 2019.* https://bpjs-kesehatan.go.id/bpjs/arsip/categories/MzA/publikasi (Original work published in Indonesian)

The Indonesia Agency of Health Research and Development. (2018). *Basic health research 2018.* Ministry of Health, Indonesia. (Original work published in Indonesian)

Torri, M. C. (2013). Knowledge and risk perceptions of traditional jamu medicine among urban consumers. *European Journal of Medicinal Plants, 3*(1), 25–39. https://doi.org/10.9734/EJMP/2013/1813

Winters, A. M., Lindberg, M., & Sol, B. G. (2012). Validation of a Dutch self-efficacy scale for adherence to fluid allowance among patients on haemodialysis. *Journal of Renal Care, 39*(1), 31–38. https://doi.org/10.1111/j.1755-6686.2012.00325.x

Wirth, J. B., & Folstein, M. F. (1982). Thirst and weight gain during maintenance hemodialysis. *Psychosomatics, 23*(11), 1134–1131. https://doi.org/10.1016/S0033-3182(82)73279-7

Wu, S.-F., Hsieh, N.-C., Lin, L.-J., & Tsai, J.-M. (2016). Prediction of self-care behaviour on the basis of knowledge about chronic kidney disease using self-efficacy as a mediator. *Journal of Clinical Nursing, 25*(17–18), 1609–1618. https://doi.org/10.1111/jocn.13305

19

Effects of Living Alone and Sedentary Behavior on Quality of Life in Patients With Multimorbidities: A Secondary Analysis of Cross-Sectional Survey Data Obtained From the National Community Database

Young Eun AHN[1] • Chin Kang KOH[2]*

ABSTRACT

Background: Having multimorbidities may increase health problems. Moreover, health-related quality of life correlates negatively with the number of chronic conditions a patient has. Living alone has been identified as a predictor of poorer quality of life, and a sedentary lifestyle is widely known to increase health problems and mortality.

Purpose: This study was designed to identify the effects of living alone and of sedentary behavior on health-related quality of life in patients with multimorbidities using nationally representative community data.

Methods: A secondary data analysis of the Korea National Health and Nutrition Examination Survey was conducted. In this study, 1,725 adult patients aged 19 years and above with two or more chronic diseases were selected for the analysis. Health-related quality of life was measured using the European Quality of Life-5 Dimensions. Multiple logistic regression was performed to identify the effects of living alone and of sedentary behavior on health-related quality of life. The statistical analyses took into account the components of the complex sampling design such as the strata, clusters, weights, and adjustment procedures, and missing data were treated in a valid manner.

Results: After adjusting for gender, age, employment status, and number of chronic diseases, it was found that the odds of having a high health-related quality of life were lower in single households than in multiperson households (odds ratio = 0.62, 95% confidence interval [0.46, 0.84]). In addition, after adjusting for gender, age, employment status, number of chronic diseases, and living arrangement, the odds of having a high health-related quality of life decreased as sedentary time increased (odds ratio = 0.93, 95% confidence interval [0.89, 0.96]).

Conclusions/Implications for Practice: To improve quality of life in patients with multimorbidities, nursing interventions that support patients who live alone and have complicated disease-related issues and that reduce sedentary behavior should be developed.

KEY WORDS:
living arrangement, multimorbidity, quality of life, sedentary behavior.

Introduction

Quality of life has been a topic of concern for many nursing researchers in recent decades. To help patients achieve a better quality of life, it is critical to identify the related factors. Although the body of literature addressing the issue of quality of life in patients with diseases has grown greatly, more research into the factors that affect quality of life in this population is required (Shofany, 2017).

Multimorbidity means having two or more chronic conditions, which include both physical and mental health problems. The prevalence of multimorbidity has been reported to broadly range from 17.1% to 72.7%. Furthermore, this prevalence appears to increase with age (Low et al., 2019; Prazeres & Santiago, 2015) and to have been on the rise for a long time (King et al., 2018; van Oostrom et al., 2016). Having multimorbidities may increase the likelihood of other health problems (Low et al., 2019; Palladino et al., 2019), which may reduce quality of life and increase mortality (McDaid et al., 2013; Nunes et al., 2016). The number of patients who have multiple chronic conditions is expected to continue to grow because of population aging. Thus, more attention should be paid by healthcare providers to patients with multimorbidities.

Having multimorbidities has been reported in a number of studies to reduce quality of life (Heyworth et al., 2009; Makovski et al., 2019), with higher numbers of concomitant chronic conditions associated with more significant decreases in quality of life (Rothrock et al., 2010; Tyack et al., 2018). Studies on quality of life in chronically ill patients have been conducted regularly. Chronic diseases such

[1]MSN, RN, Doctoral Student, College of Nursing, Seoul National University, Seoul, Republic of Korea • [2]PhD, RN, Associate Professor, College of Nursing, The Research Institute of Nursing Research, Seoul National University, Seoul, Republic of Korea.

as cardiovascular disease, respiratory disease, and diabetes are known to affect disability, self-rated health, and quality of life. Moreover, the risks of these negative health outcomes have been shown to increase with the level of multimorbidity (McDaid et al., 2013). As chronic disease treatment strategies currently focus more on management than on achieving a cure, it is important to improve quality of life by understanding its diverse aspects. Therefore, it is necessary to identify the factors that affect health-related quality of life in patients with multiple chronic conditions.

According to the Census of Population and Housing of South Korea, the proportion of single households has increased steadily in recent years, from 23.9% in 2010 to 30.2% in 2019 (Statistics Korea, 2020). Living arrangement has been identified in several studies as a factor influencing quality of life. Sun et al. (2011), using the European Quality of Life-5 Dimensions (EQ-5D) questionnaire, found living alone to be a predictor of poor mobility, pain/discomfort, and anxiety/depression in elderly individuals. Similarly, Lin et al. (2008) found that elderly people living alone reported a poorer quality of life than the general adult population. Although many research studies have examined the subject of living arrangements, most have focused on older populations. Moreover, little research has focused on the effects of living arrangement on people with multimorbidities.

A sedentary lifestyle is widely known to increase the all-cause mortality hazard ratio independent of physical activity (van der Ploeg et al., 2012). Sedentary behavior has also been shown to affect metabolic function negatively, reduce bone mineral density, and increase vascular problems, each of which has been linked to multiple health problems (Tremblay et al., 2010). In one study of sedentary behavior and quality of life, sedentary behavior was found to affect the physical dimensions of quality of life in cancer survivors (George et al., 2014). However, few studies have examined the impact of living a sedentary lifestyle on quality of life in patients with multimorbidities.

Socioeconomic factors such as age, gender, and employment status have consistently been reported to be associated with quality of life in patients with multimorbidities (Brettschneider et al., 2013; Millá-Perseguer et al., 2019). However, living alone and sedentary behavior are two factors that have been rarely examined. Therefore, this study was developed to identify the effects of living alone and of sedentary behavior on the health-related quality of life of adult patients with multiple chronic conditions in all age groups. Moreover, by utilizing nationally representative population-based data, the authors of this study intend to provide more-generalizable findings that explain the associated factors to help patients with multimorbidities achieve a better quality of life.

Methods

Study Population and Sample
This study employed a secondary analysis of the 2017 Korea National Health and Nutrition Examination Survey (KNHANES), which included the second year data of the seventh KNHANES (KNHANES VII-2). The KNHANES, which began in 1998, is a community-based national database. The data are collected and managed by the Korea Ministry of Health and Welfare. The KNHANES VII-2 includes nationally representative data on 8,127 people and covers the following three main sections: health survey, physical and laboratory tests, and nutrition survey. The 1,725 data sets from adult patients in the KNHANES VII-2 who had multiple chronic conditions were used in this study. All of the participants in this study were adult patients aged 19 years and above with two or more chronic diseases who were living in the community.

The KNHANES provides open data to researchers, which may be utilized after registration. The raw data do not include any personal identifiers and thus comply with the Personal Information Protection Act and Statistics Act. This study was exempted from review by the institutional review board of Seoul National University.

Study Variables
The variables focused on in this study included living arrangement, sedentary behavior, and health-related quality of life. The covariates addressed included gender, age, employment status, and number of chronic diseases, which have been reported in previous research as factors associated with quality of life in patients with multimorbidities (Brettschneider et al., 2013; Millá-Perseguer et al., 2019; Rothrock et al., 2010; Tyack et al., 2018). These data were obtained from the health survey section of the KNHANES VII-2.

Living arrangement was determined based on the response of survey participants to a question about the number of members in their household. Sedentary behavior was assessed in terms of the average amount of time (in hours and minutes) that survey participants reported spending sitting or lying down each day outside normal sleeping hours. For convenience, the average amount of time spent in sedentary behavior was expressed in hours only in this study.

Health-related quality of life was investigated using the EQ-5D questionnaire, with scores of 1 = *no disruption* or *no problem*, 2 = *little disruption* or *some problems*, and 3 = *cannot* or *extreme problems* used in each of the five dimensions of mobility, self-care, usual activities, pain/discomfort, and anxiety/depression. The EQ-5D index value used in this study was converted using the South Korean population-based preference weight, which was established by Y. K. Lee et al. (2009), with negative values, 0, and 1 indicating "worse than death," "death," and "full health," respectively, with higher EQ-5D scores indicating better health-related quality of life. The validity and reliability of the Korean version of EQ-5D have been confirmed in previous studies (Kim et al., 2005; S. I. Lee, 2011).

In terms of the covariates, employment status was categorized into "yes" (employed) or "no" (not employed), and the number of chronic diseases was calculated as the sum of the "currently prevalent" answers to questions about 33 diseases, including circulatory diseases (hypertension, dyslipidemia, stroke, etc.), musculoskeletal diseases (osteoarthritis, osteoporosis, etc.), respiratory diseases (pulmonary tuberculosis, asthma, etc.), endocrine and metabolic diseases (diabetes, thyroid disease), cancer, digestive diseases (hepatitis B, hepatitis C, etc.), "other" diseases (neurologic, sensory, urinary, reproductive, and dermatological), and eye and ear diseases.

Statistical Analyses

Two-stage stratified cluster sampling was used in the KNHANES VII-2. Multiple survey and sampling methods were employed to ensure the nationally representative nature of this database. If an analysis does not consider the sampling procedure when selecting subpopulations from this type of data or when deleting missing cases, the results of the analysis may be biased. Therefore, all of the statistical analyses in this study took into account the components of the complex sampling design, including strata, clusters, weights, and adjustment procedures, with missing data treated in a valid manner (Korea Centers for Disease Control and Prevention, 2019). The significance level was set to .05, and all numbers were rounded off.

Living arrangement was classified as either single household (1) or multiperson household (0). The EQ-5D index, which was used in this study to evaluate health-related quality of life and which was originally a continuous variable, was coded as a dichotomous variable based on the average score of 0.905 because of a ceiling effect in the distribution where many respondents answered "full health" (Song et al., 2018). An above-average quality of life score was coded as 1, and an average or less-than-average score was coded as 0 (2018). The mean value for the quality of life of the participants in this study was used as the cutoff point because the EQ-5D index score based on the Korean population preference weight does not provide a specific index value as a cutoff point.

Multiple logistic regression was conducted to identify the effects of living alone and of sedentary behavior on health-related quality of life. In Model 1, gender, age, employment status, and number of chronic diseases were included as independent variables. In Model 2, living arrangement was introduced and adjusted for gender, age, employment status, and number of chronic diseases. Sedentary behavior was introduced in Model 3.

Results

The sociodemographic and health-related characteristics of the participants are shown in Table 1. Of the 1,725 individuals with multiple chronic conditions in the 2017 KNHANES, 1,057 (61.3%) were female. The mean age of the sample used in this study was 60.76 years, with the ≥ 65-year-old group accounting for the largest proportion. In terms of employment

Table 1

Sociodemographic and Health-Related Characteristics of Patients With Multiple Chronic Conditions (N = 1,725)

Variable (Category)	n	%
Gender		
Male	668	38.7
Female	1,057	61.3
Age (years; M and SD)	60.76	0.56
19–29	43	2.5
30–39	54	3.1
40–49	118	6.8
50–64	566	32.8
≥ 65	944	54.7
Employment status		
Yes (employed)	775	44.9
No (not employed)	941	54.6
Nonresponse (missing)	9	0.5
Number of chronic diseases (n; M and SD)	2.80	0.03
2	860	49.9
3	458	26.6
4	245	14.2
≥ 5	162	9.4
Living arrangement		
Single household	351	20.3
Multiperson household	1,374	79.7
Sedentary behavior (hours/day; M and SD)	8.21	0.12
Health-related quality of life [a] (index score; M and SD)	0.90	0.00

[a] Using the European Quality of Life-5 Dimensions questionnaire.

status, there were slightly more unemployed individuals (54.6%) than employed individuals (44.9%). The average number of chronic diseases was 2.80, with the largest proportion of participants reporting two chronic diseases (860, 49.9%). Multiperson households (79.7%) outnumbered single households (20.3%). The average duration of sedentary behavior was 8.21 hours, and the average health-related quality of life score was 0.90. The prevalence of each chronic disease (i.e., the frequency of the "currently prevalent" answer for each disease) is shown in Table 2. Hypertension (1,058) was the most common chronic disease, followed by dyslipidemia (775), osteoarthritis (561), and diabetes (482).

The unadjusted odds ratio (OR) for higher health-related quality of life for each variable is as follows. The odds of higher health-related quality of life were greater in men than in women (OR = 2.03, 95% confidence interval [CI; 1.61, 2.56]) and greater in employed individuals than in unemployed individuals (OR = 3.50, 95% CI [2.76, 4.46]). In addition, the odds of higher health-related quality of life decreased with age (OR = 0.95, 95% CI [0.93, 0.97]) and were lower for those with more chronic diseases (OR = 0.62, 95% CI [0.55, 0.69]), who lived in single households

Table 2

Prevalence of Each Chronic Disease
(N = 1,725)

Chronic Disease	n	%
Hypertension	1,058	61.3
Dyslipidemia	775	44.9
Osteoarthritis	561	32.5
Diabetes	482	27.9
Cataract	361	20.9
Osteoporosis	360	20.9
Allergic rhinitis	305	17.7
Depression	118	6.8
Sinusitis	109	6.3
Asthma	95	5.5
Stroke	95	5.5
Angina pectoris	87	5.0
Thyroid disease	84	4.9
Rheumatoid arthritis	79	4.6
Glaucoma	73	4.2
Myocardial infarction	58	3.4
Atopic dermatitis	56	3.2
Macular degeneration	33	1.9
Other cancer 1	31	1.8
Tympanitis	30	1.7
Thyroid cancer	29	1.7
Hepatitis B	27	1.6
Liver cirrhosis	17	1.0
Renal failure	14	0.8
Breast cancer	11	0.6
Colorectal cancer	8	0.5
Gastric cancer	8	0.5
Liver cancer	6	0.3
Lung cancer	6	0.3
Hepatitis C	6	0.3
Cervical cancer	5	0.3
Pulmonary tuberculosis	2	0.1
Other cancer 2	1	0.1

Note. "Other cancer 1" indicates cancers other than thyroid, breast, colorectal, gastric, liver, lung, and cervical cancers. "Other cancer 2" indicates having one more "other" cancer.

$(OR = 0.43, 95\%$ CI $[0.32, 0.57])$, and who reported longer sedentary times $(OR = 0.90, 95\%$ CI $[0.87, 0.94])$.

Multiple logistic regression was performed to identify the effects of living arrangement and sedentary behavior on quality of life (Table 3). Model 1 is a basic regression model that included gender, age, employment status, and number of chronic diseases $(R^2 = .21, p < .001)$. The odds of high health-related quality of life were found to be greater in men than in women $(OR = 1.39, 95\%$ CI $[1.06, 1.82])$ and in employed individuals than in unemployed individuals $(OR = 2.20, 95\%$ CI $[1.59, 3.04])$. Furthermore, the odds of high health-related quality of life decreased with age $(OR = 0.97, 95\%$ CI $[0.95, 0.99])$ and in participants with more chronic diseases $(OR = 0.75, 95\%$ CI $[0.66, 0.84])$. The living arrangement variable was introduced in Model 2 $(R^2 = .21, p < .001)$. After adjusting for gender, age, employment status, and number of chronic diseases, the odds of high health-related quality of life were shown to be lower in participants living in single households than in those living in multiperson households $(OR = 0.62, 95\%$ CI $[0.46, 0.84])$. The sedentary behavior variable was introduced in Model 3 $(R^2 = .22, p < .001)$. After adjusting for gender, age, employment status, number of chronic diseases, and living arrangement, the odds of high health-related quality of life decreased as sedentary time increased $(OR = 0.93, 95\%$ CI $[0.89, 0.96])$.

Discussion

Multimorbidity has become a global health priority (Navickas et al., 2016) and is a growing issue in nursing. Research into the impact of multimorbidity on patients' lives may support nurses' daily practice (O'Connor et al., 2018). Moreover, identifying the social factors that relate to the health of patients with multimorbidities is important for nurses to help them understand the context and barriers that patients experience (Northwood et al., 2018). This study focused on the quality of life of individuals with multimorbidities and explored the related factors.

Number of chronic diseases was found to be associated with their health-related quality of life. This result is consistent with previous research. A recent review also reported that having multiple diseases is closely correlated with quality of life (Makovski et al., 2019). Moreover, in the South Korean population with multimorbidity, it has been shown that an increased number of chronic diseases is a predictor of low health-related quality of life in young adults as well as older adults (Joe et al., 2016). Adding one chronic condition causes more-complicated care issues.

In this study, living arrangement was found to be a significant predictor of health-related quality of life in patients with multiple chronic diseases, even after controlling for age, gender, employment status, and number of diseases. The effect of living alone on persons with multiple chronic diseases has rarely been studied. Nevertheless, some studies have explored the health outcomes of living alone by focusing on a single chronic condition such as cardiovascular disease, diabetes, and cancer. Ma (2018) found that older people with hypertension who live alone exhibit more depressive symptoms. It has also been reported that patients with heart failure who live alone have higher readmission rates than those who live with family members (Lu et al., 2016). Moreover, living alone is associated with lower

Table 3

Logistic Regression Analysis of Living Arrangement and Sedentary Behavior on Health-Related Quality of Life (N = 1,725)

Variable (Category)	Model 1			Model 2			Model 3		
	Adjusted *OR*	95% CI	*p*	Adjusted *OR*	95% CI	*p*	Adjusted *OR*	95% CI	*p*
Gender			.016			.023			.015
Male (ref: female)	1.39	[1.06, 1.82]		1.37	[1.05, 1.79]		1.42	[1.07, 1.87]	
Age	0.97	[0.95, 0.99]	.001	0.97	[0.95, 0.99]	.001	0.97	[0.95, 0.99]	.001
Employment status			< .001			< .001			< .001
Yes (ref: no)	2.20	[1.59, 3.04]		2.15	[1.57, 2.95]		1.99	[1.46, 2.70]	
Number of chronic diseases	0.75	[0.66, 0.84]	< .001	0.76	[0.67, 0.85]	< .001	0.79	[0.70, 0.89]	< .001
Living arrangement						.002			.013
Single household (ref: multiperson household)				0.62	[0.46, 0.84]		0.66	[0.47, 0.91]	
Sedentary behavior							0.93	[0.89, 0.96]	< .001
	Nagelkerke R^2 = .21, *p* < .001			R^2 = .21, *p* < .001			R^2 = .22, *p* < .001		

Note. OR = odds ratio; CI = confidence interval; ref = reference.

angina-related quality of life and higher mortality after myocardial infarction (Bucholz et al., 2011; Schmaltz et al., 2007). Thus, living alone has been reported as a factor associated with negative health outcomes among persons with chronic diseases. The findings of this study support this association in the population with multimorbidity.

A reason for the poorer health-related quality of life experienced by patients who live alone compared with that of those who live with family may be that they find it more difficult to manage their disease. Uchmanowicz et al. (2018) found that older adults with hypertension who live alone have a lower level of treatment adherence. As living alone affects the disease management of patients with a single chronic condition, having multiple chronic conditions may affect this even more. In addition to disease management, activities of daily living may be another issue. There may be more barriers to food preparation, which is essential for a good health condition (Miyawaki et al., 2016). Household chores that help maintain a healthy and clean environment may also be more of a burden for patients who live alone. People with multiple chronic conditions have complex care needs. Thus, the families' and carers' contributions are important for helping patients manage their disease and their daily life to maintain health (O'Connor et al., 2018).

Another reason for lower health-related quality of life may be loneliness and social isolation. Living alone has been reported to be associated with loneliness and social isolation in general, which impacts health-related quality of life, particularly in the dimension of mental health (Beutel et al., 2017; Ge et al., 2017). Various nursing interventions have been developed to prevent or reduce loneliness and social isolation, including facilitating interpersonal interactions, conducting psychological therapies with group activities, providing health and social care support, and organizing

leisure activities (Gardiner et al., 2018). More research is needed to develop and test the effects of nursing interventions that are tailored to patients with comorbidities who live alone in the community.

In this study, sedentary behavior was found to be a significant predictor of health-related quality of life after controlling for age, gender, employment status, number of diseases, and living arrangement. For patients with chronic diseases, sedentary behavior may be a factor that worsens their health conditions. Sedentary behavior in patients with rheumatoid arthritis, for example, may exacerbate inflammation, resulting in increased pain, fatigue, and depression and decreased quality of life (Fenton et al., 2018). The findings of this study are meaningful as they elucidate the association between sedentary behavior and quality of life in populations with multimorbidities.

Although sedentary behavior is a risk factor affecting quality of life in patients with multimorbidities, the average number of sedentary hours in this study of 8.2 hours per day is more than the average 6.1 hours per day among the adult population in South Korea (Park et al., 2018). More research should be performed on nursing interventions that are designed to reduce sedentary hours and encourage a more active life and are tailored for multiple chronic conditions. Moreover, nurses who work with patients with multimorbidities need to plan strategies to curtail sedentary lifestyle habits. This might help people with multimorbidities to achieve a better quality of life.

This study has several limitations. First, the sum of the "currently prevalent" answers was used as the criterion for multimorbidity instead of examining medical records. Second, the effect of sedentary behavior on health-related quality of life may vary according to the signs/symptoms or severity of disease. This issue could not be addressed in this study because of the characteristics of the data. Third, this study could not consider variables beyond what was available in the original data set, and the range of control and the application of data were limited because this was a secondary analysis. Moreover, this study divided subjects into high EQ-5D and low EQ-5D groups using the average score of all participants. Therefore, the results must be interpreted cautiously. Finally, the health-related quality of life was not classified as a dimension in this study. Future study may examine if each dimension of the health-related quality of life is more greatly affected by living arrangement or sedentary behavior.

This study was the first in South Korea to identify the effects of living arrangement and sedentary behavior on health-related quality of life in patients with multiple chronic conditions. In addition, more-generalized results were obtained regarding adults of all ages using representative data from a population-based survey.

Conclusions

Multimorbidity is a global issue. Helping people with multimorbidities experience a better quality of life is an important part of the daily practice of nurses. In addition, living alone may increase the probability of patients with multimorbidities belonging to a comparatively lower-quality-of-life group. Nursing interventions that are tailored to patients who live alone should be helpful in managing the complicated issues that arise from having more than one disease. Moreover, sedentary behavior, which is a global health risk, increases the risk of having a comparatively lower quality of life in patients with multimorbidities. Their quality of life may be improved by making an effort to reduce their sedentary behavior.

Author Contributions

Study conception and design: All authors
Data collection: All authors
Data analysis and interpretation: All authors
Drafting of the article: All authors
Critical revision of the article: All authors

References

Beutel, M. E., Klein, E. M., Brähler, E., Reiner, I., Jünger, C., Michal, M., Wiltink, J., Wild, P. S., Münzel, T., Lackner, K. J., & Tibubos, A. N. (2017). Loneliness in the general population: Prevalence,

determinants and relations to mental health. *BMC Psychiatry,* *17*(1), Article No. 97. https://doi.org/10.1186/s12888-017-1262-x

Brettschneider, C., Leicht, H., Bickel, H., Dahlhaus, A., Fuchs, A., Gensichen, J., Maier, W., Riedel-Heller, S., Schafer, I., Schon, G., Weyerer, S., Wiese, B., van den Bussche, H., Scherer, M., Konig, H. H., & MultiCare Study Group. (2013). Relative impact of multimorbid chronic conditions on health-related quality of life—Results from the multicare cohort study. *PLOS ONE, 8*(6), Article e66742. https://doi.org/10.1371/journal.pone.0066742

Bucholz, E. M., Rathore, S. S., Gosch, K., Schoenfeld, A., Jones, P. G., Buchanan, D. M., Spertus, J. A., & Krumholz, H. M. (2011). Effect of living alone on patient outcomes after hospitalization for acute myocardial infarction. *The American Journal of Cardiology, 108* (7), 943–948. https://doi.org/10.1016/j.amjcard.2011.05.023

Fenton, S. A. M., Veldhuijzen van Zanten, J. J. C. S., Duda, J. L., Metsios, G. S., & Kitas, G. D. (2018). Sedentary behaviour in rheumatoid arthritis: Definition, measurement and implications for health. *Rheumatology, 57*(2), 213–226. https://doi.org/10.1093/rheumatology/kex053

Gardiner, C., Geldenhuys, G., & Gott, M. (2018). Interventions to reduce social isolation and loneliness among older people: An integrative review. *Health and Social Care in the Community, 26*(2), 147–157. https://doi.org/10.1111/hsc.12367

Ge, L., Yap, C. W., Ong, R., & Heng, B. H. (2017). Social isolation, loneliness and their relationships with depressive symptoms: A population-based study. *PLOS ONE, 12*(8), Article e0182145. https://doi.org/10.1371/journal.pone.0182145

George, S. M., Alfano, C. M., Groves, J., Karabulut, Z., Haman, K. L., Murphy, B. A., & Matthews, C. E. (2014). Objectively measured sedentary time is related to quality of life among cancer survivors. *PLOS ONE, 9*(2), Article e87937. https://doi.org/10.1371/journal.pone.0087937

Heyworth, I. T., Hazell, M. L., Linehan, M. F., & Frank, T. L. (2009). How do common chronic conditions affect health-related quality of life? *British Journal of General Practice, 59*(568), e353–e358. https://doi.org/10.3399/bjgp09X453990

Joe, S., Lee, I., & Park, B. (2016). Factors influencing health-related quality of life of young adults and elderly with multimorbidity: A secondary analysis of the 2013 Korea Health Panel Data. *Journal of Korean Academy of Community Health Nursing, 27*(4), 358–369. https://doi.org/10.12799/jkachn.2016.27.4.358

Kim, M.-H., Cho, Y.-S., Uhm, W.-S., Kim, S., & Bae, S.-C. (2005). Cross-cultural adaptation and validation of the Korean version of the EQ-5D in patients with rheumatic diseases. *Quality of Life Research, 14*(5), 1401–1406. https://doi.org/10.1007/s11136-004-5681-z

King, D. E., Xiang, J., & Pilkerton, C. S. (2018). Multimorbidity trends in United States adults, 1988–2014. *The Journal of the American Board of Family Medicine, 31*(4), 503–513. https://doi.org/10.3122/jabfm.2018.04.180008

Korea Centers for Disease Control and Prevention. (2019). *The 11th National Health and Nutrition Examination Survey and Youth Risk Behavior Web-Based Survey Data Utilization Workshop.* Author. https://knhanes.cdc.go.kr/knhanes/sub03/sub03_07_01. do (Original work published in Korean)

Lee, S. I. (2011). *Validity and reliability evaluation for EQ-5D in Korea.* Korea Centers for Disease Control and Prevention. http://www.ndsl.kr/ndsl/commons/util/ndslOriginalView.do? cn=TRKO201300000474&dbt=TRKO (Original work published in Korean)

Lee, Y.-K., Nam, H.-S., Chuang, L.-H., Kim, K.-Y., Yang, H.-K.,

Kwon, I.-S., Kind, P., Kweon, S.-S., & Kim, Y.-T. (2009). South Korean time trade-off values for EQ-5D health states: Modeling with observed values for 101 health states. *Value in Health, 12*(8), 1187–1193. https://doi.org/10.1111/j.1524-4733.2009.00579.x

Lin, P.-C., Yen, M., & Fetzer, S. J. (2008). Quality of life in elders living alone in Taiwan. *Journal of Clinical Nursing, 17*(12), 1610–1617. https://doi.org/10.1111/j.1365-2702.2007.02081.x

Low, L. L., Kwan, Y. H., Ko, M. S. M., Yeam, C. T., Lee, V. S. Y., Tan, W. B., & Thumboo, J. (2019). Epidemiologic characteristics of multimorbidity and sociodemographic factors associated with multimorbidity in a rapidly aging Asian country. *JAMA Network Open, 2*(11), Article e1915245. https://doi.org/10.1001/jamanetworkopen.2019.15245

Lu, M. L. R., Davila, C. D., Shah, M., Wheeler, D. S., Ziccardi, M. R., Banerji, S., & Figueredo, V. M. (2016). Marital status and living condition as predictors of mortality and readmissions among African Americans with heart failure. *International Journal of Cardiology, 222*, 313–318. https://doi.org/10.1016/j.ijcard.2016.07.185

Ma, C. (2018). The prevalence of depressive symptoms and associated factors in countryside-dwelling older Chinese patients with hypertension. *Journal of Clinical Nursing, 27*(15–16), 2933–2941. https://doi.org/10.1111/jocn.14349

Makovski, T. T., Schmitz, S., Zeegers, M. P., Stranges, S., & van den Akker, M. (2019). Multimorbidity and quality of life: Systematic literature review and meta-analysis. *Aging Research Review, 53*, Article 100903. https://doi.org/10.1016/j.arr.2019.04.005

McDaid, O., Hanly, M. J., Richardson, K., Kee, F., Kenny, R. A., & Savva, G. M. (2013). The effect of multiple chronic conditions on self-rated health, disability and quality of life among the older populations of Northern Ireland and the Republic of Ireland: A comparison of two nationally representative cross-sectional surveys. *BMJ Open, 3*(6), Article e002571. https://doi.org/10.1136/bmjopen-2013-002571

Millá-Perseguer, M., Guadalajara-Olmeda, N., Vivas-Consuelo, D., & Usó-Talamantes, R. (2019). Measurement of health-related quality by multimorbidity groups in primary health care. *Health and Quality of Life Outcomes, 17*(1), Article No. 8. https://doi.org/10.1186/s12955-018-1063-z

Miyawaki, Y., Shimizu, Y., & Seto, N. (2016). Classification of support needs for elderly outpatients with diabetes who live alone. *Canadian Journal of Diabetes, 40*(1), 43–49. https://doi.org/10.1016/j.jcjd.2015.09.005

Navickas, R., Petric, V. K., Feigl, A. B., & Seychell, M. (2016). Multimorbidity: What do we know? What should we do? *Journal of Comorbidity, 6*(1), 4–11. https://doi.org/10.15256/joc.2016.6.72

Northwood, M., Ploeg, J., Markle-Reid, M., & Sherifali, D. (2018). Integrative review of the social determinants of health in older adults with multimorbidity. *Journal of Advanced Nursing, 74*(1), 45–60. https://doi.org/10.1111/jan.13408

Nunes, B. P., Flores, T. R., Mielke, G. I., Thumé, E., & Facchini, L. A. (2016). Multimorbidity and mortality in older adults: A systematic review and meta-analysis. *Archives of Gerontology and Geriatrics, 67*, 130–138. https://doi.org/10.1016/j.archger.2016.07.008

O'Connor, S., Deaton, C., Nolan, F., & Johnston, B. (2018). Nursing in an age of multimorbidity. *BMC Nursing, 17*, Article No. 49. https://doi.org/10.1186/s12912-018-0321-z

Palladino, R., Pennino, F., Finbarr, M., Millett, C., & Triassi, M. (2019). Multimorbidity and health outcomes in older adults in ten European health systems, 2006–15. *Health Affairs, 38*(4), 613–623. https://doi.org/10.1377/hlthaff.2018.05273

Park, J. H., Joh, H. K., Lee, G. S., Je, S. J., Cho, S. H., Kim, S. J., Oh, S. W., & Kwon, H. T. (2018). Association between sedentary time and cardiovascular risk factors in Korean adults. *Korean Journal of Family Medicine, 39*(1), 29–36. (Original work published in Korean)

Prazeres, F., & Santiago, L. (2015). Prevalence of multimorbidity in the adult population attending primary care in Portugal: A cross-sectional study. *BMJ Open, 5*(9), Article e009287. https://doi.org/10.1136/bmjopen-2015-009287

Rothrock, N. E., Hays, R. D., Spritzer, K., Yount, S. E., Riley, W., & Cella, D. (2010). Relative to the general US population, chronic diseases are associated with poorer health-related quality of life as measured by the Patient-Reported Outcomes Measurement Information System (PROMIS). *Journal of Clinical Epidemiology, 63*(11), 1195–1204. https://doi.org/10.1016/j.jclinepi.2010.04.012

Schmaltz, H. N., Southern, D., Ghali, W. A., Jelinski, S. E., Parsons, G. A., King, K. M., & Maxwell, C. J. (2007). Living alone, patient sex and mortality after acute myocardial infarction. *Journal of General Internal Medicine, 22*(5), 572–578. https://doi.org/10.1007/s11606-007-0106-7

Shofany, C. (2017). Quality of life among chronic disease patients. *Nursing & Care Open Access Journal, 4*(2), 385–394. https://doi.org/10.15406/ncoaj.2017.04.00103

Song, H. J., Park, S., & Kwon, J. W. (2018). Quality of life of middle-aged adults in single households in South Korea. *Quality of Life Research, 27*, 2117–2125. https://doi.org/10.1007/s11136-018-1858-8

Statistics Korea. (2020). *2019 census of population and housing (registration census method aggregation result)*. Ministry of Economy and Finance. http://kostat.go.kr/ (Original work published in Korean)

Sun, X., Lucas, H., Meng, Q., & Zhang, Y. (2011). Associations between living arrangements and health-related quality of life of urban elderly people: A study from China. *Quality of Life Research, 20*(3), 359–369. https://doi.org/10.1007/s11136-010-9752-z

Tremblay, M. S., Colley, R. C., Saunders, T. J., Healy, G. N., & Owen, N. (2010). Physiological and health implications of a sedentary lifestyle. *Applied Physiology, Nutrition, and Metabolism, 35*(6), 725–740. https://doi.org/10.1139/H10-079

Tyack, Z., Kuys, S., Cornwell, P., Frakes, K., & McPhaill, S. (2018). Health-related quality of life of people with multimorbidity at a community-based, interprofessional student-assisted clinic: Implications for assessment and intervention. *Chronic Illness, 14*(3), 169–181. https://doi.org/10.1177/1742395317724849

Uchmanowicz, B., Chudiak, A., Uchmanowicz, I., Rosinczuk, J., & Froelicher, E. S. (2018). Factors influencing adherence to treatment in older adults with hypertension. *Clinical Interventions in Aging, 13*, 2425–2441. https://doi.org/10.2147/CIA.S182881

van der Ploeg, H. P., Chey, T., Korda, R. J., Banks, E., & Bauman, A. (2012). Sitting time and all-cause mortality risk in 222,497 Australian adults. *Archives of Internal Medicine, 172*(6), 494–500. https://doi.org/10.1001/archinternmed.2011.2174

van Oostrom, S. H., Gijsen, R., Stirbu, I., Korevaar, J. C., Schellevis, F. G., Picavet, H. S. J., & Hoeymans, N. (2016). Time trends in prevalence of chronic diseases and multimorbidity not only due to aging: Data from general practices and health surveys. *PLOS ONE, 11*(8), Article e0160264. https://doi.org/10.1371/journal.pone.0160264

20

Effects of Patient Activation Intervention on Chronic Diseases

Mei-Yu LIN[1] • Wei-Shih WENG[2] • Renny Wulan APRILIYASARI[3] • Pham VAN TRUONG[4] • Pei-Shan TSAI[5]*

ABSTRACT

Background: Patient activation has been described as a potential strategy to improve chronic disease self-management. However, the effects of patient activation interventions on psychological and behavioral outcomes have not been systematically evaluated.

Purpose: This study was designed to evaluate the effects of patient activation interventions on physiological, psychological, behavioral, and health-related quality of life outcomes in patients with chronic diseases.

Methods: We systematically searched four databases (PubMed, Cochrane, CINAHL, and Embase) from inception to September 1, 2017. We identified English- and Chinese-language published reports of randomized controlled trials that evaluated the effects of patient activation interventions for adults with chronic diseases. Study selection, data extraction, and quality assessment were performed by two reviewers independently. We summarized the intervention effects with Hedges's g values and 95% confidence intervals using a random-effects model. We used the Cochrane Handbook to assess the methodological quality of the randomized controlled trials.

Results: Twenty-six randomized controlled trials were included in the qualitative synthesis and meta-analysis. In terms of overall study quality, most of the included studies were affected by performance and detection bias. Patient activation interventions produced significant effects on outcomes related to physiological, psychological, behavioral, and health-related quality of life in the context of chronic diseases. The following effect sizes were obtained: (a) physiological, namely, glycated hemoglobin = −0.31 ($p < .01$), systolic blood pressure = −0.20 ($p < .01$), diastolic blood pressure = −0.80 ($p = .02$), body weight = −0.12 ($p = .03$), and low-density lipoprotein = −0.21 ($p = .01$); (b) psychological, namely, depression = −0.16 ($p < .01$) and anxiety = −0.25 ($p = .01$); (c) behavioral, namely, patient activation = 0.33 ($p < .01$) and self-efficacy = 0.57 ($p < .01$); and (d) health-related quality of life = 0.25 ($p = .01$).

Conclusions: Patient activation interventions significantly improve patients' physiological, psychosocial, and behavioral health statuses. Healthcare providers should implement patient activation interventions that tailor support to the individual patients' level of patient activation and strengthen the patients' role in managing their healthcare to improve chronic-disease-related health outcomes.

KEY WORDS:
chronic disease, meta-analysis, depression, anxiety, self-efficacy.

Introduction

Patient activation, which is defined as having the knowledge, skill, and confidence to manage one's health, emphasizes patients' willingness and ability to take independent actions to manage their health and care (Hibbard et al., 2004). Patient activation, or engaging patients in their own care, has been described as a potential strategy to improve chronic disease self-management (Hibbard et al., 2007). Raising levels of patient activation is desirable because patients who are more activated are more likely to engage in self-management behaviors that improve health (Hibbard et al., 2007; Jacobson et al., 2018). Patient activation is a critical component of management strategies for patients with chronic diseases and is the least well-developed intervention within chronic disease care (Hibbard et al., 2007). Patient activation interventions have focused specifically on a tailored approach to improve patients' motivation, knowledge, skills, and confidence to manage their health (Hibbard et al., 2004; Young et al., 2016). For example, health coaching is a patient-oriented intervention that activates patients to change their behavior (Bennett et al., 2010; Olsen, 2014). Empowerment is an intervention to help people make behavior changes to adhere to a care plan. Patients are empowered when they have the necessary knowledge, skills, attitudes, and self-awareness to change both their behavior and the behavior of others to improve their quality of life (Funnell et al., 1991; Tol et al., 2015). Self-management programs that focus on skill development, problem solving, and/or peer support are believed to increase the activation levels of patients (Greene & Hibbard, 2012). Strategies

[1]*PhD, RN, Postdoctoral Fellow, School of Nursing, College of Nursing, Taipei Medical University, Taiwan, ROC* • [2]*MSN, RN, Department of Nursing, Tri-Service General Hospital, Taiwan, ROC* • [3]*MSN, Doctoral Student, School of Nursing, College of Nursing, Taipei Medical University, Taiwan, ROC; and Nursing Lecturer, Sekolah Tinggi Ilmu Kesehatan Cendekia Utama Kudus, Indonesia* • [4]*MSN, Doctoral Student, School of Nursing, College of Nursing, Taipei Medical University, Taiwan, ROC* • [5]*PhD, RN, Professor, School of Nursing, College of Nursing, Taipei Medical University; Department of Nursing, & Center for Nursing and Healthcare Research in Clinical Practice Application, Wan Fang Hospital, Taipei Medical University; and Sleep Research Center, Taipei Medical University Hospital, Taiwan, ROC.*

commonly used in patient activation interventions include problem solving, feedback, individualized care plans, peer support, lay health advisors, theory-based counseling, and skill building (Bolen et al., 2014).

Noncommunicable diseases, also known as chronic diseases, are defined by the World Health Organization as diseases that have a long duration, have generally slow progression, and are not passed from person to person. Diseases of this type are a leading global health problem and a significant cause of premature death (World Health Organization, 2018). Patients with chronic diseases must become their own principal caregiver and take responsibility for daily disease management, behavioral changes, management of emotions, and accurate reporting on disease status (Holman & Lorig, 2004). Therefore, important outcomes for the self-management of chronic diseases include physiologic, psychological, and behavioral outcomes.

Patient activation has been associated with outcomes of care for patients with chronic conditions (Hibbard et al., 2007; Mosen et al., 2007). Patient activation is strongly related to a broad range of health-related outcomes, and related interventions have great potential and must be examined to assess their effectiveness (Greene & Hibbard, 2012). In addition, emerging evidence suggests that patient activation is a factor that may predict the health status of patients with chronic diseases (Hibbard & Greene, 2013). A previous meta-analysis revealed that patient activation interventions were associated with improvements in clinical outcomes such as glycated hemoglobin (HbA1C), systolic blood pressure (SBP), body weight, and low-density lipoprotein (LDL) in adults with diabetes mellitus (Bolen et al., 2014). The effects of patient activation interventions on psychological and behavioral outcomes have not been evaluated systematically. Thus, despite widespread research into interventions to improve patient activation, the effect of patient activation interventions on chronic conditions remains unclear. No systematic review or meta-analysis has been conducted since 2014 on the effect of patient activation interventions on patients with chronic diseases. Cardiovascular disease, cancer, chronic respiratory diseases, and diabetes mellitus are the largest causes of death worldwide (World Health Organization, 2018). Therefore, we conducted a meta-analysis of randomized controlled trials to quantify the outcomes of physiological, psychological, behavioral, and health-related quality of life (HRQOL) for patient activation interventions across these four chronic disease categories.

Methods

This study conformed to the Preferred Reporting Items for Systematic Reviews and Meta-Analyses statement.

Search Strategy

Four electronic databases (PubMed, Cochrane, CINAHL, and Embase) were searched from their inception to September 1, 2017, using the following strings of keywords:

("cardiovascular" OR "coronary heart disease" OR "coronary artery disease" OR "heart failure" OR "hypertension" OR "blood pressure" OR "peripheral vessel disease" OR "cancer" OR "neoplasm" OR "tumor" OR "malignancy" OR "oncology" OR "neoplasm" OR "carcinoma" OR "diabetes" OR "diabetes mellitus" OR "DM" OR "chronic obstructive pulmonary disease" OR "COPD" OR "chronic respiratory disease" OR "lung" OR "pulmonary" OR "asthma" OR "noncommunicable diseases") AND ("patient activation" OR "activation intervention" OR "PAM" OR "empowerment" OR "patient engagement" OR "patient participation" OR "coaching" OR "motivational interviewing" OR "self-management") AND ("randomized controlled trial" OR "controlled clinical trial" OR "random allocation" OR "randomization" OR "RCT"). Furthermore, references from the retrieved articles were reviewed to identify additional, potentially relevant studies.

Study Eligibility

Reports of randomized controlled trials published in either English or Chinese that enrolled adults aged 18 years or older with a diagnosis of cardiovascular disease, cancer, chronic respiratory disease, or diabetes mellitus and used an intervention (i.e., health coaching, empowerment, self-management programs, or patient activation programs) to increase patients' knowledge, skills, and confidence to self-manage their health were eligible for inclusion. Outcomes of interest were physiological (i.e., HbA1C, SBP, diastolic blood pressure [DBP], body weight, and LDL), psychosocial (i.e., depression, anxiety, and HRQOL), and behavioral (i.e., patient activation and self-efficacy).

Study Selection

The initial screening was performed by two reviewers who independently screened the titles and abstracts of potentially relevant studies. Full texts of the studies that met the inclusion criteria were retrieved and evaluated independently for inclusion by the two reviewers. Any disagreements were resolved by discussion, and if necessary, a third reviewer was involved.

Data Extraction

Data regarding the study design, participant characteristics, interventions, and outcome measures were extracted independently by the same two reviewers. A self-developed data extraction form was used to extract data. We contacted the authors of primary reports to request any unpublished data. If no response or additional data were received from an author, the available data only were used in the analysis.

Quality Assessment

The two reviewers independently assessed the methodological quality of the included randomized controlled trials using the Cochrane Handbook for assessing the risk of bias (Higgins et al., 2011). We evaluated random sequence generation, allocation concealment, blinding of participants and personnel, blinding of outcome assessment, incomplete outcome data, and selective reporting. Disagreements were resolved through discussion and by consultation with the third reviewer.

Statistical Analysis

All statistical analyses were performed using Comprehensive Meta-Analysis software 2.0. Hedges's g was used to interpret the values of effect sizes established for our pooled estimates. Furthermore, 95% confidence intervals were assessed using a random-effects model. A two-sided p value of < .05 was used to indicate statistical significance.

Egger's regression was used to assess publication bias, and I^2 or Q value was used to assess the statistical heterogeneity and inconsistency of study results. Subgroup and moderator analyses according to type of intervention, type of disease, intervention delivery mode, and intervention duration were conducted to explore possible sources of heterogeneity in the effect sizes. We conducted subgroup analyses when at least two studies could be included in each subgroup. Moderator variables were analyzed using an analog to the analysis of variance for categorical moderators that compare within- and between-group heterogeneity using the Q statistic. Age and gender are associated with health-related behaviors (Deeks et al., 2009). Therefore, we examined the impact of age and gender on the estimates of treatment effect. We conducted a meta-regression analysis on mean age and percentage of female participants as independent variables, using heterogeneous outcomes as the dependent variables.

Results

Search Retrievals

The search of electronic databases identified an initial set of 5,761 publications. After removing duplicates, 3,293 titles and abstracts were screened and 47 full-text articles were retrieved for full-text assessment. The selection process is illustrated in Figure 1.

Study Characteristics

In total, 26 published studies assessing the effects of a patient activation intervention on patients with chronic diseases were included. We performed a qualitative synthesis and meta-analysis of 26 randomized controlled trials. All of the studies were published between 2005 and 2017. Sixteen studies assessed HbA1C, nine studies assessed SBP, seven studies assessed DBP, five studies assessed body weight, eight studies assessed LDL, eight studies assessed depression, three studies assessed anxiety, five studies assessed patient activation, 11 studies assessed self-efficacy, and nine studies assessed HRQOL. Thirteen studies were conducted in the United States; four, in Europe; two, in Taiwan; two, in Iran; two, in China; one, in South Korea; one, in Australia; and one, in

Thailand. The detailed information, including participant and design characteristics, of the 26 included studies are summarized in Table 1.

Publication Bias

The results of Egger's regression analyses were not significant in any of the outcomes assessed.

Quality Assessment

In terms of overall study quality, most of the included studies were subject to performance bias and detection bias. Table 2 illustrates the risk of bias of each study.

Physiological Effects: Glycated Hemoglobin

The effects of patient activation interventions on patients' HbA1C were evaluated in 16 studies, and the pooled effect was statistically significant. The study population included patients with diabetes mellitus and patients with cardiovascular disease. The effect on HbA1C had an effect size of −0.31 (p < .01), which indicated a small effect (Table 3). The studies were moderately heterogeneous (I^2 = 74.12, p < .01). The moderator analysis indicated no significant differences in effect sizes for HbA1C among the three types of interventions (p = .20; Table 4), suggesting that the size of the effect for HbA1C was not influenced by intervention type. Interventions varied in length from 6 weeks to 18 months. The moderator analysis indicated no significant differences in effect sizes for HbA1C among the three intervention durations, suggesting that the size of the effect for HbA1C was not influenced by intervention duration (p = .25; Table 4). The intervention delivery mode was face-to-face plus telephone support in 10 studies, face-to-face only in three studies, and telephone support only in three studies. The moderator analysis indicated no significant differences in effect sizes for HbA1C among the three intervention delivery modes, suggesting that the size of the effect for HbA1C was not influenced by intervention delivery mode (p = .26; Table 4). Meta-regression results showed a significant association between mean age and the effect size of HbA1C (p = .01; Table 5). No significant association was found between the effect size of HbA1C and the percentage of female participants (p = .83; Table 5).

Physiological Effects: Systolic Blood Pressure

The effects of patient activation interventions on patients' SBP were evaluated in nine studies, and the pooled effect was statistically significant. The study population included patients with diabetes mellitus and patients with cardiovascular disease. The effect on SBP had an effect size of −0.20 (p < .01), which indicated a small effect (Table 3). The studies were unlikely to be heterogeneous (I^2 < 0.01, p = .44). Although significant heterogeneity in the effect sizes of SBP was not found, a moderator analysis was performed, which indicated no significant

Figure 1

Preferred Reporting Items for Systematic Reviews and Meta-Analyses Flowchart for Study Selection

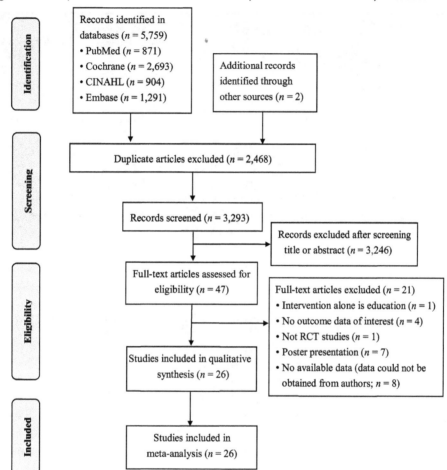

differences in effect sizes for SBP among the three intervention types (p = .09; Table 4). Interventions varied in length from 5 weeks to 15 months. The moderator analysis indicated no significant differences in effect sizes for SBP among the three intervention durations (p = .71; Table 4). The intervention delivery mode was face-to-face plus telephone support in six studies, face-to-face only in one study, and telephone support only in two studies. The moderator analysis indicated no significant differences in effect sizes for SBP between the two intervention delivery modes, suggesting that SBP effect size was not influenced by intervention delivery mode (p = .19; Table 4).

Physiological Effects: Diastolic Blood Pressure

The effects of patient activation interventions on patients' DBP were evaluated in seven studies, and the pooled effect was statistically significant. The study population included patients with diabetes mellitus and patients with cardiovascular disease. The effect on DBP had an effect size of –0.80 (p = .02), indicating a large effect (Table 3). The studies were highly heterogeneous (I^2 = 97.34, p < .01). The moderator analysis showed no significant

differences in effect sizes for DBP between intervention types (p = .63; Table 4), suggesting that type of intervention is unable to explain the source of heterogeneity in the effect sizes for DBP. The duration of the interventions ranged from 5 weeks to 15 months. The moderator analysis showed no significant differences in effect sizes for DBP among the three intervention durations (p = .60; Table 4), suggesting that intervention duration is unable to explain the source of heterogeneity in the effect sizes for DBP. The intervention delivery mode was face-to-face plus telephone support in five studies, face-to-face only in one study, and telephone support only in one study. Meta-regression results showed no significant association between the effect size of DBP and mean age (p = .20; Table 5) or between the effect size of DPB and the percentage of female participants (p = .45; Table 5).

Physiological Effects: Body Weight

The effects of patient activation interventions on patients' body weight were evaluated in five studies, and the pooled effect was statistically significant. The study population included patients with diabetes mellitus and patients with

Table 1

Characteristics of the Studies Included in the Meta-Analysis

Author (Year)/ Location	Study Population	No. of Patients	Mean Age	Intervention		
				Type	Duration	Mode of Delivery
1. Yun et al. (2017)/ South Korea	Cancer	EG: 134 CG: 72	EG: 50.52 ± 10.21 CG: 51.04 ± 7.55	Health coaching	6 months	Face-to-face Telephone
2. Moein et al. (2017)/ Iran	DM	EG: 47 CG: 49	NA	Empowerment program	4 weeks	Face-to-face
3. Cortez et al. (2017)/ United States	DM	EG:127 CG:111	EG: 58.00 ± 9.20 CG: 57.50 ± 9.70	Empowerment program	Over 12 months	Face-to-face Telephone
4. Young et al. (2016)/ United States	HF	EG: 51 CG: 49	EG: 68.70 ± 11.80 CG: 71.80 ± 12.60	Patient activation	3 months	Face-to-face Telephone
5. Pauley et al. (2016)/ United States	DM	EG: 47 CG: 47	EG: 65.10 ± 13.20 CG: 66.90 ± 11.70	Self-management coaching	6 weeks	Face-to-face
6. Odnoletkova et al. (2016)/ Europe	DM	EG:287 CG:287	EG: 63.80 ± 8.70 CG:62.40 ± 8.90	Health coaching	6 months	Telephone
7. Meng et al. (2016)/ Europe	HF	EG: 248 CG: 227	EG: 61.20 ± 11.70 CG: 61.90 ± 11.20	Self-management	Not specified	Face-to-face
8. Ebrahimi et al. (2016)/ Iran	DM	EG: 53 CG: 53	EG: 46.97 ± 5.54 CG: 48.15 ± 6.52	Empowerment program	8 weeks	Face-to-face
9. Safford et al. (2015)/ United States	DM	EG: 168 CG: 192	EG: 59.20 ± 11.80 CG: 61.10 ± 12.40	Health coaching	10 months	Telephone
10. Chen et al. (2015)/ Taiwan, ROC	DM	EG: 36 CG: 36	EG: 62.12 ± 7.51 CG: 61.72 ± 8.79	Empowerment program	3 months	Face-to-face Telephone
11. Jonsdottir et al. (2015)/ Europe	COPD	EG: 48 CG: 52	EG: 59.41 ± 4.66 CG: 58.67 ± 4.39	Self-management	6 months	Face-to-face Telephone
12. García et al. (2015)/ United States	DM	EG: 39 CG: 33	EG: 50.00 ± 8.70 CG: 49.10 ± 9.70	Self-management	6 months	Face-to-face Telephone
13. Lynch et al. (2014)/ United States	DM and HT	EG: 30 CG: 31	EG: 53.40 ± 11.40 CG: 54.80 ± 8.50	Self-management	6 months	Face-to-face Telephone
14. Thom et al. (2013)/ United States	DM	EG: 148 CG: 151	EG: 56.30 ± 10.30 CG: 54.10 ± 10.40	Health coaching	6 months	Face-to-face Telephone
15. Shao et al. (2013)/ Taiwan, ROC	HF	EG: 54 CG: 54	EG: 72.20 ± 5.66 CG: 71.87 ± 5.34	Self-management	3 months	Face-to-face Telephone
16. Blackberry et al. (2013)/ Australia	DM	EG: 236 CG: 237	EG: 63.60 ± 10.40 CG: 61.90 ± 10.50	Empowerment-based health coaching	15 months	Face-to-face Telephone
17. Van der Wulp et al. (2012)/ Europe	DM	EG: 59 CG: 60	NA	Self-management coaching	3 months	Face-to-face Telephone
18. Li et al. (2012)/ China	DM	EG: 123 CG: 125	65.34 ± 12.25	Self-management	18 months	Face-to-face Telephone
19. Tousman et al. (2011)/ United States	Asthma	EG: 21 CG: 24	EG: 51.40 ± 14.70 CG: 55.00 ± 10.00	Self-management	7 weeks	Face-to-face
20. McGowan (2011)/ United States	DM	EG: 82 CG: 152	EG: 55.00 ± 12.00 CG: 59.00 ± 12.00	Self-management	6 weeks	Face-to-face
21. Wolever et al. (2010)/ United States	DM	EG: 30 CG: 26	EG: 53.10 ± 8.29 CG: 52.80 ± 7.64	Health coaching	6 months	Telephone

(continues)

Table 1

Characteristics of the Studies Included in the Meta-Analysis, Continued

Author (Year)/ Location	Study Population	No. of Patients	Mean Age	Intervention		
				Type	Duration	Mode of Delivery
22. Lorig et al. (2009)/ United States	DM	EG: 186 CG: 159	EG: 67.70 ± 11.90 CG: 65.40 ± 11.40	Self-management	6 weeks	Face-to-face
23. Anderson et al. (2009)/ United States	DM	EG: 156 CG: 154	EG: 55.50 ± 11.30 CG: 55.70 ± 11.50	Empowerment-based self-management	24 months	Face-to-face Telephone
24. Xue et al. (2008)/ China	HT	EG: 70 CG: 70	EG: 57.50 ± 6.96 CG: 57.40 ± 6.95	Self-management	5 weeks	Face-to-face
25. Keeratiyutawong et al. (2006)/ Thailand	DM	EG: 45 CG: 45	NA	Self-management	5 months	Face-to-face Telephone
26. Anderson et al. (2005)/ United States	DM	EG: 125 CG: 114	61.00 ± 11.40	Empowerment program	6 weeks	Face-to-face Telephone

Note. EG = experimental group; CG = control group; DM = diabetes mellitus; NA = not available; HF = heart failure; COPD = chronic obstructive pulmonary disease; HT = hypertension.

hypertension disease. The effect on body weight had an effect size of −0.12 ($p = .03$), indicating a small effect (Table 3). The studies were unlikely to be heterogeneous ($I^2 < 0.01, p = .86$). Although significant heterogeneity in the effect sizes of body weight was not found, a moderator analysis was performed. The duration of interventions ranged from 6 weeks to 15 months. The moderator analysis showed no significant differences in effect sizes for body weight between intervention durations ($p = .52$; Table 4).

Physiological Effects: Low-Density Lipoprotein

The effects of patient activation interventions on patients' LDL were evaluated in the population with diabetes in eight studies, and the pooled effect was statistically significant. The effect on LDL had an effect size of −0.21 ($p = .01$), indicating a small effect (Table 3). The studies were moderately heterogeneous ($I^2 = 61.60, p = .01$). The moderator analysis indicated no significant differences in effect sizes for LDL among the three types of interventions ($p = .60$; Table 4), suggesting that the size of the effect for LDL was not influenced by intervention type. Interventions varied in length from 6 weeks to over 12 months. The moderator analysis indicated no significant differences in effect sizes for LDL among the three intervention durations, suggesting that the size of the effect for LDL was not influenced by intervention duration ($p = .13$; Table 4). The intervention delivery mode was face-to-face plus telephone support in four studies, face-to-face only in two studies, and telephone support only in two studies. The moderator analysis indicated no significant differences in effect sizes for LDL among the three intervention delivery modes, suggesting that the size of the effect for LDL was not influenced by intervention delivery mode ($p = .80$; Table 4). Meta-regression results showed a significant association between mean age and the effect size of LDL ($p = .03$;

Table 5). No significant association was found between the effect size of LDL and the percentage of female participants ($p = .68$; Table 5).

Psychological Effects: Depression

The effects of patient activation interventions on patients' depression were evaluated in eight studies, and the pooled effect was statistically significant. The study population included patients with cancer, chronic respiratory diseases, and diabetes mellitus. The effect on depression had an effect size of −0.16 ($p < .01$), indicating a small effect (Table 3). The studies were unlikely to be heterogeneous ($I^2 < 0.01, p = .65$). Although significant heterogeneity in the effect sizes of depression was not found, a moderator analysis was performed, which found no significant differences in effect sizes for depression between types of disease ($p = .80$; Table 4). The duration of interventions ranged from 6 weeks to 24 months. The moderator analysis showed no significant differences in effect sizes for depression among the three intervention durations ($p = .51$; Table 4). The intervention delivery mode was face-to-face plus telephone support in five studies and face-to-face only in three studies. The moderator analysis showed no significant differences in effect sizes for depression between the two intervention delivery modes ($p = .11$; Table 4).

Psychological Effects: Anxiety

The effects of patient activation interventions on patients' anxiety were evaluated in three studies, and the pooled effect was statistically significant. The study population included patients with cancer, chronic respiratory diseases, and diabetes mellitus. The effect on anxiety had an effect size of −0.25 ($p = .01$), indicating a small effect (Table 3). The studies were unlikely to be heterogeneous ($I^2 < 0.01$, $p = .49$). Interventions varied in length from 6 weeks to 6 months. The intervention delivery mode was face-to-face

Risk of Bias Summary of Methodological Quality for Each Included Study

Author (Year)	Selection Bias		Performance Bias	Detection Bias		Attrition Bias	Reporting Bias
	Random Sequence Generation	Allocation Concealment	Blinding of Participants and Personnel	Blinding of Outcome Assessment (Patient-Reported Outcome)	Blinding of Outcome Assessment (Objective Outcome)	Incomplete Outcome Data	Selective Reporting
Yun et al. (2017)	+	?	?	−	−	+	+
Moein et al. (2017)	+	?	−	−	?	+	+
Cortez et al. (2017)	+	?	−	−	+	−	+
Young et al. (2016)	+	+	−	−	+	+	+
Pauley et al. (2016)	+	?	−	−	?	+	+
Odnoletkova et al. (2016)	+	?	−	?	+	+	+
Meng et al. (2016)	+	+	−	−	?	+	+
Ebrahimi et al. (2016)	+	?	+	?	+	+	+
Safford et al. (2015)	+	?	−	−	+	+	+
Chen et al. (2015)	+	+	−	+	+	+	+
Jonsdottir et al. (2015)	+	?	−	−	?	−	+
García et al. (2015)	?	?	−	+	+	+	+
Lynch et al. (2014)	+	+	?	−	+	+	+
Thom et al. (2013)	?	+	−	?	+	+	+
Shao et al. (2013)	+	+	+	−	?	+	+
Blackberry et al. (2013)	+	+	−	−	+	+	+
Van der Wulp et al. (2012)	+	+	−	+	?	+	+
Li et al. (2012)	?	?	−	?	+	?	+
Tousman et al. (2011)	?	?	−	−	+	+	+
McGowan (2011)	+	+	−	−	+	+	+
Wolever et al. (2010)	?	?	−	−	+	+	+
Lorig et al. (2009)	+	?	−	−	+	+	+
Anderson et al. (2009)	+	+	−	−	+	−	+
Xue et al. (2008)	+	+	−	−	+	+	+
Keeratiyutawong et al. (2006)	?	+	−	−	+	+	+
Anderson et al. (2005)	?	?	−	−	+	+	+

Note. + = low risk of bias; − = high risk of bias; ? = uncertain risk of bias.

Table 3

Effect Sizes for Studies Measuring Patient Activation Intervention on Outcomes

Study (Year)	Statistic for Each Study				Hedges's *g* and 95% CI
	Hedges's *g*	SE	Variance	*p*	
1. HbA1C					
Cortez et al. (2017)	−0.31	0.13	0.02	.02	
Odnoletkova et al. (2016)	−0.20	0.09	0.01	.02	
Ebrahimi et al. (2016)	−0.60	0.20	0.04	.00	
Safford et al. (2015)	−0.05	0.12	0.01	.68	
Chen et al. (2015)	−0.38	0.25	0.06	.12	
García et al. (2015)	−1.97	0.29	0.08	.00	
Lynch et al. (2014)	−0.45	0.27	0.07	.10	
Thom et al. (2013)	−0.26	0.13	0.02	.04	
Blackberry et al. (2013)	−0.04	0.10	0.01	.64	
Li et al. (2012)	−0.52	0.13	0.02	.00	
McGowan (2011)	−0.34	0.14	0.02	.01	
Wolever et al. (2010)	−0.38	0.27	0.07	.16	
Lorig et al. (2009)	−0.06	0.12	0.01	.60	
Anderson et al. (2009)	−0.15	0.13	0.02	.24	
Keeratiyutawong et al. (2006)	−0.06	0.22	0.05	.79	
Anderson et al. (2005)	−0.10	0.13	0.02	.43	
Total (95% CI)	−0.31	0.07	0.01	.00	
2. SBP					
Cortez et al. (2017)	−0.32	0.13	0.02	.01	
Odnoletkova et al. (2016)	−0.12	0.09	0.01	.16	
Safford et al. (2015)	−0.07	0.12	0.01	.59	
García et al. (2015)	−0.37	0.24	0.06	.12	
Lynch et al. (2014)	−0.16	0.27	0.07	.54	
Thom et al. (2013)	−0.20	0.13	0.02	.11	
Blackberry et al. (2013)	−0.20	0.10	0.01	.05	
Xue et al. (2008)	−0.57	0.17	0.03	.00	
Anderson et al. (2005)	−0.16	0.13	0.02	.24	
Total (95% CI)	−0.20	0.04	0.00	.00	
3. DBP					
Cortez et al. (2017)	−2.89	0.19	0.03	.00	
Odnoletkova et al. (2016)	−0.11	0.09	0.01	.21	
García et al. (2015)	−1.60	0.27	0.07	.00	
Lynch et al. (2014)	−0.30	0.27	0.07	.26	
Blackberry et al. (2013)	−0.10	0.10	0.01	.34	
Xue et al. (2008)	−0.57	0.17	0.03	.00	
Anderson et al. (2005)	−0.11	0.13	0.02	.42	
Total (95% CI)	−0.80	0.34	0.11	.02	
4. Body weight					
Odnoletkova et al. (2016)	−0.14	0.09	0.01	.12	
Lynch et al. (2014)	−0.37	0.27	0.07	.17	
Blackberry et al. (2013)	−0.10	0.10	0.01	.35	
McGowan (2011)	−0.11	0.14	0.02	.40	
Anderson et al. (2005)	−0.04	0.14	0.02	.78	
Total (95% CI)	−0.12	0.05	0.00	.03	

(continues)

Table 3

Effect Sizes for Studies Measuring Patient Activation Intervention on Outcomes, Continued

Study (Year)	Statistic for Each Study				Hedges's *g* and 95% CI
	Hedges's *g*	SE	Variance	*p*	
5. LDL					
Cortez et al. (2017)	−0.03	0.13	0.02	.84	
Odnoletkova et al. (2016)	−0.24	0.09	0.01	.01	
Ebrahimi et al. (2016)	−0.48	0.20	0.04	.02	
Safford et al. (2015)	−0.11	0.12	0.01	.35	
García et al. (2015)	−1.03	0.25	0.06	.00	
Thom et al. (2013)	−0.09	0.13	0.02	.51	
Blackberry et al. (2013)	−0.05	0.10	0.01	.65	
McGowan (2011)	−0.19	0.14	0.02	.16	
Total (95% CI)	−0.21	0.08	0.01	.01	
6. Depression					
Yun et al. (2017)	−0.03	0.15	0.02	.83	
Pauley et al. (2016)	−0.13	0.20	0.04	.52	
Jonsdottir et al. (2015)	−0.19	0.20	0.04	.34	
Blackberry et al. (2013)	−0.13	0.10	0.01	.19	
Van der Wulp et al. (2012)	−0.07	0.18	0.03	.69	
Tousman et al. (2011)	−0.05	0.29	0.09	.87	
Lorig et al. (2009)	−0.39	0.12	0.01	.00	
Anderson et al. (2009)	−0.12	0.13	0.02	.34	
Total (95% CI)	−0.16	0.05	0.00	.00	
7. Anxiety					
Yun et al. (2017)	−0.36	0.15	0.02	.01	
Pauley et al. (2016)	−0.06	0.21	0.04	.77	
Jonsdottir et al. (2015)	−0.23	0.20	0.04	.24	
Total (95% CI)	−0.25	0.10	0.01	.01	
8. Patient activation					
Young et al. (2016)	0.44	0.20	0.04	.03	
Safford et al. (2015)	0.25	0.12	0.01	.04	
Tousman et al. (2011)	0.41	0.30	0.09	.17	
Wolever et al. (2010)	0.70	0.27	0.07	.01	
Lorig et al. (2009)	0.28	0.12	0.01	.02	
Total (95% CI)	0.33	0.07	0.01	.00	
9. Self-efficacy					
Moein et al. (2017)	0.98	0.21	0.05	.00	
Young et al. (2016)	0.28	0.20	0.04	.16	
Pauley et al. (2016)	0.20	0.22	0.05	.37	
Meng et al. (2016)	0.00	0.10	0.01	1.00	
Chen et al. (2015)	0.97	0.26	0.07	.00	
García et al. (2015)	2.26	0.31	0.10	.00	
Shao et al. (2013)	1.39	0.23	0.05	.00	
Blackberry et al. (2013)	0.11	0.10	0.01	.27	
Van der Wulp et al. (2012)	0.12	0.18	0.03	.51	
McGowan (2011)	0.12	0.14	0.02	.39	
Lorig et al. (2009)	0.39	0.12	0.01	.00	
Total (95% CI)	0.57	0.15	0.02	.00	

(continues)

Table 3

Effect Sizes for Studies Measuring Patient Activation Intervention on Outcomes, Continued

Study (Year)	Statistic for Each Study				Hedges's *g* and 95% CI
	Hedges's *g*	SE	Variance	*p*	
10. HRQOL					
Yun et al. (2017)	0.11	0.15	0.02	.45	
Meng et al. (2016)	0.09	0.10	0.01	.38	
Safford et al. (2015)	0.06	0.12	0.01	.63	
Chen et al. (2015)	1.04	0.26	0.07	.00	
Jonsdottir et al. (2015)	0.05	0.21	0.04	.79	
Blackberry et al. (2013)	0.11	0.10	0.01	.27	
Tousman et al. (2011)	0.07	0.29	0.09	.82	
Wolever et al. (2010)	0.23	0.28	0.08	.42	
Keeratiyutawong et al. (2006)	0.92	0.23	0.05	.00	
Total (95% CI)	0.25	0.10	0.01	.01	

Note. HbA1C = glycated hemoglobin; SBP = systolic blood pressure; DBP = diastolic blood pressure; LDL = low-density lipoprotein; HRQOL = health-related quality of life.

plus telephone support in two studies and face-to-face only in one study.

Behavioral Effects: Patient Activation

The effects of patient activation interventions on patients' activation were evaluated in five studies, and the pooled effect size was statistically significant. The study population included patients with cardiovascular disease, chronic respiratory diseases, and diabetes mellitus. The effect on patient activation had an effect size of 0.33 ($p < .01$), indicating a small effect (Table 3). The studies were unlikely to be heterogeneous ($I^2 < 0.01$, $p = .60$). The moderator analysis showed no significant differences in effect sizes for patients' activation between intervention types ($p = .65$; Table 4). The interventions varied in length from 6 weeks to 10 months. The intervention delivery mode was face-to-face plus telephone support in one study, face-to-face only in two studies, and telephone support only in two studies. The moderator analysis showed no significant differences in effect sizes for patient activation between the face-to-face and telephone modes ($p = .65$; Table 4).

Behavioral Effects: Self-Efficacy

The effects of patient activation interventions on patients' self-efficacy were evaluated in 11 studies, with the pooled effect size found to be statistically significant. The study population included patients with diabetes mellitus and patients with cardiovascular disease. The effect on self-efficacy had an effect size of 0.57 ($p < .01$), indicating a medium effect (Table 3). The studies were highly heterogeneous ($I^2 = 89.53$, $p < .01$). The moderator analysis indicated no significant differences in the effect sizes for self-efficacy between intervention types ($p = .53$; Table 4) or between types of disease ($p = .91$; Table 4), suggesting that intervention and disease types did not affect the size of the effect for self-efficacy. The interventions varied in length from 4 weeks to

15 months. The intervention delivery mode was face-to-face plus telephone support in six studies and face-to-face only in five studies. The moderator analysis indicated no significant differences in the effect sizes for self-efficacy between the two intervention delivery modes ($p = .12$; Table 4), suggesting that mode of intervention delivery did not affect the size of the effect for self-efficacy. Meta-regression results showed no significant association between the effect size of self-efficacy and mean age ($p = .24$; Table 5) or between the effect size of self-efficacy and the percentage of female participants ($p = .15$; Table 5).

Effects on Health-Related Quality of Life

The effects of patient activation interventions on patients' HRQOL were evaluated in nine studies, and the pooled effect size was statistically significant. The study population included patients with cancer, diabetes mellitus, chronic respiratory diseases, and cardiovascular disease. The effect on HRQOL had an effect size of 0.25 ($p = .01$), indicating a small effect (Table 3). The studies were moderately heterogeneous ($I^2 = 66.58$, $p < .01$). The moderator analysis showed no significant differences in effect sizes for HRQOL between intervention types ($p = .41$) or between types of disease ($p = .14$; Table 4), suggesting that the size of the effect for HRQOL was not influenced by either different types of interventions or different types of disease. The interventions varied in length from 7 weeks to 15 months. The moderator analysis showed no significant differences in effect sizes for HRQOL among the three intervention durations ($p = .38$; Table 4), suggesting that the size of the effect for HRQOL was not influenced by differences in intervention durations. The intervention delivery mode was face-to-face plus telephone support in six studies, telephone support only in one study, and face-to-face only in two studies. The moderator analysis showed no significant differences in effect sizes for HRQOL between the face-to-face plus

Table 4

Summary of Results for Moderator Analyses

Group	No. of RCT	Hedges's g	95% CI	p	Between-Group p
Types of intervention					
1. HbA1C					.20
Health coaching	4	−0.19	[−0.31, −0.07]	< .01	
Empowerment	4	−0.31	[−0.51, −0.11]	< .01	
Self-management	6	−0.52	[−0.92, −0.13]	.01	
2. SBP					.09
Health coaching	3	−0.13	[−0.25, −0.01]	.04	
Empowerment	2	−0.24	[−0.43, −0.06]	.01	
Self-management	3	−0.43	[−0.67, −0.19]	< .01	
3. DBP					.63
Empowerment	2	−1.50	[−4.23, 1.23]	.28	
Self-management	3	−0.81	[−1.51, −0.12]	.02	
4. LDL					.60
Health coaching	3	−0.17	[−0.29, −0.04]	.01	
Empowerment	2	−0.23	[−0.67, 0.21]	.31	
Self-management	2	−0.59	[−1.41, 0.24]	.16	
5. Patient activation					.65
Health coaching	2	0.41	[−0.01, 0.83]	.06	
Self-management	2	0.30	[0.08, 0.51]	.01	
6. Self-efficacy					.53
Empowerment	2	0.98	[0.66, 1.30]	< .01	
Self-management	5	0.77	[0.20, 1.34]	.01	
7. HRQOL					.41
Health coaching	3	0.09	[−0.08, 0.27]	.29	
Self-management	4	0.27	[−0.11, 0.64]	.16	
Types of disease					
1. Depression					.80
Respiratory diseases	2	−0.15	[−0.47, 0.18]	.39	
Diabetes mellitus	5	−0.19	[−0.31, −0.07]	< .01	
2. Self-efficacy					.91
Cardiovascular	3	0.54	[−0.23, 1.31]	.17	
Diabetes mellitus	8	0.59	[0.23, 0.94]	< .01	
3. HRQOL					.14
Respiratory diseases	2	0.06	[−0.27, 0.39]	.73	
Diabetes mellitus	5	0.43	[0.07, 0.79]	.02	
Intervention duration					
1. HbA1C					.25
≤ 3 months	5	−0.25	[−0.44, −0.07]	.01	
> 3 months but ≤ 6 months	5	−0.61	[−1.07, −0.14]	.01	
>6 months	6	−0.19	[−0.35, −0.03]	.02	
2. SBP					.71
≤ 3 months	2	−0.35	[−0.75, 0.05]	.09	
> 3 months but ≤ 6 months	4	−0.17	[−0.30, −0.04]	.01	
> 6 months	3	−0.19	[−0.33, 0.06]	.01	
3. DBP					.60
≤ 3 months	2	−0.32	[−0.77, 0.12]	.16	
> 3 months but ≤ 6 months	2	−0.65	[−1.51, 0.21]	.14	
> 6 months	2	−1.49	[−4.23, 1.25]	.29	
4. Body weight					.52
≤ 3 months	2	−0.08	[−0.27, 0.11]	.43	
> 3 months but ≤ 6 months	2	−0.16	[−0.32, 0.01]	.06	

(continues)

Table 4

Summary of Results for Moderator Analyses, Continued

Group	No. of RCT	Hedges's *g*	95% CI	*p*	Between-Group *p*
5. LDL				.13	
≤ 3 months	2	−0.30	[−0.57, −0.03]	.03	
> 3 months but ≤ 6 months	3	−0.38	[−0.77, 0.01]	.05	
> 6 months	3	−0.06	[−0.19, 0.07]	.36	
6. Depression					.51
≤ 3 months	4	−0.24	[−0.41, −0.07]	.01	
> 3 months but ≤ 6 months	2	−0.09	[−0.32, 0.15]	.47	
> 6 months	2	−0.13	[−0.29, 0.03]	.11	
7. HRQOL					.38
≤ 3 months	2	0.56	[−0.39, 1.52]	.25	
> 3 months but ≤ 6 months	4	0.31	[−0.07, 0.69]	.11	
> 6 months	2	0.09	[−0.06, 0.25]	.25	
Intervention delivery mode					
1. HbA1C					.26
Face-to-face plus telephone support	10	−0.37	[−0.59, −0.15]	< .01	
Face-to-face	3	−0.30	[−0.59, −0.01]	.04	
Telephone support	3	−0.16	[−0.30, −0.03]	.02	
2. SBP					.19
Face-to-face plus telephone support	6	−0.22	[−0.34, −0.11]	< .01	
Telephone support	2	−0.11	[−0.24, 0.04]	.14	
3. LDL					.80
Face-to-face plus telephone support	4	−0.23	[−0.53, 0.08]	.14	
Face-to-face	2	−0.30	[−0.57, −0.03]	.03	
Telephone support	2	−0.19	[−0.34, −0.05]	.01	
4. Depression					.11
Face-to-face plus telephone support	5	−0.11	[−0.23, 0.01]	.08	
Face-to-face	3	−0.30	[−0.48, −0.11]	< .01	
5. Patient activation					.65
Face-to-face	2	0.30	[0.08, 0.51]	.01	
Telephone support	2	0.41	[−0.01, 0.83]	.06	
6. Self-efficacy					.12
Face-to-face plus telephone support	6	0.82	[0.24, 1.40]	.01	
Face-to-face	5	0.31	[0.02, 0.60]	.04	
7. HRQOL					.16
Face-to-face plus telephone support	6	0.32	[0.05, 0.60]	.02	
Face-to-face	2	0.09	[−0.10, 0.27]	.37	

Note. DBP = diastolic blood pressure; HbA1C = glycated hemoglobin; HRQOL = health-related quality of life; LDL = low-density lipoprotein; RCT = randomized controlled trial; SBP = systolic blood pressure.

telephone support and face-to-face only by delivery modes (p = .16; Table 4), suggesting that the size of the effect for HRQOL was not influenced by different intervention delivery modes. Meta-regression results found no significant association between the effect size of HRQOL and mean age (p = .79; Table 5) or between the effect size of HRQOL and the percentage of female participants (p = .64; Table 5).

Discussion

Improving the level of activation in patients is desirable because patients who are more activated are more likely to engage in self-management behaviors perceived as effective in improving health (Hibbard et al., 2007; Jacobson et al., 2018). This meta-analysis of 26 studies determined the effects of patient activation interventions for patients with chronic diseases. The patient activation interventions were found to improve patients' physiological, psychosocial, and behavioral health statuses as well as HRQOL.

Bolen et al. (2014) found that patient activation interventions reduced slightly the intermediate outcomes for HbA1C, SBP, body weight, and LDL in patients with diabetes mellitus. However, the effects of patient activation interventions on psychological and behavioral contexts remain unclear. Depression, anxiety, and physical illness commonly co-occur, and depression and anxiety are prevalent in patients with chronic diseases (Clarke & Currie, 2009; Yohannes et al., 2010). Individuals with multiple comorbidities experience difficulties participating in care planning and self-management (Jowsey et al., 2009). Anxiety and depression are associated with poor disease self-management (Fredericks et al., 2012) and nonadherence to medications (Grenard et al., 2011). The data presented in this study show the effect of patient activation interventions on the psychological and behavioral aspects of chronic-disease-related outcomes as well as on physiological outcomes. Significant improvements in HbA1C, SBP, DBP, body weight, LDL, depression, anxiety, patient activation, and self-efficacy were observed, supporting implementing patient activation programs for patients with chronic diseases. Patient-reported outcomes such as HRQOL are important disease-specific clinical outcomes (Grimm & Grünwald, 2017). The salient finding from this study is that patient activation interventions were effective in improving self-reported HRQOL in patients with chronic diseases.

In this study, the evaluation of physiological, psychosocial, and quality of life outcomes in relation to patient activation interventions found only small effects because of several reasons. First, patient characteristics may affect, at least in part, the effect of patient activation on physiological outcomes, as the effect sizes for HbA1C and LDL were found to be larger in older adults. Second, more intensive management of chronic diseases, including various types of patient activation interventions, possibly led to increased feelings of burden and subsequent negative effects on psychological outcomes and quality of life. Third, given the complex nature of chronic diseases, a multimodal approach to disease management may be necessary to affect care outcomes in patients with chronic diseases substantively (Kim et al., 2014).

The evidence indicates that interventions that are tailored to an individual's level of activation effectively increase patient activation as an intermediate outcome of care that is linked to improved outcomes (Hibbard & Greene, 2013). In addition, the results of previous research suggest that interventions enhance self-management support by addressing the suggested areas of knowledge, improving information sharing, and providing tangible support (Donald et al., 2019). Therefore, healthcare providers should regularly assess patients' activation levels related to their self-management of chronic diseases. Appropriate patient activation interventions may be used to increase patient activation in clinical settings, which in turn may improve health outcomes.

This study was affected by several limitations. First, some relevant studies were possibly not included in the meta-analysis because relevant databases were not used because of their lack of medical subject headings. Second, the limited effect that the patient activation interventions had on self-management behavior may be because of an insufficient number of relevant studies overall. Third, because of varying intervention designs and types of disease, significant heterogeneity existed among the included studies. Thus, moderator analyses were performed to explore whether the differences in types of disease, types of interventions, intervention duration, and intervention delivery mode accounted for the observed heterogeneity. The effect sizes for HbA1C, DBP, body weight, LDL, self-efficacy, and HRQOL were found to be unaffected by intervention type, intervention duration, disease type, or mode of intervention delivery. Meta-regression revealed that age influenced the effects of patient activation interventions on HbA1C and LDL. Unfortunately, we were unable to identify other moderator variables that explained the heterogeneity.

Table 5

Summary of Results for Meta-Regression Analyses

Parameter	No. of RCT	Coefficient	Standard Error	p
1. HbA1C				
Age	15	0.04	0.01	.01
%Female	16	−0.00	0.01	.83
2. DBP				
Age	7	0.10	0.08	.20
%Female	7	−0.02	0.03	.45
3. LDL				
Age	8	0.03	0.01	.03
%Female	8	−0.00	0.01	.68
4. Self-efficacy				
Age	9	−0.04	0.04	.24
%Female	11	0.02	0.01	.15
5. HRQOL				
Age	8	0.00	0.01	.79
%Female	9	0.00	0.01	.64

Note. RCT = randomized controlled trial; HbA1C = glycated hemoglobin; DBP = diastolic blood pressure; LDL = low-density lipoprotein; HRQOL = health-related quality of life.

Conclusions

The results of the meta-analysis show patient activation interventions to be effective in improving the health status and quality of life in patients with chronic diseases. Therefore, healthcare providers should assess patients' activation levels in the self-management of chronic diseases regularly. Furthermore, healthcare providers should implement patient activation interventions that tailor support to the individual's level of patient activation and strengthen the role of patients in managing their healthcare to improve chronic-disease-related health outcomes.

Author Contributions

Study conception and design: PST, MYL
Data collection: MYL, WSW, RWA, PVT
Data analysis and interpretation: PST, MYL
Drafting of the article: All authors
Critical revision of the article: PST

References

*References marked with an asterisk indicate studies included in the meta-analysis.

*Anderson, R. M., Funnell, M. M., Aikens, J. E., Krein, S. L., Fitzgerald, J. T., Nwankwo, R., Tannas, C. L., & Tang, T. S. (2009). Evaluating the efficacy of an empowerment-based self-management consultant intervention: Results of a two-year randomized controlled trial. *Therapeutic Patient Education, 1*(1), 3–11. https://doi.org/10.1051/tpe/2009002

*Anderson, R. M., Funnell, M. M., Nwankwo, R., Gillard, M. L., Oh, M., & Fitzgerald, J. T. (2005). Evaluating a problem-based empowerment program for African Americans with diabetes: Results of a randomized controlled trial. *Ethnicity & Disease, 15*(4), 671–678. https://doi.org/10.2337/diacare.18.7.943

Bennett, H. D., Coleman, E. A., Parry, C., Bodenheimer, T., & Chen, E. H. (2010). Health coaching for patients with chronic illness. *Family Practice Management, 17*(5), 24–29. https://doi.org/10.1093/nq/175.18.315a

*Blackberry, I. D., Furler, J. S., Best, J. D., Chondros, P., Vale, M., Walker, C., Dunning, T., Segal, L., Dunbar, J., Audehm, R., Liew, D., & Young, D. (2013). Effectiveness of general practice based, practice nurse led telephone coaching on glycaemic control of type 2 diabetes: The patient engagement and coaching for health (PEACH) pragmatic cluster randomised controlled trial. *BMJ (Clinical Research Ed.), 347*, f5272. https://doi.org/10.1136/bmj.f5272

Bolen, S. D., Chandar, A., Falck-Ytter, C., Tyler, C., Perzynski, A. T., Gertz, A. M., Sage, P., Lewis, S., Cobabe, M., Ye, Y., Menegay, M., & Windish, D. M. (2014). Effectiveness and safety of patient activation interventions for adults with type 2 diabetes: Systematic review, meta-analysis, and meta-regression. *Journal of General Internal Medicine, 29*(8), 1166–1176. https://doi.org/10.1007/s11606-014-2855-4

*Chen, M. F., Wang, R. H., Lin, K. C., Hsu, H. Y., & Chen, S. W. (2015). Efficacy of an empowerment program for Taiwanese patients with type 2 diabetes: A randomized controlled trial. *Applied Nursing Research, 28*(4), 366–373. https://doi.org/10.1016/j.apnr.2014.12.006

Clarke, D. M., & Currie, K. C. (2009). Depression, anxiety and their relationship with chronic diseases: A review of the epidemiology, risk and treatment evidence. *The Medical Journal of Australia, 190*(7, Suppl.), S54–S60. https://doi.org/10.5694/j.1326-5377.2009.tb02471.x

*Cortez, D. N., Macedo, M. M., Souza, D. A., Dos Santos, J. C., Afonso, G. S., Reis, I. A., & Torres, H. C. (2017). Evaluating the effectiveness of an empowerment program for self-care in type 2 diabetes: A cluster randomized trial. *BMC Public Health, 17*(1), 41. https://doi.org/10.1186/s12889-016-3937-5

Deeks, A., Lombard, C., Michelmore, J., & Teede, H. (2009). The effects of gender and age on health related behaviors. *BMC Public Health, 9*, 213. https://doi.org/10.1186/1471-2458-9-213

Donald, M., Beanlands, H., Straus, S., Ronksley, P., Tam-Tham, H., Finlay, J., MacKay, J., Elliott, M., Herrington, G., Harwood, L., Large, C. A., Large, C. L., Waldvogel, B., Sparkes, D., Delgado, M., Tong, A., Grill, A., Novak, M., James, M. T., Hemmelgarn, B. R. (2019). Identifying needs for self-management interventions for adults with CKD and their caregivers: A qualitative study. *American Journal of Kidney Diseases, 74*(4), 474–482. https://doi.org/10.1053/j.ajkd.2019.02.006

*Ebrahimi, H., Sadeghi, M., Amanpour, F., & Vahedi, H. (2016). Evaluation of empowerment model on indicators of metabolic control in patients with type 2 diabetes, a randomized clinical trial study. *Primary Care Diabetes, 10*(2), 129–135. https://doi.org/10.1016/j.pcd.2015.09.003

Fredericks, S., Lapum, J., & Lo, J. (2012). Anxiety, depression, and self-management: A systematic review. *Clinical Nursing Research, 21*(4), 411–430. https://doi.org/10.1177/1054773812436681

Funnell, M. M., Anderson, R. M., Arnold, M. S., Barr, P. A., Donnelly, M., Johnson, P. D., Taylor-Moon, D., & White, N. H. (1991). Empowerment: An idea whose time has come in diabetes education. *The Diabetes Educator, 17*(1), 37–41. https://doi.org/10.1177/014572179101700108

*García, A. A., Brown, S. A., Horner, S. D., Zuñiga, J., & Arheart, K. L. (2015). Home-based diabetes symptom self-management education for Mexican Americans with type 2 diabetes. *Health Education Research, 30*(3), 484–496. https://doi.org/10.1093/her/cyv018

Greene, J., & Hibbard, J. H. (2012). Why does patient activation matter? An examination of the relationships between patient activation and health-related outcomes. *Journal of General Internal Medicine, 27*(5), 520–526. https://doi.org/10.1007/s11606-011-1931-2

Grenard, J. L., Munjas, B. A., Adams, J. L., Suttorp, M., Maglione, M., McGlynn, E. A., & Gellad, W. F. (2011). Depression and medication adherence in the treatment of chronic diseases in the United States: A meta-analysis. *Journal of General Internal Medicine, 26*(10), 1175–1182. https://doi.org/10.1007/s11606-011-1704-y

Grimm, M. O., & Grünwald, V. (2017). Health-related quality of life as a prognostic measure of clinical outcomes in renal cell carcinoma: A review of the checkmate 025 trial. *Oncology and Therapy, 5*(1), 75–78. https://doi.org/10.1007/s40487-017-0042-6

Hibbard, J. H., & Greene, J. (2013). What the evidence shows about patient activation: Better health outcomes and care experiences; fewer data on costs. *Health Affairs (Project Hope), 32*(2), 207–214. https://doi.org/10.1377/hlthaff.2012.1061

Hibbard, J. H., Mahoney, E. R., Stock, R., & Tusler, M. (2007). Do increases in patient activation result in improved self-management behaviors? *Health Services Research, 42*(4), 1443–1463. https://doi.org/10.1111/j.1475-6773.2006.00669.x

Hibbard, J. H., Stockard, J., Mahoney, E. R., & Tusler, M. (2004). Development of the patient activation measure (PAM): Conceptualizing and measuring activation in patients and consumers. *Health Services Research, 39*(4, Pt. 1), 1005–1026. https://doi.org/10.1111/j.1475-6773.2004.00269.x

Higgins, J. P., Altman, D. G., Gøtzsche, P. C., Jüni, P., Moher, D., Oxman, A. D., Savović, J., Schulz, K. F., Weeks, L., Sterne, J. A. C., Cochrane Bias Methods Group; Cochrane Statistical Methods Group. (2011). The Cochrane Collaboration's tool for assessing risk of bias in randomised trials. *BMJ (Clinical Research Ed.), 343*, d5928. https://doi.org/10.1136/bmj.d5928

Holman, H., & Lorig, K. (2004). Patient self-management: A key to effectiveness and efficiency in care of chronic disease. *Public Health Reports, 119*(3), 239–243. https://doi.org/10.1016/j.phr. 2004.04.002

Jacobson, A. F., Sumodi, V., Albert, N. M., Butler, R. S., DeJohn, L., Walker, D., Dion, K., Tai, H. L., & Ross, D. M. (2018). Patient activation, knowledge, and health literacy association with self-management behaviors in persons with heart failure. *Heart & Lung, 47*(5), 447–451. https://doi.org/10.1016/j.hrtlng. 2018.05.021

*Jonsdottir, H., Amundadottir, O. R., Gudmundsson, G., Halldorsdottir, B. S., Hrafnkelsson, B., Ingadottir, T. S., Jonsdottir, R., Jonsson, J. S., Sigurjonsdottir, E. D., & Stefansdottir, I. K. (2015). Effectiveness of a partnership-based self-management programme for patients with mild and moderate chronic obstructive pulmonary disease: A pragmatic randomized controlled trial. *Journal of Advanced Nursing, 71*(11), 2634–2649. https://doi.org/10.1111/jan.12728

Jowsey, T., Jeon, Y. H., Dugdale, P., Glasgow, N. J., Kljakovic, M., & Usherwood, T. (2009). Challenges for co-morbid chronic illness care and policy in Australia: A qualitative study. *Australia and New Zealand Health Policy, 6*, 22. https://doi.org/10.1186/1743-8462-6-22

*Keeratiyutawong, P., Hanucharurnkul, S., Melkus, G. D. E., Panpakdee, O., & Vorapongsathorn, T. (2006). Effectiveness of a self-management program for Thais with type 2 diabetes: An integrative review. *Thai Journal of Nursing Research, 10*(2), 85–97. https://doi:10.1016/j.ijnss.2018.12.002

Kim, K. B., Han, H. R., Huh, B., Nguyen, T., Lee, H., & Kim, M. T. (2014). The effect of a community-based self-help multimodal behavioral intervention in Korean American seniors with high blood pressure. *American Journal of Hypertension, 27*(9), 1199–1208. https://doi.org/10.1093/ajh/hpu041

*Li, X., Zhou, Q., Zou, F., Wu, L., Chen, H., & Liu, Z. (2012). Effectiveness of systematic self-management education on blood sugar level of patients in the community with type 2 diabetes. *Journal of Central South University: Medical Sciences, 37*(4), 355–358. https://doi.org/10.3969/j.issn.1672-7347.2012.04.006 (Original work published in Chinese)

*Lorig, K., Ritter, P. L., Villa, F. J., & Armas, J. (2009). Community-based peer-led diabetes self-management: A randomized trial. *Diabetes Educator, 35*(4), 641–651. https://doi.org/10.1177/0145721709335006

*Lynch, E. B., Liebman, R., Ventrelle, J., Avery, E. F., & Richardson, D. (2014). A self-management intervention for African Americans with comorbid diabetes and hypertension: A pilot randomized controlled trial. *Preventing Chronic Disease, 11*, E90. https://doi.org/10.5888/pcd11.130349

*McGowan, P. (2011). The efficacy of diabetes patient education and self-management education in type 2 diabetes. *Canadian Journal of Diabetes, 35*(1), 46–53. https://doi.org/10.1016/S1499-2671(11)51008-1

*Meng, K., Musekamp, G., Schuler, M., Seekatz, B., Glatz, J., Karger, G., Kiwus, U., Knoglinger, E., Schubmann, R., Westphal, R. & Faller, H. (2016). The impact of a self-management patient education program for patients with chronic heart failure undergoing inpatient cardiac rehabilitation. *Patient Education and Counseling, 99*(7), 1190–1197. https://doi.org/10.1016/j.pec.2016.02.010

*Moein, M., Aghajani, M., Ajorpaz, N. M., & Khorasanifar, L.

(2017). Effect of an empowerment program on self-efficacy of patients with type 2 diabetes. *Iranian Red Crescent Medical Journal, 19*(1), e29252. https://doi.org/10.5812/ircmj.29252

Mosen, D. M., Schmittdiel, J., Hibbard, J., Sobel, D., Remmers, C., & Bellows, J. (2007). Is patient activation associated with outcomes of care for adults with chronic conditions? *The Journal of Ambulatory Care Management, 30*(1), 21–29. https://doi.org/10.1097/00004479-200701000-00005

*Odnoletkova, I., Goderis, G., Nobels, F., Fieuws, S., Aertgeerts, B., Annemans, L., & Ramaekers, D. (2016). Optimizing diabetes control in people with type 2 diabetes through nurse-led telecoaching. *Diabetic Medicine, 33*(6), 777–785. https://doi.org/10.1111/dme.13092

Olsen, J. M. (2014). Health coaching: A concept analysis. *Nursing Forum, 49*(1), 18–29. https://doi.org/10.1111/nuf.12042

*Pauley, T., Gargaro, J., Chenard, G., Cavanagh, H., & McKay, S. M. (2016). Home-based diabetes self-management coaching delivered by paraprofessionals: A randomized controlled trial. *Home Health Care Services Quarterly, 35*(3–4), 137–154. https://doi.org/10.1080/01621424.2016.1264339

*Safford, M. M., Andreae, S., Cherrington, A. L., Martin, M. Y., Halanych, J., Lewis, M., Patel, A., Johnson, E., Clark, D., Gamboa, C., & Richman, J. S. (2015). Peer coaches to improve diabetes outcomes in rural Alabama: A cluster randomized trial. *The Annals of Family Medicine, 13*(1, Suppl.), S18–S26. https://doi.org/10.1370/afm.1798

*Shao, J. H., Chang, A. M., Edwards, H., Shyu, Y. I., & Chen, S. H. (2013). A randomized controlled trial of self-management programme improves health-related outcomes of older people with heart failure. *Journal of Advanced Nursing, 69*(11), 2458–2469. https://doi.org/10.1111/jan.12121

*Thom, D. H., Ghorob, A., Hessler, D., De Vore, D., Chen, E., & Bodenheimer, T. A. (2013). Impact of peer health coaching on glycemic control in low-income patients with diabetes: A randomized controlled trial. *Annals of Family Medicine, 11*(2), 137–144. https://doi.org/10.1370/afm.1443

Tol, A., Alhani, F., Shojaeazadeh, D., Sharifirad, G., & Moazam, N. (2015). An empowering approach to promote the quality of life and self-management among type 2 diabetic patients. *Journal of Education and Health Promotion, 4*, 13. https://doi.org/10.4103/2277-9531.154022

*Tousman, S. A., Zeitz, H., Bond, D., Stewart, D., Rackow, R., Greer, R., Hatfield, S., Layman, K., & Ganjwala, P. (2011). A randomized controlled behavioral trial of a new adult asthma self-management program. *Journal of Asthma and Allergy Educators, 2*(2), 91–96. https://doi.org/10.1177/2150129710395752

*Van der Wulp, I., de Leeuw, J. R., Gorter, K. J., & Rutten, G. E. (2012). Effectiveness of peer-led self-management coaching for patients recently diagnosed with type 2 diabetes mellitus in primary care: A randomized controlled trial. *Diabetic Medicine, 29* (10), e390–e397. https://doi.org/10.1111/j.1464-5491.2012.03629.x

*Wolever, R. Q., Dreusicke, M., Fikkan, J., Hawkins, T. V., Yeung, S., Wakefield, J., Duda, L., Flowers, P., Cook, C., & Skinner, E. (2010). Integrative health coaching for patients with type 2 diabetes: A randomized clinical trial. *Diabetes Educator, 36*(4), 629–639. https://doi.org/10.1177/0145721710371523

World Health Organization. (2018). *Noncommunicable diseases.* https://www.who.int/en/news-room/fact-sheets/detail/noncommunicable-diseases

*Xue, F., Yao, W., & Lewin, R. J. (2008). A randomised trial of a 5 week,

manual based, self-management programme for hypertension delivered in a cardiac patient club in Shanghai. *BMC Cardiovascular Disorders, 8*, 10. https://doi.org/10.1186/1471-2261-8-10

Yohannes, A. M., Willgoss, T. G., Baldwin, R. C., & Connolly, M. J. (2010). Depression and anxiety in chronic heart failure and chronic obstructive pulmonary disease: Prevalence, relevance, clinical implications and management principles. *International Journal of Geriatric Psychiatry, 25*(12), 1209–1221. https://doi.org/10.1002/gps.2463

*Young, L., Hertzog, M., & Barnason, S. (2016). Effects of a home-based activation intervention on self-management adherence and readmission in rural heart failure patients: The PATCH randomized controlled trial. *BMC Cardiovascular Disorders, 16*(1), 176. https://doi.org/10.1186/s12872-016-0339-7

*Yun, Y. H., Kim, Y. A., Lee, M. K., Sim, J. A., Nam, B. H., Kim, S., Lee, E. S., Noh, D. Y., Lim, J. Y., Kim, S., Kim, S. Y., Cho, C. H., Jung, K. H., Chun, M., Lee, S. N., Park, K. H., & Park, S. (2017). A randomized controlled trial of physical activity, dietary habit, and distress management with the leadership and coaching for health (LEACH) program for disease-free cancer survivors. *BMC Cancer, 17*(1), 298. https://doi.org/10.1186/s12885-017-3290-9

21

Effects of Auricular Acupressure in Patients on Hemodialysis

Eun Sook JUNG[1] • Ae Kyung CHANG[2]*

ABSTRACT

Background: Although studies on the effectiveness of self-management in limiting fluid intake in patients on hemodialysis have been conducted extensively, xerostomia, which is a powerful stimulus of fluid intake, has received scarce attention.

Purpose: The purpose of this study was to examine the effects of a 4-week auricular acupressure treatment on xerostomia, salivary flow rate, interdialytic weight gain, constipation, and diet-related quality of life in patients on hemodialysis in Korea.

Methods: This was a randomized controlled trial. Sixty patients on hemodialysis were randomly assigned to either the experimental group ($n = 30$) or the control group ($n = 30$). The experimental group received an auricular acupressure intervention, which included the application of skin tape with a *Semen vaccariae* seed on the five auricular acupoints, including the large intestine (CO7), San Jiao (CO17), middle triangular fossa (TF3), spleen (CO13), and upper tragus (TG1), for 4 weeks. The control group received only the application of skin tape without a seed on the same auricular acupoints for the same period. The outcome variables were as follows: xerostomia, measured using the visual analog scale; salivary flow rate, measured using the unstimulated whole saliva absorbed in oral cotton; interdialytic weight gain; the constipation assessment scale score; and the Quality of Life Related to Dietary Change Questionnaire results.

Results: The experimental group scored significantly better than the control group in terms of xerostomia ($p = .004$), salivary flow rate ($p = .010$), constipation ($p = .009$), and diet-related quality of life ($p < .001$).

Conclusions/Implications for Practice: Auricular acupressure may be an important tool for alleviating the negative symptoms of xerostomia and for improving quality of life in patients on hemodialysis. Nurses caring for patients on hemodialysis with both xerostomia and constipation may teach auricular acupressure to help patients self-manage their discomfort.

KEY WORDS:
auricular acupressure, xerostomia, interdialytic weight gain, constipation, quality of life.

Introduction

Studies on the efficacy of self-management in limiting the fluid intake of patients on hemodialysis have been conducted extensively. However, xerostomia (dry mouth), which is a powerful stimulus of fluid intake, has received little attention. Xerostomia is one of the most common complaints of patients on hemodialysis, with up to 78% experiencing this symptom (Bossola, Pepe, & Vulpio, 2018; Kara, 2016). Xerostomia is caused by a lower rate of salivary flow in these patients (Bossola & Tazza, 2012). Although xerostomia is a subjective feeling, it may negatively affect the social activities and personal lives of these patients; may engender difficulties in tasting, chewing, and swallowing; and may cause bad breath (G. Yang et al., 2017). In particular, xerostomia causes patients on hemodialysis to feel thirsty and to drink more water, which may lead to failure to comply with fluid restriction regimens. It has been estimated that only 25%–30% of patients on hemodialysis reduce their dietary fluid intake to 1 liter per day or less (Howren et al., 2015). Poor adherence to fluid restriction has been associated with interdialytic weight gain (IDWG), which may lead to serious complications such as hypertension, congestive heart failure, and death (Kalantar-Zadeh et al., 2009). Prior strategies for alleviating xerostomia include salivary substitutes such as oral pilocarpine and mechanical stimulation of the salivary gland (e.g., chewing gum). However, salivary substitutes may cause hot flashes, chest tightness, or dyspnea, and chewing gum may not have a significant effect on xerostomia and may overwork the masticatory muscles and teeth (Bossola & Tazza, 2012). Thus, a valid and standardized therapy for controlling xerostomia in patients on hemodialysis remains to be introduced.

Constipation is a highly prevalent gastrointestinal problem (40%–73%) that adversely affects the physical and mental well-being of patients on hemodialysis (Tvistholm, Munch, & Danielsen, 2017). Fluid and food intake restrictions that are necessary to maintain the patient's "dry weight" are the main causes of constipation and xerostomia. Common remedies for constipation are the intake of dietary fiber and water and increased physical activity. However, these methods are

[1]MSN, RN, Graduate School, Kyung Hee University, Seoul, Republic of Korea • [2]PhD, RN, Associate Professor, College of Nursing Science & East-West Nursing Research Institute, Kyung Hee University, Seoul, Republic of Korea.

not always suitable for patients on hemodialysis, who must instead rely on laxatives (Y. M. Lee et al., 2006). The long-term use of laxatives may worsen constipation because it may alter the intestinal mucosa, weaken muscle tension, and reduce normal bowel reflexes. Moreover, previous studies have reported that laxatives are ineffective for 23%–45% of patients with constipation (Li, Lee, & Suen, 2014). Therefore, a more effective management strategy for constipation should be developed.

Unless they receive a kidney transplant, it is essential for patients to receive dialysis two or three times per week. Patients experience physical and emotional stress from not only the dialysis but also the strict and complex therapeutic regimen, which may significantly decrease their quality of life (Morganstein, 2005). Eating is a basic human desire, a source of joy, and an important social activity that is closely linked to life quality (Delahanty, Hayden, Ammerman, & Nathan, 2002). It is desirable for patients on hemodialysis to gain satisfaction and pleasure from eating despite their dietary restrictions and limitations. However, their diet-related quality of life is often reduced by the burden of and dissatisfaction with their diet therapy (J. Lee, Kim, & Kim, 2013) as well as gastrointestinal symptoms such as xerostomia and constipation (E. K. Yang & Kim, 2016). Therefore, nursing interventions should aim not only to alleviate constipation and xerostomia but also to enhance quality of life.

Auricular acupressure (AA) is one of the most popular complementary therapies, as it stimulates specific auricular acupoints to manage physical and psychological health. Several different theories have been developed to provide a framework for understanding the mechanisms that underlie AA (Oleson, 2014). AA was first documented in a classical Chinese medical book, *The Yellow Emperor's Classic of Internal Medicine*, in which the ear is posited to share a close relationship with the meridians and internal organs in the human body (Y. Wang, 2008). According to this book, the six yang meridians enter the ear directly or distribute to areas surrounding the ear (Y. Wang, 2008), whereas the six yin meridians connect to the ear indirectly through their corresponding yang meridians (Oleson, 2014). The compression of the auricular acupoints helps activate the meridians, balance yin and yang, and control the circulation of vital energy (Qi), with the aim of resolving health problems and restoring health (Yeh et al., 2014). Traditional Chinese medicine holds that the ear is closely connected with a number of internal organs, including the five Zang organs (liver, heart, spleen, lungs, and kidneys) and the six Fu organs (gall bladder, small intestine, stomach, large intestine, bladder, and triple energizer). Pathological changes in a person's organs are reflected in the external ear. Therefore, acupuncture or acupressure on the ear treats ailments of these organs (Oleson, 2014; Y. Wang, 2008). The World Health Organization acknowledged AA as the most scientifically developed method of the microacupuncture systems (Working Group on Auricular Acupuncture Nomenclature & World Health Organization Traditional Medicine Unit, 1991).

Unlike acupuncture, AA is noninvasive, safe, and easy to implement. Therefore, it is well suited for application in clinical practice to alleviate discomfort and distress (Li et al., 2014). AA has been found to effectively alleviate physical and psychological symptoms in patients on hemodialysis, including fatigue, uremic pruritus, constipation, and depression (Li et al., 2014; S. Wang et al., 2014). AA may stimulate the vagus nerve, which triggers residual salivary secretory capacity (G. Yang et al., 2017). Application of pressure to auricular acupoints may also stimulate secretion of neuropeptides such as neuropeptide Y and neurokinin A, which increase salivary flow (Bossola et al., 2018). However, the effect of AA on xerostomia in patients on hemodialysis has not been adequately investigated. One study on 28 patients on hemodialysis found that acupressure significantly reduced thirst and increased salivary flow rates in comparison with placebo acupressure, which was applied before the actual acupressure (L. Y. Yang, Yates, Chin, & Kao, 2010). However, practice effects because of the within-group repeated measurements may have affected the internal validity of this investigation. Another study showed that a 4-week AA reduced xerostomia in maintenance patients on hemodialysis (G. Yang et al., 2017). However, the lack of a control group negatively affected the validity of that study's findings.

The objective of this randomized, placebo-controlled trial was to examine the effects of AA on physical and mental health in patients on hemodialysis. Applying AA was expected to reduce xerostomia and constipation in patients on hemodialysis, leading to a decrease in IDWG, which would, in turn, enhance the diet-related quality of life of these patients. This study tested the following hypotheses: (a) The experimental group receiving the 4-week AA therapy intervention will have significantly less xerostomia and IDWG and a significantly higher salivary flow rate than the control group, (b) constipation will decrease significantly more in the experimental group than in the control group, and (c) diet-related quality of life will improve significantly more in the experimental group than in the control group.

Methods

Design and Participants

This single-blinded, randomized, and placebo-controlled study was conducted between October and November 2017. The study sites were two hemodialysis centers in a metropolitan city in South Korea that were similar in size, staff composition, number of patients, and operational status. In each center, patients on hemodialysis were randomly divided into an experimental group and a control group. The selection process and the study procedure are shown in Figure 1. An advertisement regarding the research program was posted on the message board of two hemodialysis centers. Seventy-five patients expressed interest in the study. Of these, 60 met the selection criteria and were randomly assigned to one of the two groups (Center A: experimental group, *n* = 12;

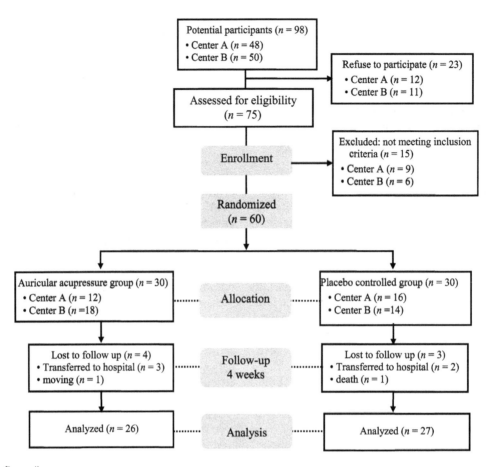

Figure 1. Study flow diagram.

control group, $n = 16$, Center B: experimental group, $n = 18$; control group, $n = 14$) by tossing a coin (heads: experimental group; tails: control group). Patients aged $\geq$ 20 years who were on regular hemodialysis three times a week, had experienced xerostomia in the last month, had IDWG $\geq$ 1 kg at the beginning of the study, and had fulfilled the Rome III diagnostic criteria for constipation were included in the study. A patient was considered to have fulfilled the Rome III diagnostic criteria if two or more of the following six criteria were met for more than 25% of defecations in at least 3 of the previous 6 months: straining, lumpy or hard stools, sensation of incomplete evacuation, sensation of anorectal obstruction/blockage, application of manual maneuvers, and fewer than three defecations per week (Longstreth et al., 2006).

The exclusion criteria were as follows: patients with a skin condition (e.g., ulcer or rash) on the AA site; patients taking medication such as tricyclic antidepressants, anticholinergics, antihistamines, or beta-blockers that could cause xerostomia (patients were asked to stop taking this type of medication at least 1 week before participation); and patients currently participating in a bowel-training program. The sample size was calculated using G*Power 3.1 (Heinrich Heine University, Dusseldorf, Germany). The study of G. Yang et al. (2017) was referenced to determine sample size. A sample size of 52 (26 in each group) was identified as necessary to detect a large effect

size ($d = 0.80$) between two independent sample means at $\alpha = .05$ with a power = 0.80.

Intervention and procedures

This study was preceded by a 4-week pilot investigation to test the feasibility of AA. In the pilot test, AA was applied to two patients on hemodialysis who met the inclusion criteria. The results of the pilot test indicated the feasibility of applying AA to a larger group.

The experimental group received AA, which included the application skin tape with a *Semen vaccariae* seed for 4 weeks, and the control group received only the skin tape (without a *Semen vaccariae* seed) on the same auricular acupoints and for the same period. The *Semen vaccariae* seeds used in this study have been shown in previous studies on patients on hemodialysis to be safe and effective for xerostomia treatment (G. Yang et al., 2017). An AA protocol was developed based on a review of the literature (Li et al., 2014; National Department of Meridian Acupoints, 2000; G. Yang et al., 2017; L. Y. Yang et al., 2010) and in consultation with an AA specialist. The intervention lasted 4 weeks and was conducted by a master's-prepared registered nurse who had been trained for this study by the researcher. All of the participants in the experimental group received AA on five auricular acupoints, including the large intestine (CO7), San Jiao

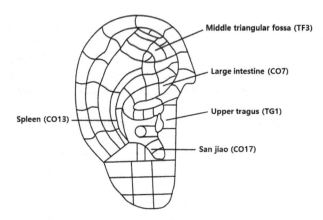

Figure 2. A map of the five auricular acupoints used in this study.

(CO17), middle triangular fossa (TF3), spleen (CO13), and upper tragus (TG1; Figure 2). According to the meridian and Zang–Fu theories, the large intestine, San Jiao, middle triangular fossa, and spleen points help alleviate constipation, whereas stimulation of the upper tragus point is effective in increasing saliva secretion and reducing thirst (Li et al., 2014; G. Yang et al., 2017). For AA to be effective, auricular acupoints should be pressed until the subject feels dullness, pressure, or distention (L. Y. Yang et al., 2010). We defined the force of finger pressure as 0.3–0.5 kg during the pilot test, and the same pressure range was used in the main study. AA was applied while the participants were receiving hemodialysis. The area to which AA was applied was sterilized using 70% alcohol. A section of tape to which one *Semen vaccariae* seed was attached was applied to each acupoint and maintained for 4 weeks. The participants were asked to press each seed four times per day or whenever they experienced thirst. To avoid skin irritation, the ears were treated alternately for 1 week each. Stickers were replaced at each dialysis session, and participant AA performance was evaluated. Outcomes were measured at baseline and after the 4-week intervention period in both groups.

Ethical Considerations

This study was approved by the institutional review board at the host institution (K-1709-001-009). The researchers explained the study purpose and procedures to the participants and obtained written informed consent. Participants in the control group received AA treatment after the study had ended.

Measures

General characteristics

Demographic and clinical data collected on the participants included age, gender, socioeconomic status, drinking status, smoking status, regular exercise status, years on hemodialysis, comorbidities, diabetes mellitus history, and use of laxatives. To measure exercise status, a criterion introduced by the investigator was used. A participant was classified as a "regular exerciser" if they exercised for 20 minutes at least 3 days per week for more than 6 months and a "nonexerciser" if they did not exercise on a regular basis.

Xerostomia

Participants rated their xerostomia using a visual analog scale ranging from 0 = *no thirst* to 10 = *extreme thirst*.

Salivary flow rate

Salivary flow rate was measured using the amount of unstimulated saliva absorbed in oral cotton. Participants refrained from eating, drinking, and oral care at least 1 hour before this measurement, and saliva was collected for 5 minutes without stimulation. The collected saliva was measured to a sensitivity of 0.0001 g using a CAS electric scale 120 (Seoul, Korea). The weight of the collected saliva was converted to a secretion-per-minute value (ml/min).

Interdialytic weight gain

IDWG, defined as the difference in predialysis and postdialysis body weights, is calculated as the weight difference (kilograms) between the body weight immediately before and the body weight immediately after a consecutive hemodialysis treatment. In this study, body weight was measured using a CAS electronic scale 200B (Seoul, Korea). Pre- and post-IDWG were measured before (baseline) and after the 4-week intervention. IDWG was calculated by averaging the weekly IDWG values.

Constipation

The constipation assessment scale (CAS) was used to assess constipation. The CAS was originally developed by McMillan and Williams (1989) and translated into Korean by S. Yang (1992). The CAS comprises eight items, respectively scored on a 3-point Likert scale (0 = *no problem*, 1 = *slight problem*, 2 = *serious problem*), and is used to determine constipation-related discomfort and ease of bowel movement. A higher CAS score indicates greater constipation severity. The reliability of the scale at the time of development was Cronbach's α = .70, and the reliability in this study was Cronbach's α = .73.

Diet-related quality of life

Diet-related quality of life was assessed using the Quality of Life Related to Dietary Change Questionnaire, which was developed by Delahanty et al. (2002) and modified by J. Lee et al. (2013). The questionnaire comprises three subcategories ("quality of life-related to dietary change," "satisfaction," and "dietary impact"), each of which includes 13, seven, and four items, respectively. Each item is measured using a 5-point scale, with higher scores indicating higher diet-related quality of life. The Cronbach's α coefficient was .79 in the study by J. Lee et al. and .87 in this study.

Statistical Analysis

Data were analyzed using IBM SPSS Statistics Version 23.0 (IBM, Inc., Armonk, NY, USA). The homogeneity in general characteristics and in the variables of interest between the two groups was analyzed using the chi-square test, Fisher's exact test, and t test. All data were normally distributed, as tested using the Kolmogorov–Smirnov test. A two-way, repeated-measures analysis of variance was used to investigate the main effect of AA over time according to group. Within-group analyses were conducted using paired t tests. The significance level was set at $p < .05$ for all analyses.

Results

Demographic and Baseline Characteristics

Four participants in the experimental group withdrew because of hospitalization (three participants) and moving to another area (one participant), and three participants in the control group withdrew because of hospitalization (two participants) and death (one participant), resulting in a dropout rate of 11.7%. Thus, data from 53 participants (experimental group, $n = 26$; control group, $n = 27$) were used in data analysis.

Mean participant age was 64.4 ± 1.31 years, and 56.6% of the participants were men. Furthermore, 47.2% of the participants reported their economic status as "low," mean duration of dialysis was 66.7 ± 56.21 months, nearly all of the participants (98.1%) had concomitant diseases, 52.8% had diabetes, 30.2% were smokers, and 77.4% drank alcohol. Half of the participants were regular exercisers (52.8%), 56.6% experienced bowel movements fewer than three times per week, and 22.6% regularly took laxatives. In the pretest, no significant difference was identified between the experimental group and the control group in terms of xerostomia, salivary flow rates, IDWG, constipation, or diet-related quality of life (all $ps > .05$; Table 1).

Intervention Effects

The xerostomia scores of the experimental group decreased at posttest ($t = 6.08$, $p < .001$). A significant interaction effect between time and group on xerostomia scores was evident ($F = 8.91$, $p = .004$). Salivary flow rates increased from baseline to posttest (4 weeks later) in the experimental group

TABLE 1.
Comparison of Participants' General Characteristics

Characteristic	All ($N = 53$) n	All ($N = 53$) %	Experimental Group ($n = 26$) n	Experimental Group ($n = 26$) %	Control Group ($n = 27$) n	Control Group ($n = 27$) %	χ^2/ t	p
Age (years; M and SD)	64.40	1.31	67.30	10.60	61.50	1.31	1.64	.108
Gender (male)	30	56.6	12	46.2	18	66.7	2.27	.132
Economic status							1.36	.508
High	12	22.6	7	26.9	5	18.5		
Middle	16	30.2	6	23.1	10	37.0		
Low	25	47.2	13	50.0	12	44.4		
Alcohol (yes)	41	77.4	20	76.9	21	77.8	1.90	.247
Smoking (yes)	16	30.2	7	26.9	9	33.3	0.26	.611
Comorbidities (yes)	52	98.1	25	96.2	27	100.0	1.06	.304
Diabetes mellitus (yes)	28	52.8	10	38.5	18	66.7	4.23	.056
Duration of hemodialysis (months; M and SD)	66.70	56.21	61.04	63.36	72.15	48.94	0.71	.480
Regular exercise (yes)	28	52.8	11	42.3	17	63.0	2.27	.132
Frequency of bowel movements (per week)								
< 3	30	56.6	18	69.2	12	44.4	33.17	.069
Regular prescribed laxative usage (yes)	12	22.6	4	15.4	8	29.6	1.54	.327
	M	SD	M	SD	M	SD		
Xerostomia	5.77	2.37	5.65	2.08	5.89	2.65	−0.36	.720
Salivary flow rates (ml/minute)	0.48	0.49	0.53	0.49	0.44	0.50	0.64	.523
Interdialytic weight gain (kg)	3.00	1.19	3.10	1.30	2.89	1.09	0.64	.525
Constipation	4.96	3.30	4.31	2.92	5.59	3.57	−1.44	.157
Diet-related quality of life	68.57	12.08	67.46	13.76	69.63	10.35	−0.65	.521

(t = –7.07, p < .001). In addition, there was a significant Time × Group interaction effect on salivary flow rates (F = 7.19, p = .010). The mean IDWG score improved in the experimental group (t = 3.02, p = .006), whereas the control group remained largely unchanged (t = 0.28, p = .785). However, there was no significant interaction effect between time and group on IDWG scores (F = 3.18, p = .081).

The experimental group had significantly lower constipation scores (t = 5.08, p < .001) at posttest than at baseline. In addition, a significant interaction was identified between time and group for the constipation score (F = 7.35, p = .009).

The diet-related quality of life scores increased between baseline and posttest in the experimental group only (t = –9.25, p < .001). There was a significant interaction between time and group in diet-related quality of life (F = 52.89, p < .001; Table 2).

Discussion

The AA intervention executed in this study successfully improved xerostomia, salivary flow rate, constipation, and diet-related quality of life in patients on hemodialysis. The results of this study are meaningful because AA was shown to effectively alleviate common discomfort and improve mental well-being in patients on hemodialysis. This is important, as the number of patients on hemodialysis has been increasing at a rate of 5%–8% per year in South Korea (Korean Society of Nephrology, 2019). AA was shown to be effective in terms of significantly lowering xerostomia scores and increasing saliva secretion. These results are consistent with the results of a pilot observational study that conducted a 4-week AA intervention on patients on hemodialysis, in which xerostomia and saliva secretion significantly improved from baseline values (G. Yang

et al., 2017). Xerostomia was likely improved because of the increase in saliva secretion, which was induced by the activation of the parasympathetic nervous system caused by the selective stimulus on the thirst auricular acupoint (Bossola & Tazza, 2012). Previous studies have shown the beneficial effects of acupuncture on the ears as a complementary treatment to alleviate xerostomia in patients who had received head and neck radiation therapy (Homb, Wu, Tarima, & Wang, 2014; Morganstein, 2005). Although these previous reports employed invasive acupuncture in different settings and patient populations, similar effects were found because both acupuncture and AA apply pressure to auricular acupoints to stimulate the circulation of Qi and restore normal bodily functions (National Department of Meridian Acupoints, 2000). Recent studies have recommended acupuncture for alleviating xerostomia using four acupoints (three on each ear and one on each index finger; Morganstein, 2005; G. Yang et al., 2017; L. Y. Yang et al., 2010). However, significantly increased salivary secretion from 0.53 to 1.17 ml/m was found in this study when pressure was applied to only one acupoint on the ear (TG1). Therefore, this simplified protocol may be sufficient to alleviate xerostomia, with the advantage of reducing skin discomfort by targeting fewer acupoints. Further studies are necessary to provide more concrete evidence for the efficacy of this protocol.

The mean IDWG of the participants before the experiment was 2.99 kg, which was higher than the 1.3 kg reported for Italian patients on hemodialysis (Bellomo, Coccetta, Pasticci, Rossi, & Selvi, 2015) and the 2.45 kg previously observed in Taiwanese patients (L. Y. Yang et al., 2010). This IDWG value is alarming because previous studies have consistently reported IDWG values greater than 1.5 kg to be

TABLE 2.
Effect of the Intervention on Outcomes

Variable	n	Pretest		Posttest		Time Effect × Group		Group × Time Effect	
		Mean	SD	Mean	SD	t	p	F	p
Xerostomia								8.91	.004
Experimental group	26	5.65	2.08	2.96	2.01	6.08	< .001		
Control group	27	5.89	2.65	5.15	1.68	1.55	.134		
Salivary flow rates (ml/minute)								7.19	.010
Experimental group	26	0.53	0.49	1.17	0.49	–7.07	< .001		
Control group	27	0.44	0.50	0.58	0.88	–0.91	.371		
Interdialytic weight gain (kg)								3.18	.081
Experimental group	26	3.10	1.30	2.60	0.95	3.02	.006		
Control group	27	2.89	1.09	2.84	1.37	0.28	.785		
Constipation								7.35	.009
Experimental group	26	4.31	2.92	1.69	1.93	5.08	< .001		
Control group	27	5.59	3.57	4.89	3.51	1.46	.157		
Diet-related quality of life								52.89	< .001
Experimental group	26	67.46	13.76	84.73	7.57	–9.25	< .001		
Control group	27	69.63	10.35	70.33	12.27	–0.53	.601		

[a]By paired t tests. [b]By two-way repeated-measures analysis of variance.

significantly related to mortality (Kalantar-Zadeh et al., 2009) and increases or decreases of 1% in body weight as strongly related to mortality in patients on hemodialysis (Cabezas-Rodriguez et al., 2013). However, the results of this study failed to support the hypothesis that AA therapy reduces IDWG. This may be because of the 4-week duration of the study, which may have been too short to alter the water intake habits of the participants. However, IDWG decreased significantly after the intervention in the experimental group, which suggests that AA has beneficial effects on dietary fluid restriction by alleviating the symptoms of xerostomia. This finding should be verified using a longer duration of treatment. It has been emphasized in previous studies that symptom management should be prioritized to improve the effectiveness of a therapeutic regimen in patients on hemodialysis (G. Yang et al., 2017). Undoubtedly, AA is a safe method for these patients to self-manage xerostomia simply by pressing a specific point on the ear. Thus, AA may be a strategy with the potential to help patients on dialysis adhere to dietary fluid restrictions.

Furthermore, AA significantly reduced constipation in the experimental group. This result is similar to those of previous studies with regard to constipation (Li et al., 2014) and fecal impaction (Mojalli, Abbasi, Kianmehr, & Zamani, 2016) in patients on hemodialysis. Four of the acupoints used in this study (CO7, CO17, TF3, and CO13) promote bowel movement by regulating the circulation of blood, increasing intestinal peristalsis, and reducing the desiccation and hardening of stools (National Department of Meridian Acupoints, 2000). The participants in the experimental group reported easier passing and softening of their stools. A study conducted in South Korea revealed that patients on hemodialysis had a significantly longer transit time in the right and rectosigmoid colon than patients with chronic constipation (Y. M. Lee et al., 2006). Therefore, AA may be a suitable intervention for patients on hemodialysis who need to restrict fluid and dietary fiber intake and to shorten the duration of passage through the colon.

The diet-related quality of life score of the experimental group improved significantly, whereas that of the control group did not. These results concur with previous findings that AA improved the life quality in patients with diabetes and chronic kidney disease (S. Wang et al., 2014). Furthermore, this result supports findings that acupressure is helpful for managing symptoms such as sleep disturbances in patients on hemodialysis, resulting in enhanced health-related quality of life (Arab et al., 2016). Alleviation of constipation and increased chewing and swallowing ease because of the mitigation of xerostomia may improve diet-related quality of life. J. Lee et al. (2013) showed that diet-related quality-of-life scores in patients on hemodialysis were lower than those in patients with diabetes or hypercholesterolemia. In particular, patients with gastrointestinal symptoms, including constipation, had significantly lower scores for dietary-related quality of life than those without symptoms in that study. According to a phenomenological study of Korean patients on hemodialysis (E. K. Yang & Kim, 2016), participants perceived eating as a "painful" activity because they had been required to give up their favorite foods,

could not eat as much as they would have liked, and found it difficult to taste or swallow foods. Therefore, it is strongly advised to include AA in nursing care to increase saliva secretion and decrease the discomfort associated with eating, with the goal of significantly improving quality of life in patients on hemodialysis (Kim & Kim, 2004; J. Lee et al., 2013).

This study is affected by several limitations. First, the small sample size may have resulted in Type II errors. Second, as data were collected 4 weeks after treatment only, no information regarding the long-term effects of AA is available. Finally, the recruitment of participants was restricted to South Korea, and thus the findings may not be generalizable to other populations.

Conclusions

AA decreases xerostomia and constipation and improves salivary flow rate and diet-related quality of life. AA acts through the stimulation of the acupuncture points of the ear to prevent disease, improve health, and enhance quality of life. Therefore, AA may be an important tool to alleviate negative symptoms and improve overall quality of life in patients on hemodialysis. In addition, because of its noninvasive nature, AA is recommended for use as an effective, independent nursing intervention.

Implications for Clinical Practice

On the basis of the findings of this study, nurses in hemodialysis centers should consider AA as a strategy to enhance the physical and mental well-being of patients on hemodialysis. Nurses may teach AA as an intervention to help patients with xerostomia and constipation to manage their discomfort. Therefore, AA may help patients on hemodialysis better control fluid ingestion and blood pressure and reduce their risk of developing cardiovascular disease.

Author Contributions

Study conception and design: AKC
Data collection: ESJ
Data analysis and interpretation: All authors
Drafting of the article: All authors
Critical revision of the article: AKC

References

Arab, Z., Shariati, A., Asayesh, H., Vakili, M., Bahrami-Taghanaki, H., & Azizi, H. (2016). A sham-controlled trial of acupressure on the quality of sleep and life in haemodialysis patients. *Acupuncture in Medicine, 34*(1), 2–6. https://doi.org/10.1136/acupmed-2014-010369

Bellomo, G., Coccetta, P., Pasticci, F., Rossi, D., & Selvi, A. (2015). The effect of psychological intervention on thirst and interdialytic weight gain in patients on chronic hemodialysis: A randomized controlled trial. *Journal of Renal Nutrition, 25*(5), 426–432. https://doi.org/10.1053/j.jrn.2015.04.005

Bossola, M., Pepe, G., & Vulpio, C. (2018). The frustrating attempt to limit the interdialytic weight gain in patients on chronic hemodialysis: New insights into an old problem. *Journal of Renal Nutrition, 28*(5), 293–301. https://doi.org/10.1053/j.jrn.2018.01.015

Bossola, M., & Tazza, L. (2012). Xerostomia in patients on chronic hemodialysis. *Nature Reviews Nephrology, 8*(3), 176–182. https://doi.org/10.1038/nrneph.2011.218

Cabezas-Rodriguez, I., Carrero, J. J., Zoccali, C., Qureshi, A. R., Ketteler, M., Floege, J., ... Cannata-Andia, J. B. (2013). Influence of body mass index on the association of weight changes with mortality in hemodialysis patients. *Clinical Journal of the American Society of Nephrology, 8*(10), 1725–1733. https://doi.org/10.2215/CJN.10951012

Delahanty, L., Hayden, D., Ammerman, A., & Nathan, D. (2002). Medical nutrition therapy for hypercholesterolemia positively affects patient satisfaction and quality of life outcomes. *Annals of Behavioral Medicine, 24*(4), 269–278. https://doi.org/10.1207/S15324796ABM2404_03

Homb, A., Wu, H., Tarima, S., & Wang, D. (2014). Improvement of radiation-induced xerostomia with acupuncture: A retrospective analysis. *Acupuncture and Related Therapies, 2*(2), 34–38. https://doi.org/10.1016/j.arthe.2014.02.001

Howren, M. B., Kellerman, Q. D., Hillis, S. L., Cvengros, J., Lawton, W., & Christensen, A. J. (2015). Effect of a behavioral self-regulation intervention on patient adherence to fluid-intake restrictions in hemodialysis: A randomized controlled trial. *Annals of Behavioral Medicine, 50*(2), 167–176. https://doi.org/10.1007/s12160-015-9741-0

Kalantar-Zadeh, K., Regidor, D. L., Kovesdy, C. P., Van Wyck, D., Bunnapradist, S., Horwich, T. B., & Fonarow, G. C. (2009). Fluid retention is associated with cardiovascular mortality in patients undergoing long-term hemodialysis. *Circulation, 119*(5), 671–679. https://doi.org/10.1161/CIRCULATIONAHA.108.807362

Kara, B. (2016). Determinants of thirst distress in patients on hemodialysis. *International Urology and Nephrology, 48*(9), 1525–1532. https://doi.org/10.1007/s11255-016-1327-7

Kim, E. Y., & Kim, J. S. (2004). Predictors of quality of life among hemodialysis patients. *Journal of Korean Academy of Adult Nursing, 16*(4), 597–607. (Original work published in Korean)

Korean Society of Nephrology. (2019). *Current renal replacement therapy in Korea: Insan Memorial Dialysis Registry 2018.* Seoul, ROK: Author.

Lee, J., Kim, J. M., & Kim, Y. (2013). Association of diet-related quality of life with dietary regimen practice, health-related quality of life, and gastrointestinal symptoms in end-stage renal disease patients with hemodialysis. *Korean Journal of Nutrition, 46*(2), 137–146. https://doi.org/10.4163/kjn.2013.46.2.137 (Original work published in Korean)

Lee, Y. M., Jeong, S. W., Ju, H. J., Shim, H., Kim, Y. S., Shi, J. H., ... Park, O. R. (2006). Colonic transit time in maintenance hemodialysis patients with constipation. *Kidney Research and Clinical Practice, 25*(2), 289–294. (Original work published in Korean)

Li, M., Lee, T. D., & Suen, K. L. (2014). Complementary effects of auricular acupressure in relieving constipation symptoms and promoting disease-specific health-related quality of life: A randomized placebo-controlled trial. *Complementary Therapies in Medicine, 22*(2), 266–277. https://doi.org/10.1016/j.ctim.2014.01.010

Longstreth, F., Thompson, W. G., Chey, W. D., Houghton, L. A., Mearin, F., & Spiller, R. C. (2006). Functional bowel disorders. *Gastroenterology, 130*(5), 1480–1491. https://doi.org/10.1053/j.gastro.2005.11.061

McMillan, S. C., & Williams, F. A. (1989). Validity and reliability of the constipation assessment scale. *Cancer Nursing, 12*(3), 183–188.

Mojalli, M., Abbasi, P., Kianmehr, M., & Zamani, S. (2016). Effect of acupressure on fecal impaction in hemodialysis patients. *Journal of Mazandaran University of Medical Sciences, 26*(136), 18–25.

Morganstein, W. M. (2005). Auricular acupuncture in the treatment of xerostomia. *Journal of Chinese Medicine, 79,* 5–8.

National Department of Meridian Acupoints. (2000). *Acupuncture.* Seoul, ROK: Gypmundang.

Oleson, T. (2014). *Auriculotherapy manual: Chinese and western systems of ear acupuncture* (4th ed.). Edinburgh, Scotland: Churchill Livingstone Elsevier.

Tvistholm, N., Munch, L., & Danielsen, A. K. (2017). Constipation is casting a shadow over everyday life—A systematic review on older people's experience of living with constipation. *Journal of Clinical Nursing, 26*(7–8), 902–914. https://doi.org/10.1111/jocn.13422

Wang, S., Chen, Z., Fu, P., Zang, L., Wang, L., Zhai, X., ... Zhang, Y. (2014). Use of auricular acupressure to improve the quality of life in diabetic patients with chronic kidney diseases: A prospective randomized controlled trial. *Evidence-Based Complementary and Alternative Medicine, 2014.* Article ID 343608. https://doi.org/10.1155/2014/343608

Wang, Y. (2008). *Micro-acupuncture in practice* (1st ed.). St. Louis, MO: Churchill Livingstone Elsevier.

Working Group on Auricular Acupuncture Nomenclature & World Health Organization Traditional Medicine Unit. (1991). *Report on the working group on auricular acupuncture nomenclature, Lyon, France, 28–30 November 1990.* Retrieved from https://apps.who.int/iris/handle/10665/60870

Yang, E. K., & Kim, I. O. (2016). Hemodialysis patients' experience of adapting to dietary therapy. *Korean Journal of Adult Nursing, 28*(3), 323–333. https://doi.org/10.7475/kjan.2016.28.3.323 (Original work published in Korean)

Yang, G., Lin, S., Wu, Y., Zhang, S., Wu, X., Liu, X., ... Lin, Q. (2017). AA helps alleviate xerostomia in maintenance patients on hemodialysis: A pilot study. *The Journal of Alternative and Complementary Medicine, 23*(4), 278–284. https://doi.org/10.1089/acm.2016.0283

Yang, L. Y., Yates, P., Chin, C. C., & Kao, T. K. (2010). Effect of acupressure on thirst in patients on hemodialysis. *Kidney & Blood Pressure Research, 33*(4), 260–265. https://doi.org/10.1159/000317933

Yang, S. (1992). *Effects on fluid intake, dietary fiber supplement and abdominal muscle exercise on antipsychotic drug-induced constipation in schizophrenics* (Unpublished doctoral dissertation). Seoul, ROK: Catholic University of Korea. (Original work published in Korean)

Yeh, C. H., Chien, L. C., Albers, K. M., Ren, D., Huang, L. C., Cheng, B., ... Suen, L. K. (2014). Function of auricular point acupressure in inducing changes in inflammatory cytokines during chronic low-back pain: A pilot study. *Medical Acupuncture, 26*(1), 31–39. https://doi.org/10.1089/acu.2013.1015

22

The Frequency and Perceived Effectiveness of Pain Self-Management Strategies Used by Individuals With Migraine

Hao-Yuan CHANG[1]* • Chih-Chao YANG[2] • Mark P. JENSEN[3] • Yeur-Hur LAI[4]

ABSTRACT

Background: Migraine is ranked among the most important causes of disability worldwide. Some effective migraine treatments have been identified. However, little is known regarding the treatment strategies used by patients with migraine to manage pain or their efficacy.

Purpose: This study was designed to (a) investigate the pain management strategies used by migraineurs and their perceived effectiveness and (b) evaluate the association between the number of strategies used and their overall perceived effectiveness.

Methods: A cross-sectional design with consecutive sampling was used in a medical center in Taiwan. Individuals with migraine (*N* = 174) completed self-administered questionnaires and in-depth interviews to assess the frequency and perceived effectiveness of a variety of pain management strategies.

Results: Most participants reported using prescription medications (56%) and over-the-counter medications (51%), which were rated as having good efficacy rates of 78% and 81%, respectively. Traditional Chinese medicine (17%) and folk remedies (13%) were used less frequently and rated as relatively less effective at 65% and 48%, respectively. About half (47%) reported using more than one pain management strategy. Significantly more of those who reported using multiple pain management strategies reported at least "some effect" than those who reported using one strategy only (73% vs. 27%, *p* = .001).

Conclusions: Prescription medications showed good usage rate and good perceived efficacy. However, about half of the participants used multiple pain management strategies, supporting the need for further research to evaluate the efficacy of combination treatments and to identify those combinations that may have the most additive and/or synergistic effects. Furthermore, the findings indicate that continued use of medications for migraine management is appropriate for many individuals because of the relatively high rates of perceived efficacy for this strategy found in this study.

KEY WORDS:
migraine, pain management, self-management, perceived effectiveness.

Introduction

Migraine is one of the most important causes of disability worldwide, affecting estimated 1.04 billion people worldwide in 2016 (Stovner et al., 2018). Moreover, migraine-related disability and missed workdays cause significant human downtime (an estimated 45.1 million years of life lived with disability globally in 2016; Stovner et al., 2018) and a significant financial cost (an estimated loss of $13 billion dollars a year in the United States; Hu et al., 1999; Silberstein & Marmura, 2015). Headache is a universal health problem, even in nurse populations (Ko et al., 2018), further supporting the importance of appropriate migraine management.

Research has identified a number of effective migraine treatments, including abortive medications (e.g., triptans, nonsteroidal anti-inflammatory drugs; Dodick, 2018; Macone & Perloff, 2017) and preventive medications (e.g., beta-blockers, calcium channel blockers; Mayans & Walling, 2018). However, little is known regarding how patients with migraine actually manage their pain and how they perceive the efficacy of their pain management/treatment strategies. In addition, little is known regarding the association between the number of pain management strategies used and overall effectiveness.

Research to address these knowledge gaps would clarify the extent to which migraineurs use the management strategies that have been identified as effective in the literature. Such research could potentially identify new or understudied management approaches that warrant additional research to

[1]PhD, RN, Assistant Professor, School of Nursing, College of Medicine, National Taiwan University, and Adjunct Supervisor, Department of Nursing, National Taiwan University Hospital, Taiwan, ROC • [2]MD, Attending Physician, Department of Neurology, National Taiwan University Hospital, Taiwan, ROC • [3]PhD, Professor, Department of Rehabilitation Medicine, University of Washington, Seattle, WA, USA • [4]PhD, RN, FAAN, Professor, School of Nursing, College of Medicine, National Taiwan University, and Director, Department of Nursing, National Taiwan University Cancer Center, Taipei, Taiwan, ROC.

evaluate their efficacy. Moreover, knowledge in this area could provide insights for clinical professionals to facilitate their consulting with patients regarding management strategies that may be most effective.

Given these considerations, the purposes of this study were to (a) investigate the frequency of use and perceived efficacy of different pain management strategies actually used by migraineurs seeking treatment by physicians and (b) evaluate the association between the number of pain management strategies used and overall effectiveness.

We hypothesized that pain management strategies with the most solid empirical support (e.g., medications) would emerge as being used most frequently and also rated as the most effective, relative to other migraine pain management strategies. However, we also sought to determine if there were additional pain management strategies used that were rated as being effective by at least some individuals with migraine and thus potentially worthy of further empirical study. Moreover, considering the potential synergistic effects of different treatments when used in combination, we also hypothesized that the number of pain management strategies adopted by migraineurs would relate positively to overall effectiveness.

Methods

Design

A cross-sectional design was adopted to address the study aims. Consecutive sampling was adopted to maximize sample representation. Consecutive sampling refers to the sampling method in which all members of an identified population are approached and invited to participate over a fixed period (Polit & Beck, 2017).

Setting and Participants

Patients were diagnosed as having migraine by four board-certified neurologists based on International Headache Society criteria. We recruited participants from nine different clinics (seven neurology clinics and two general medicine clinics) of a large medical center in Taiwan from September 2015 through July 2016. Inclusion criteria were (a) being 20–65 years old and (b) having a migraine diagnosis based on International Headache Society criteria, including migraine without aura (International Classification of Headache Disorders [ICHD] Code 1.1) and migraine with typical aura (ICHD 1.2.1). Exclusion criteria were being diagnosed with (a) a rare migraine type, basilar-type migraine (ICHD Code 1.2.2), including hemiplegic migraine (ICHD Code 1.2.3), retinal migraine, and other migraine types (ICHD Codes 1.2.4–1.2.6 and 1.3–1.5) or (b) a mixed headache type, for example, combination of migraine and tension-type headache. Medication overuse headache (ICHD Code 8.2), defined as a headache attributed to a substance or its withdrawal, was also excluded.

Patients who met the inclusion/exclusion criteria were referred to our research team. When these potential participants returned to the clinic for a subsequent visit, a research assistant described the study to them and invited them to participate. Those who agreed to participate were asked to sign the informed consent form before any data were collected.

The estimated sample size was calculated using G*Power Version 3.1.9.2. For an effect size $f = .25$, alpha = .05, power = .80, and number of groups = 3, the estimated sample size was set at a minimum of 159. From September 2015 through July 2016, we approached 214 potential participation patients who met the inclusion criteria. Thirteen (6%) declined to participate, 25 (12%) did not return to the clinic again, and two (1%) withdrew from the study after completing the interview. This left valid information from 174 participants (81% of those who were eligible) in the final data set.

Ethical Considerations

All of the study procedures were approved by the institutional review board at National Taiwan University Hospital (201505065RIND). Signed informed consent was obtained from participants before data collection. Data were collected by three trained research assistants who followed a standardized assessment procedure.

Measures

The data presented in this article were collected as part of a survey study on a group of patients with migraine that used semistructured questionnaires and in-depth interviews to survey patient perspectives (Polit & Beck, 2017). Domains assessed included pain management strategies used, the perceived effectiveness of these strategies, pain intensity, migraine-related disability, and demographic information. The Migraine-Specific Quality of Life Chinese Version 2.1 (MSQv2.1-C) was also administered to this group, and the findings related this measure have already been reported (Chang et al., 2019). No overlap in study aims exist between Chang et al. and this study.

Pain management strategies and perceived effectiveness

Participants answered questions regarding "headache pain management" and perceived effectiveness, including "pain relief" and "effect duration." The first, open-ended question was "What pain management strategies have you ever used for your migraine?" Participants were then asked to describe each pain management strategy they had used in as much detail as possible. Each strategy was then was coded into specific pain management categories, including prescription medicine, over-the-counter (OTC) medicine, traditional Chinese medicine (TCM), folk remedy, and other management strategies.

The second question was "Please circle the percentage amount to indicate how much pain relief you obtained using this treatment." This question assessed the amount of pain relief that the participant achieved using each pain management strategy. The respondent could circle one of 11 response options along a graded scale ranging from 0% (*no relief*) to 100% (*total relief*). Some of the participants asked if they could indicate a pain relief level between two response options (e.g., 55% or 65%), which was allowed.

The third question was "How long did the pain relief last?" Participants were asked to choose one response for each pain management strategy used on a 4-point Likert scale: 1 = *no effect*, 2 = *less than 1 day*, 3 = *more than 1 day*, and 4 = *I have not had a migraine episode since this treatment*. For prescription medications, "treatment" reflected the dose and frequency of use as, although the immediate effects of most prescription medications are short-lived (i.e., less than 24 hours), treatment often lasts for an extended period.

Demographic and pain-related data

Basic demographic information (age, education level, and marital status) were provided by the participants for descriptive purposes. Average pain intensity during the past 3 months and worst pain intensity in the last migraine episode were measured using a 0–10 numerical rating scale, with 0 = *no pain at all* and 10 = *worst pain I can imagine*.

Migraine-related disability was measured using the Migraine Disability Assessment (MIDAS; Hung et al., 2006; Stewart et al., 1999). The MIDAS measures three aspects of daily life: employment (work/school), household work, and nonwork activities. On the MIDAS, respondents are asked to indicate the number of days that five different activities were limited by migraine. Total possible MIDAS scores range from 0 to 270, with the result used to classify respondents into four grades of migraine-related disability: (a) 0–5, little or no disability; (b) 6–10, mild disability; (c) 11–20, moderate disability; and (d) ≥ 21, severe disability.

The MIDAS was developed by Stewart et al. (1999) and has shown good reliability and validity, with a 21-day test–retest reliability of .67–.73 for the items and .84 for the total scale. Internal consistency reliability (Cronbach's alpha) was found to be .83 and .79, respectively, in the original scale development sample and in this study. MIDAS scores have been shown to differ between migraineurs and nonmigraineurs, supporting the discriminant validity of the measure (Stewart et al., 1999). The MIDAS has been translated from English into other languages, including traditional Chinese (Hung et al., 2006), Japanese (Iigaya et al., 2003), and Turkish (Ertas et al., 2004). All of the translated versions of this scale have shown good reliability and validity.

Data Analysis

Descriptive statistics were first computed with the demographic, migraine/pain history, and disability measures to describe the sample. Next, the frequency, percentage, means, and standard deviations of the responses to the pain management use and effectiveness questions were calculated. Chi-square analysis was used to examine the association between the number of strategies used and overall effectiveness. Analysis of variance using Scheffe's post hoc test was used to examine the association between attack severity and usage of multiple pain management strategies. IBM SPSS Version 21.0 (IBM, Armonk, NY, USA) was used for all statistical analyses, and the level of significance was set as .05.

Results

Description of the Participants

Demographic and pain-related data for the sample are shown in Table 1. The average age was 38.5 years (SD = 11.8), and most held a college degree (66%) and were married (53%). The mean worst pain intensity score for the most recent migraine episode was 6.3/10 (SD = 2.1), and the mean average pain intensity score of migraine headaches during the past 3 months was 5.5/10 (SD = 2.1). The plurality of disability grade was "minimal or infrequent" (48%).

Use and Perceived Effectiveness of Pain Management Strategies

As shown in Table 2, most participants used physician-prescribed medications (56%, e.g., Imigran, Cafergot, Inderal), 51% used OTC medications (e.g., acetaminophen, acetaminophen plus caffeine, caffeine plus ergotamine, or nonsteroidal anti-inflammatory drugs), 17% used TCM, and 13% used a folk remedy (e.g., massage or "gua sha," an instrument-assisted massage that induces cutaneous petechiae). During the interviews, the participants indicated that gua sha was usually used during acute pain episodes. Some of the participants indicated that they were given gua sha massages by their friends or relatives, and some reported that they were given gua sha massages by masseurs. Other, significantly less-frequently used strategies included rest/sleep, coffee, and essential oils applied to the body.

Of the listed pain management strategies, 8%–37% were reported to be totally ineffective, with prescribed medications reported as ineffective the least often (prescription medications: 8%; OTC medications: 10%; TCM: 37%; folk remedies: 23%; other strategies: 16%). Twenty-five (14%) of the participants reported all of the pain management strategies used as totally ineffective.

Two themes emerged from the interviews: (a) considering both Western and Chinese medicine and (b) managing the headache.

Considering both Western and Chinese medicine

The three subthemes that emerged under this theme were (a) uncertainty regarding the effects of treatment, (b) using a combination of Chinese and Western medicine approaches, and (c) using Western medicine as a last resort.

Uncertainty regarding the effects of treatment: Whatever the pain treatment, participants reported uncertainty regarding its effects. For example, "*Painkillers are not always effective*" (Case 69). Because of this uncertainty, the participants sought other pain management strategies for their migraine. For example, "*Panadol Extra is not effective, so I went for*

Table 1

Demographics and Pain-Related Data of the Participants (N = 174)

Variable	n	%	Mean	SD	Range
Age (years)			38.5	11.8	20–65
20–30	49	28			
31–40	57	33			
41–50	35	20			
51–60	26	15			
61–65	6	3			
Missing (refuse to provide)	1	1			
Body mass index			22.6	3.9	15.0–40.1
Education					
High school or less	32	18			
College	115	66			
Graduate school	27	16			
Marital status					
Unmarried	75	43			
Married	92	53			
Ever married	7	4			
Average pain intensity			5.5	2.1	0–10
Mild (1–4)	55	32			
Moderate (5–6)	59	34			
Severe (7–10)	60	34			
Worst pain intensity			6.3	2.1	1–10
Mild (1–4)	33	20			
Moderate (5–6)	47	28			
Severe (7–10)	85	52			
Disability (MIDAS)			16.0	33.3	0–270
Minimal or infrequent (0–5)	84	48			
Mild (6–10)	32	18			
Moderate (11–20)	27	16			
Severe (21 or above)	31	18			
Number of pain management strategies used					
One	93	53			
Two	48	28			
More than three	33	19			

Note. MIDAS = Migraine Disability Assessment.

Chinese medicine" (Case 48), "*Traditional Chinese medicine was effective one month ago, but now, it is gone. The effect is not immediate; the effect is uncertain*" (Case 41), and "*I went to seek a physician's help because I found the OTC was not effective for my headache*" (Case 97).

Using a combination of Chinese and Western medicine approaches: Some participants choose to use both Chinese and Western medicine (Cases 56, 98, and 99). For example, "*I take Western medicine in the morning and evening and take Chinese medicine after meals three times a day. If the pain persists, I take OTC medicine*" (Case 56) and "*When it hurts as much as a 2 (Numerical Rating Scales pain scale), I take Western medicine (acetaminophen). I also take Chinese medicine four times a day*" (Case 99).

Using Western medicine as a last resort: The timing of taking pain medicine was polarized. Only seven participants

reported that they "*Take medicine as soon as it hurts*" (n = 8; Cases 65, 82, 141, 149, 151, 154, 159, and 161), whereas 27 participants reported: "*I take the medicine when I cannot endure the pain*" (n = 27; Cases 7, 17, 19, 21, 23–25, 30, 35, 38, 72, 77, 86, 96, 133, 135, 136, 140, 148, 152, 153, 158, 160, 163, 167, 170, and 176). Some reported trying massage first and taking medicine only if the pain persisted (n = 5; Cases 22, 148, 153, 160, and 163): "*It hurts, but I need to work. Thus, I took Panadol*" (Case 6).

Managing the headache

The four subthemes that emerged under this theme were (a) seeking to identify a "protocol" suitable for their headache, (b) avoiding aggravating factors and triggers, (c) adopting regular prevention, and (d) adopting passive coping.

Table 2

Pain Management and Relief Ratings Reported by the Participants (N = 174)

Pain Management	n	%	Pain Relief M	SD	[Median, Mode]	Effective Rate [a] (%)	No effect n	%	≤ 1 Day n	%	> 1 Day n	%	No Attack n	%	Missing [b] n	%
Prescription medicine	98	56	65	31.0	[70, 100]	78	8	8	13	13	49	50	13	13	15	15
Abortive [c]	80	46	69	27.6	[70, 100]	82	5	6	11	14	40	50	11	14	13	16
Rescue [d]	24	14	53	34.8	[60, 0 & 80]	67	3	13	2	8	11	46	3	13	5	21
Preventive [e]	29	17	66	32.3	[65, 100]	80	1	3	5	17	10	34	4	14	9	31
Over-the-counter medicine [f]	89	51	70	31.0	[80, 100]	81	9	10	20	22	32	36	23	26	5	6
Acetaminophen	36	21	64	32.2	[70, 100]	79	4	11	6	17	13	36	10	28	3	8
Analgesics (unknown)	23	13	70	35.3	[80, 100]	73	3	13	7	30	7	30	6	26	–	–
NSAIDs	22	13	80	20.2	[85, 100]	90	–	–	5	23	9	41	7	32	1	5
Acetaminophen + caffeine	8	5	52	43.2	[60, 0]	67	2	25	2	25	3	38	–	–	1	13
Traditional Chinese medicine	30	17	52	27.7	[60, 60 & 70]	65	11	37	5	17	6	20	2	7	6	20
Chinese herbs	19	11	49	26.2	[60, 60]	67	10	53	1	5	4	21	1	5	3	16
Acupuncture	7	4	68	26.8	[80, 40 & 80]	60	–	–	3	43	1	14	1	14	2	29
Herbs + acupuncture	4	2	40	36.1	[50, 0 & 50 & 70]	67	1	25	1	25	1	25	–	–	1	25
Folk remedy	22	13	49	32.1	[40, 30]	48	5	23	8	36	5	23	2	9	2	9
Massage	20	11	45	31.0	[40, 30]	42	5	25	7	35	5	25	1	5	2	10
"Gua sha" therapy	4	2	63	28.7	[55, 40]	50	1	25	2	50	–	–	1	25	–	–
Hot packing	1	< 1	30	0.0	[30, 30]	0	–	–	–	–	1	100	–	–	–	–
Electronic therapy	1	< 1	40	0.0	[40, 40]	0	1	100	–	–	–	–	–	–	–	–
Other management	32	18	57	33.1	[60, 60 & 100]	64	5	16	8	25	12	38	3	9	4	13
Rest/sleep	11	6	64	36.0	[70, 100]	70	1	9	2	18	4	36	3	27	1	9
Hot coffee	11	6	51	36.7	[60, 0 & 60]	64	2	18	3	27	6	55	–	–	–	–
Essential oil (applied to body)	6	3	26	24.0	[40, 0 & 40]	20	3	50	2	33	1	17	–	–	–	–
Healthy supplement	1	< 1	100	0.0	[100, 100]	100	–	–	–	–	1	100	–	–	–	–
Meditation	1	< 1	90	0.0	[90, 90]	100	–	–	–	–	1	100	–	–	–	–
Pray	1	< 1	70	0.0	[70]	100	–	–	1	100	–	–	–	–	–	–
Emetic by finger	1	< 1	60	0.0	[60]	100	–	–	1	100	–	–	–	–	–	–
Beating head	1	< 1	30	0.0	[30, 30]	0	1	100	–	–	–	–	–	–	–	–

Note. NSAIDs = nonsteroidal anti-inflammatory drugs.
[a] Treatments that provided a 50% or greater amount of pain relief were defined as effective. Effective rate refers to the proportion of respondents endorsing effective pain relief among those who used the pain management approach; [b] Participants who find that a pain management approach is not consistently effective are not able to rate the duration of effect for that approach; [c] Abortive (e.g., triptans, ergotamine tartrate plus caffeine, nonsteroidal anti-inflammatory drugs, antiemetics); [d] Rescue (e.g., tramadol plus acetaminophen, benzodiazepine, anxiolytics, muscle relaxant, anticoagulants); [e] Preventive (e.g., β-blocker, antidepressant, anticonvulsant, calcium channel blockers); [f] Over-the-counter medicine refers to the medicine bought from pharmacy.

Seeking to identify a "protocol" suitable for their headache: For example, "*I have coffee every day. When it hurts, I take Naposin as soon as possible, and then sit and do not move. If it still hurts after one hour, I will take Imigran*" (Case 65) and "*If my pain score is only 5, I take Panadol Extra (acetaminophen plus caffeine). If my pain scale is 8, I will take Imigran. If Imigran is not effective, I will take Panadol Extra six hours later*" (Case 18).

Avoiding aggravating factors and triggers: The participants reported avoiding aggravating factors and triggers such as cold environments, high stress, fatigue, cheese products, and pungent smells: "*I try to find the source of my headache such as being in environments with large temperature differences, high stress, or fatigue*" (Case 11), "*I know that my headache will become more severe after drinking coffee*" (Case 10), and

"*I avoid cheese products and other strange smells such as smoke, betel nut, and pungent perfume*" (Case 27).

Adopting regular prevention such as drinking coffee every day or taking preventive medication: For example, "*Drinking coffee during the day and ginger tea at night*" (Case 26), "*I take Inderal daily. When I have an attack, I will take Imigran with Paramol, Ibuprofen, or Naposin. Otherwise, I have a cup of coffee every day*" (Case 27), and "*If I do not have a cup of coffee, I will have a headache that day*" (Case 63).

Adopting passive coping: Some participants reported that they do not take medicine, receive massage, or engage in other active management measures but rather wait for improvement: "*I just lie on my bed and wait for relief...because...I think it's useless to take medicine. You know that...during a (migraine) attack I will vomit. Even if I take medicine, I will vomit it out"* (Case 11).

Summary of qualitative findings

Many participants viewed Western medication approaches as a last resort. The participants reported holding some concerns regarding the possible side effects of medications (such as the hepatotoxicity of Panadol) and preferred using approaches that do not involve prescription medications (such as massage, coffee, and Chinese medicine) to manage their pain. However, when these approaches did not effectively reduce pain, many then used Western pain medicines because of their perceived high efficacy. Furthermore, the participants often adopted multiple strategies to manage their migraine.

Nearly half (47%) of the participants reported using more than one pain management strategy. These combined treatments and their level of pain relief are listed in Table 3. From the perspective of the participants, "OTC only," "OTC + other management," and "OTC + folk remedy (massage) + other management" were rated as the most effective (combined) treatments. Moreover, the efficacy (i.e., pain relief) of "single" pain management strategies (except for TCM) was found to be better than that of combined treatment strategies (Table 3).

Of those participants who reported using two or more pain management strategies, significantly more reported the effectiveness to be at least "some effect" (73% vs. 27%, χ^2 (2) = 14.6, p = .001; Table 4). Use of multiple pain management strategies was associated with attack severity (F = 5.94, p = .003; Scheffe's post hoc: worst pain intensity 7.3 [three or more pain management strategies] vs. 5.8 [one strategy], p = .004).

Discussion

To the best of our knowledge, this was the first study to examine from the perspective of patients how patients manage their migraine. As hypothesized, prescription and OTC medications were used most often and rated as being most effective. Furthermore, almost half of the participants reported using more than one pain management strategy. These findings have important clinical and research implications.

Prescription and Over-the-Counter Medications

Triptans are effective in managing migraine for many people (Dodick, 2018; Macone & Perloff, 2017) in terms of providing total pain relief within 2 hours and continued pain relief for at least 24 hours (Lipton et al., 2017). Consistent with this finding, prescription medications, including triptans, were shown in this study to provide better efficacy (a larger proportion of participants reporting them as effective) and effect duration than other migraine pain management strategies. Prescription (65%) and OTC (70%) medications were identified as providing more pain relief than the other three pain

Table 3

Pain Relief Provided by Each Pain Management Combination, by Ranking (N = 174)

Combination	n	Mean (%) [a]	Rank
OTC	30	75	1
OTC + OM	6	69	2
OTC + FR (massage) + OM	2	68	3
FR (massage [2]/gua sha [3])	5	66	4
OTC + FR (massage)	3	63	5
PM	42	62	6
PM + OTC + TCM	8	61	7
OM	11	58	8
PM + OTC	23	55	9
PM + OTC + FR + OM	1	55	10
PM + OTC + TCM + OM	3	54	11
PM + OTC + OM	2	53	12
PM + OTC + FR	5	51	13
PM + OTC + TCM + FR	4	50	14
PM + TCM + FR	3	42	15
PM + TCM	7	41	16
PM + FR + OM	3	41	17
PM + OTC + TCM + FR + OM	1	40	18
PM + OM	3	35	19
PM + FR	5	32	20
OTC + TCM	1	28	21
TCM + OM	1	20	22
None	3	0	23
TCM	2	0	23

Note. OTC = over-the-counter medicine; OM = other management; FR = folk remedy; PM = prescription medicine; TCM = traditional Chinese medicine.
[a] Mean scores were calculated as the average of the pain relief scores of the pain management combination. For example, for the two participants who chose the combination "OTC + FR (massage) + OM," one reported pain relief scores for OTC, FR, and OM as 80%, 30%, and 50%, respectively (i.e., average pain relief for this combination = 53%), whereas the other reported pain relief scores for OTC, FR, and OM as 100%, 70%, and 80%, respectively (i.e., average pain relief for this combination = 83%). Thus, the mean score for the combination "OTC + FR (massage) + OM" is 68% (the average of 53% and 83%).

management options (49%–57%). These findings suggest that OTC medications may be the most effective pain management approaches used from the patients' perspective.

From the perspective of the participants, "OTC only," "OTC + other management," and "OTC + folk remedy (massage) + other management" were rated as the most effective combined treatments. These results may explain why patients with migraine use OTC medication so often. OTC medications are easy to obtain and provide good pain relief. However, for patients experiencing severe levels of migraine pain, the potential of developing medication overuse headache should be considered as a risk of using OTC drugs.

Table 4

Association Between Average Effectiveness and Number of Pain Management Strategies Used

Average Effectiveness [a]	Number of Pain Management Strategies Used				Total		Chi-Square	p
	One		≥ Two					
	n	%	*n*	%	*n*	%		
Totally ineffective (0)	17	68	8	32	25	100	14.6	.001
Some effect (1.0–4.9)	11	27	29	73	40	100	(*df* = 2)	
Effective (5.0 or above)	65	60	44	40	109	100		
Total	93	53	81	47	174	100		

[a] Average effectiveness (possible range: 0–10) = sum of pain relief score / sum of the number of pain management strategies used.

Traditional Chinese Medicine

TCM treats migraine as a symptom of imbalance in the "Qi" and insufficient blood perfusion in organs (Xiao et al., 2015). TCM doctors typically prescribe Chinese herbs/formulas to balance the Qi, promoting blood circulation and reducing stasis (Xiao et al., 2015). Consistent with research supporting the efficacy of TCM (Luo et al., 2020), the participants in this study rated herbs as being effective more often than not (67%). Thus, the findings in this study concur with the TCM perspective with respect to the perceived efficacy of related treatments.

Acupuncture is primarily used for prevention and has been shown to reduce pain intensity and improve quality of life (Jiang et al., 2018). In this study, the substantial effectiveness of acupuncture was shown to be highly effective (effective rate: 68%), although it was also found that the benefits of acupuncture lasted for less than 1 day in most participants. Thus, the findings suggest an important potential limitation of using acupuncture to manage acute pain attacks and may help explain why so few participants chose this approach (only 6% in our sample). The findings indicate that future acupuncture research should examine the duration of treatment benefits more closely. If the maintenance of benefits is found to be limited, as suggested in this study, research may be needed to identify strategies to enhance the maintenance of gains such as teaching patients to self-administer acupressure using, for example, a self-acupressure pillow (Vernon et al., 2015) or ear acupuncture (Murakami et al., 2017).

Folk Remedies

Although traditional massage has been found to be effective in reducing migraine pain, it is not widely used and has not been reported to be as effective as lymphatic drainage massage (Happe et al., 2016). Echoing the findings of prior research, folk remedies were found in this study to be not as effective as pain management strategies backed by greater empirical support for efficacy (e.g., prescription or OTC medications, TCM). Specifically, traditional massage was rated as relatively low in effectiveness (42%) and was reported as having a short duration of efficacy (67% reported no effect

or benefits lasting less than 1 day). However, the finding of a 50% effectiveness rate for gua sha therapy represents a new and consequential finding and suggests that gua sha warrants future study as a potentially effective traditional approach to migraine pain relief.

Other Approaches to Migraine Management

In this study, sleep was found to be effective in alleviating migraine, with a very high effectiveness rating of 70%. This is consistent with the findings of previous research supporting the importance of sleep in migraine management. Insufficient sleep is known to be associated with an increased frequency of migraine attacks (Kim et al., 2017), and treating insomnia may reduce the frequency of migraine attacks (Sullivan et al., 2019). The findings of this study contribute to the literature further by indicating that the benefits of good sleep on migraine may persist for more than 1 day. This finding supports the need to further evaluate the efficacy of treatments that improve sleep quality in individuals with migraine, especially those reporting sleep problems, as a potential way to reduce migraine headache frequency and severity.

Drinking an adequate amount of coffee intermittently has also been cited as an effective strategy to alleviating migraine (Lee et al., 2016; Nehlig, 2016). Caffeine may also enhance the beneficial effects of analgesics on migraine (Nehlig, 2016), although in some cases, caffeine may aggravate migraine severity (Mostofsky et al., 2019). Consistent with the findings of previous studies, in this study, drinking coffee was found to be fairly effective in alleviating migraine (64%) over an extended duration (55% reported an effect greater than 1 day). Clinicians may find this information useful and incorporate it into recommendations for patients with migraine.

Seeking Multiple Ways to More Effectively Manage Migraine

A new finding highlighted in this study is that a substantial subgroup of individuals with migraine (14% in this study) receives no significant effect from current pain management strategies. This underscores the need to identify additional and effective treatment options for people with migraine and to explore whether individuals in this subgroup are not using potentially effective management strategies.

Interestingly, and inconsistent with one of the study hypotheses, the participants who reported the greatest success in managing their migraine (i.e., perceived their means as "totally effective") tended to use a single strategy only. Thus, rather than using a "shotgun" approach to target multiple causative factors, it may be that the most effective strategy is for individuals to identify a single approach that is most effective for their particular problem or situation if their headache responds well to just one treatment. Consistent with our hypothesis, those who reported the poorest results in managing their migraine (i.e., perceived their means as "totally ineffective") were also more likely to report using a single treatment approach than their more-successful peers (Table 4). People may try to use the least medication possible, so one may expect a mild attack to be treated by one approach and a more severe attack by multiple approaches. Moreover, a second approach may be initiated later than the first approach, with the time gap affecting overall treatment efficacy. In pain management practice, multitherapy approaches have generally shown better effectiveness than single therapy approaches. For example, "acupuncture plus tui-na massage" showed better effect than "acupuncture only" in patients with migraine (Nie et al., 2019). In addition, "massage plus acupressure" showed to be relatively more effective than "massage only" or "acupressure only" on relieving labor pain (Gönenç & Terzioğlu, 2020). Thus, a multitherapy approach may be the future direction for research.

Study Limitations

Several limitations should be considered when interpreting the findings of this study. First, the use of specific pain management approaches and their effectiveness were self-reported as recalled by the participants. Although the sample size was large and saturation seems to have been achieved, it is possible that management approaches used by some individuals with migraine were not reported here.

Second, a cross-sectional design was used in this study. Thus, it is not possible to draw conclusions regarding causal relationships among the study variables. Future researchers may use longitudinal designs and a headache diary to evaluate how changes in pain management approach are associated with and precede changes in headache activity. In addition, well-designed and adequately powered clinical trials will be necessary to confirm, for example, the superior effect of Western medicine (e.g., triptans) and TCM (e.g., acupuncture) over placebos in treating migraine pain.

Summary and Conclusions

Despite its limitations, this study provides new and important knowledge regarding the use of pain management strategies in individuals with migraine. Our findings suggest the unmet needs in the pain management of migraine. As self-reported by the participants, all of whom were currently being treated by physicians, OTC medications (rather than prescription medications) were identified as most effective, with the highest prevalence and highest perceived efficacy. The findings also support the need to identify and evaluate the efficacy of additional treatment options for individuals with migraine so that all who are at risk of migraine may develop and use a management plan that is most effective for them.

Acknowledgments

The authors thank the Ministry of Science and Technology, Taiwan, for supporting this research under a financial grant (MOST-104-2314-B-002-071).

Author Contributions

Study conception and design: HYC, YHL, CCY
Data collection: HYC, CCY
Data analysis and interpretation: HYC, MPJ, YHL
Drafting of the article: HYC
Critical revision of the article: All authors

References

Chang, H.-Y., Jensen, M. P., Yang, C.-C., & Lai, Y.-H. (2019). Migraine-Specific Quality of Life Questionnaire Chinese version 2.1 (MSQv2.1-C): Psychometric evaluation in patients with migraine. *Health and Quality of Life Outcomes, 17*(1), Article No. 108. https://doi.org/10.1186/s12955-019-1169-y

Dodick, D. W. (2018). Migraine. *The Lancet, 391*(10127), 1315–1330. https://doi.org/10.1016/S0140-6736(18)30478-1

Ertas, M., Siva, A., Dalkara, T., Uzuner, N., Dora, B., Inan, L., Idiman, F., Sarica, Y., Selçuki, D., Sirin, H., Oğuzhanoğlu, A., Irkeç, C., Ozmenoğlu, M., Ozbenli, T., Oztürk, M., Saip, S., Neyal, M., & Zarifoğlu, M., Turkish MIDAS Group. (2004). Validity and reliability of the Turkish Migraine Disability Assessment (MIDAS) questionnaire. *Headache, 44*(8), 786–793. https://doi.org/10.1111/j.1526-4610.2004.04146.x

Gönenç, I. M., & Terzioğlu, F. (2020). Effects of massage and acupressure on relieving labor pain, reducing labor time, and increasing delivery satisfaction. *The Journal of Nursing Research, 28*(1), Article e68. https://doi.org/10.1097/jnr.0000000000000344

Happe, S., Peikert, A., Siegert, R., & Evers, S. (2016). The efficacy of lymphatic drainage and traditional massage in the prophylaxis of migraine: A randomized, controlled parallel group study. *Neurological Sciences, 37*(10), 1627–1632. https://doi.org/10.1007/s10072-016-2645-3

Hu, X. H., Markson, L. E., Lipton, R. B., Stewart, W. F., & Berger, M. L. (1999). Burden of migraine in the United States: Disability and economic costs. *Archives of Internal Medicine, 159*(8), 813–818. https://doi.org/10.1001/archinte.159.8.813

Hung, P. H., Fuh, J. L., & Wang, S. J. (2006). Validity, reliability and application of the Taiwan version of the Migraine Disability Assessment questionnaire. *Journal of the Formosan Medical Association, 105*(7), 563–568. https://doi.org/10.1016/S0929-6646(09)60151-0

Iigaya, M., Sakai, F., Kolodner, K. B., Lipton, R. B., & Stewart, W. F. (2003). Reliability and validity of the Japanese Migraine Disability Assessment (MIDAS) Questionnaire. *Headache, 43*(4), 343–352. https://doi.org/10.1046/j.1526-4610.2003.03069.x

Jiang, Y., Bai, P., Chen, H., Zhang, X.-Y., Tang, X.-Y., Chen, H.-Q., Hu, Y.-Y., Wang, X.-L., Li, X.-Y., Li, Y.-P., & Tian, G.-H. (2018). The effect of acupuncture on the quality of life in patients with migraine: A systematic review and meta-analysis. *Frontiers in Pharmacology, 9*, Article 1190. https://doi.org/10.3389/fphar.2018.01190

Kim, J., Cho, S. J., Kim, W. J., Yang, K. I., Yun, C. H., & Chu, M. K. (2017). Insufficient sleep is prevalent among migraineurs: A population-based study. *The Journal of Headache and Pain, 18*(1), Article No. 51. https://doi.org/10.1186/s10194-017-0756-8

Ko, H.-K., Chin, C.-C., & Hsu, M.-T. (2018). Moral distress model reconstructed using grounded theory. *The Journal of Nursing Research, 26*(1), 18–26. https://doi.org/10.1097/jnr.0000000000000189

Lee, M. J., Choi, H. A., Choi, H., & Chung, C.-S. (2016). Caffeine discontinuation improves acute migraine treatment: A prospective clinic-based study. *The Journal of Headache and Pain, 17*(1), Article No. 71. https://doi.org/10.1186/s10194-016-0662-5

Lipton, R. B., Munjal, S., Buse, D. C., Bennett, A., Fanning, K. M., Burstein, R., & Reed, M. L. (2017). Allodynia is associated with initial and sustained response to acute migraine treatment: Results from the american migraine prevalence and prevention study. *Headache, 57*(7), 1026–1040. https://doi.org/10.1111/head.13115

Luo, Y., Wang, C.-Z., Sawadogo, R., Tan, T., & Yuan, C.-S. (2020). Effects of herbal medicines on pain management. *American Journal of Chinese Medicine, 48*(1), 1–16. https://doi.org/10.1142/s0192415x20500019

Macone, A. E., & Perloff, M. D. (2017). Triptans and migraine: Advances in use, administration, formulation, and development. *Expert Opinion on Pharmacotherapy, 18*(4), 387–397. https://doi.org/10.1080/14656566.2017.1288721

Mayans, L., & Walling, A. (2018). Acute migraine headache: Treatment strategies. *American Family Physician, 97*(4), 243–251.

Mostofsky, E., Mittleman, M. A., Buettner, C., Li, W., & Bertisch, S. M. (2019). Prospective cohort study of caffeinated beverage intake as a potential trigger of headaches among migraineurs. *American Journal of Medicine, 132*(8), 984–991. https://doi.org/10.1016/j.amjmed.2019.02.015

Murakami, M., Fox, L., & Dijkers, M. P. (2017). Ear acupuncture for immediate pain relief—A systematic review and meta-analysis of randomized controlled trials. *Pain Medicine, 18*(3), 551–564. https://doi.org/10.1093/pm/pnw215

Nehlig, A. (2016). Effects of coffee/caffeine on brain health and disease: What should I tell my patients? *Practical Neurology, 16*(2), 89–95. https://doi.org/10.1136/practneurol-2015-001162

Nie, L., Cheng, J., Wen, Y., & Li, J. (2019). The effectiveness of acupuncture combined with tuina therapy in patients with migraine. *Complementary Medicine Research, 26*(3), 182–194. https://doi.org/10.1159/000496032

Polit, D. F., & Beck, C. T. (2017). *Essentials of nursing research: Appraising evidence for nursing practice* (9th ed.). Lippincott Williams & Wilkins.

Silberstein, S. D., & Marmura, M. J. (2015). Acute migraine treatment. *Headache, 55*(1), 1–2. https://doi.org/10.1111/head.12504

Stewart, W. F., Lipton, R. B., Kolodner, K., Liberman, J., & Sawyer, J. (1999). Reliability of the Migraine Disability Assessment score in a population-based sample of headache sufferers. *Cephalalgia, 19*(2), 107–114. https://doi.org/10.1046/j.1468-2982.1999.019002107.x

Stovner, L. J., Nichols, E., Steiner, T. J., Abd-Allah, F., Abdelalim, A., Al-Raddadi, R. M., Ansha, M. G., Barac, A., Bensenor, I. M., Doan, L. P., Edessa, D., Endres, M., Foreman, K. J., Gankpe, F. G., Gopalkrishna, G., Goulart, A. C., Gupta, R., Hankey, G. J., Hay, S. I., & Murray, C. J. L. (2018). Global, regional, and national burden of migraine and tension-type headache, 1990–2016: A systematic analysis for the Global Burden of Disease Study 2016. *The Lancet Neurology, 17*(11), 954–976. https://doi.org/10.1016/S1474-4422(18)30322-3

Sullivan, D. P., Martin, P. R., & Boschen, M. J. (2019). Psychological sleep interventions for migraine and tension-type headache: A systematic review and meta-analysis. *Scientific Reports, 9*(1), Article No. 6411. https://doi.org/10.1038/s41598-019-42785-8

Vernon, H., Borody, C., Harris, G., Muir, B., Goldin, J., & Dinulos, M. (2015). A randomized pragmatic clinical trial of chiropractic care for headaches with and without a self-acupressure pillow. *Journal of Manipulative and Physiological Therapeutics, 38*(9), 637–643. https://doi.org/10.1016/j.jmpt.2015.10.002

Xiao, Y., Yuan, L., Liu, Y., Sun, X., Cheng, J., Wang, T., Li, F., Luo, R., & Zhao, X. (2015). Traditional Chinese patent medicine for prophylactic treatment of migraine: A meta-analysis of randomized, double-blind, placebo-controlled trials. *European Journal of Neurology, 22*(2), 361–368. https://doi.org/10.1111/ene.12581

23

Validity and Reliability of the Korean Version of the Watson Caritas Patient Score

SookBin IM[1] • MiKyoung CHO[2] • MyoungLyun HEO[3]*

ABSTRACT

Background: The increasing use of information technology in healthcare settings has reduced human contact with healthcare providers and is hampering human-centered intrinsic nursing work associated with patient discomfort, emotional distress, and desire. The caring attitude of nurses affects patient compliance with medication instructions as well as the promotion of health behaviors and patient satisfaction.

Purpose: This study was designed to develop a Korean version of the Watson Caritas Patient Score (WCPS) developed by Watson and then verify its reliability and validity.

Methods: This was a methodological study. Data were collected from 240 patients in wards of the departments of internal medicine and surgery of a general hospital with more than 500 beds in Kunsan City between May 1 and June 8, 2017. Exploratory factor analysis and confirmatory factor analysis were used to verify the construct validity and model fit. The Patient Perception of Hospital Experience with Nursing was used to confirm convergence validity. Data were analyzed using descriptive analysis, Cronbach's alpha, factor analysis, and Pearson's product–moment correlation analysis.

Results: The internal consistency of the Korean version of the WCPS assessed using Cronbach's alpha was .94. The content validity index for each of the five items was 1.0. The communality ranged from .75 to .87, and the overall model fit was good. In addition, the average variance extracted was .61, the composite reliability was .89, and the convergent validity was .72 ($p < .001$).

Conclusions/Implications for Practice: The original English version and the Korean version of the WCPS both address a single factor, which confirmed the reliability and good fit of the model and showed both convergent and criterion-related validity. The Korean version of the WCPS is expected to contribute to improving the quality of nursing care in Korea by providing a simple scale that assesses patient perceptions of nursing care easily and accurately.

KEY WORDS:
caring, nurse, patient-centered care, patients' experience, validity.

Introduction

Many information-technology-based healthcare applications have been developed in recent years, and the effects of the fourth industrial revolution based on big data in the medical sector are expected to accelerate the utilization of robots and artificial intelligence in diagnosis and surgical equipment. However, although this trend has provided patients with faster and more accurate diagnoses and treatments, it has reduced human contact with healthcare providers and hampered human-centered intrinsic nursing work, which has subsequently increased patient discomfort, emotional distress, and desires (Edvardsson, Watt, & Pearce, 2017; McGilton et al., 2017). In addition to professional competencies that combine scientific and medical knowledge and skills, nurses must also have personal and esthetic attitudes that allow them to provide high-quality nursing services (Rhodes, Morris, & Lazenby, 2011). Nursing may be defined by the answer of "caring" to the question "What do you do for the patient?" (Lee, 1996).

The caring attitude of nurses affects their degree of compliance with medication instructions, the promotion of health behaviors, and patient satisfaction, which determines whether patients will select the same hospital in the future (Lee, Lee, Cho, & Seol, 1998; Paik & Kim, 2014). It has been reported that wait time, convenience of procedures, and smoothness and appropriateness of workflows affect the satisfaction of patients. Kindness and respect as well as information provided to patients by nurses affect the satisfaction of hospitalized patients and their intention to return to a hospital (Jung, 2005; Lee et al., 1998). Therefore, identifying how well nurses care for patients is very important for improving the quality of nursing care and increasing patient satisfaction. This situation has led to various studies of caring by nurses in Korea. However, few validated instruments for measuring caring have been developed and used in Korea (Park & Kim, 2016).

Jean Watson, a nursing theorist, emphasized the importance of caring science and argued that nursing should shift away from an industrial model and toward a creative and mature professional model that views patients as spirit-filled people

[1]PhD, RN, Professor, College of Nursing, Eulji University, Daejeon, ROK • [2]PhD, RN, Assistant Professor, Department of Nursing Science, College of Medicine, Chungbuk National University, Cheongju, ROK • [3]PhD, RN, Assistant Professor, Jeonju University, Jeonju, ROK.

rather than only patients (Watson, 2016). Watson and Woodward (2010) proposed 10 caritas factors and processes based on respect for human beings and developed the Watson Caritas Patient Score (WCPS), a five-item measure of the care provided by nurses as perceived by acute care and rehabilitation ward inpatients, with item scores given on a 7-point scale (Brewer & Watson, 2015). The WCPS scale has been translated into five different languages and is used worldwide (Watson et al., 2010). However, the instrument cannot be used in Korea, as no research has verified its reliability and validity on Korean subjects. This instrument is well suited for busy clinical practices because it is easy to apply and comprises easy-to-understand and concise items that reflect both the care provided by nurses and the experience of patients.

Research Aims

The purposes of this study were to (a) translate the WCPS and (b) estimate the reliability and validity of the translated instrument. The aim was to contribute to the improvement of the quality of nursing care by developing a simple scale that can easily and accurately assess nursing care as perceived by patients.

Methods

Participants and Data Collection Methods

This study used a methodological research design. The participants in this study were able to communicate in Korean, had been hospitalized in the wards of the departments of internal medicine and surgery of a general hospital with more than 500 beds in Kunsan City, and voluntarily agreed to participate. The minimum number of participants required for an exploratory factor analysis (EFA) is five times the number of variables (Kim, 2010). Using the criterion that a sample of 200 would be required for a confirmatory factor analysis (CFA; Moon, 2009), data were collected from 250 participants based on an anticipated maximum dropout rate of 20%.

After obtaining approval from the institutional review board of Kunsan College of Nursing, the researcher applied for permission to perform the study and provided information regarding the study purpose, procedures, methods, and questionnaire content to the hospital director. Advanced cooperation was obtained from the nursing department, and data were collected between May 1 and June 8, 2017. The questionnaire was distributed by the research assistant, who explained the content and confidentiality of the research as well as the method of administering the questionnaire and collected written informed consent from each participant. The questionnaire was composed of nine sociodemographic items (age, gender, religion, marital status, education, occupation, hospitalization experience, hospitalization period, and inpatient ward), five WCPS items, and 15 Patient Perception of Hospital Experience with Nursing (PPHEN) items. The

total time required to complete the questionnaire was about 10 minutes. Two hundred forty questionnaires were used in the final analysis because 10 of the submitted questionnaires were not complete.

Research Tools

Watson caritas patient score

The WCPS was developed by Brewer and Watson (2015) based on caritas factors and caritas processes, which encompass the formation of a humanistic altruistic system of value; instillation of faith and hope; cultivation of sensitivity to self and others; development of a helping-trust relationship; promotion and acceptance of the expression of positive and negative feelings; systematic use of the scientific problem-solving method for decision making; promotion of interpersonal teaching and learning; provision for supportive, protective, and corrective mental, physical, sociocultural, and spiritual environments; assistance with gratification of human needs; and allowance for existential–phenomenological forces. The questionnaire consists of the following five items: deliver my care with loving kindness; meet my basic human needs with dignity; have helping and trusting relationships with me; create a caring environment that helps me heal; and value my personal beliefs and faith, allowing for hope. The WCPS items are each scored on a 7-point scale, ranging from "not at all" (1) to "very much" (7), with a higher score indicating better nursing care. The reliability was confirmed in the original study by the developer of the tool with a Cronbach's α of .90 (Brewer & Watson, 2015).

Patient perception of hospital experience with nursing

The PPHEN was developed by Dozier, Kitzman, Ingersoll, Holmberg, and Schultz (2001) to gather self-reported patient responses on quality of care. The instrument was composed of 15 items that are scored on a 5-point Likert scale. It was developed using a conceptual framework of caring. The quality of nursing is measured from the patient's point of view, and this instrument was used in this study to confirm the criterion-related validity of the WCPS. The reliability of the PPHEN has been supported by Cronbach's α values ranging from .85 to .95 (Dozier et al., 2001; Ipek Coban & Kasikci, 2010; Heo & Im, 2019), with the highest value (.95) found in a study that was conducted in Korea (Heo & Im, 2019).

Research Procedure

Translation of the Watson Caritas Patient Score

Written approval was received from Jean Watson, the developer of the WCPS. The translation and application process for the tool was carried out in accordance with World Health Organization guidelines (World Health Organization, 2017) in the order of primary translation, expert panel assessment, back-translation, preliminary investigation, and final completion. The primary translation was carried out by a bilingual nursing professor who has both clinical practice and education experience in English-speaking countries and is familiar with the terms used in the original instrument. To check for discrepancies between the original text and the translation and in the expressions used because of cultural differences, a panel composed of three expert nursing professors and one professor of English language and literature corrected the instrument.

Item 1 raised the most discussion among members of the expert panel. The first translation process resulted in this being phrased as "to take care sincerely," with the majority opinion stating that this constituted overinterpretation. Thus, this phrase was modified to "to take care with affection and kindness" to make it easier for the layperson to understand. The other items were subject to simple modifications only (e.g., using the active rather than the passive tense), and no modifications in meaning were made. This process included the back-translation of the final version by an English-language professor who is bilingual and has an English-speaking doctoral degree. The back-translated version was subsequently accepted based on the opinion that its meaning was the same as the original text.

Preliminary investigation

The Korean version of the translated WCPS was initially administered to 30 patients who were hospitalized in one ward of the departments of internal medicine and surgery of the general hospital in May 2017 to test the clarity of content, ease of understanding, time required for responses, and potential problems in completing the questionnaire. The questionnaire content and respondent understanding of phrases were generally considered to be appropriate, and approximately 1 minute was required to complete the questionnaire. Thus, none of the items was revised (Figure 1).

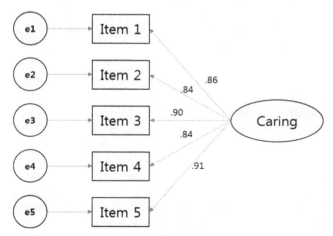

Figure 1. Path diagram of the revised version of translated Watson Caritas Patient Score.

Ethical considerations

The institutional ethics review committee of the researcher's educational institution approved this study (IRB No. 2017-04-HR-02) based on the opinion that the study involved applying a very low-risk and concise questionnaire to adult inpatients at the minimum-risk stage. Patients who voluntarily agreed to participate were given explanations of the purpose, content, and procedures of the study; of their anonymity as participants; and of their right to withdraw at any time. All of those willing to enroll as participants completed a written consent form.

Data analysis methods

The collected data were analyzed using IBM SPSS Statistics Version 22.0 and AMOS 21.0 (IBM Inc., Armonk, NY, USA). Questionnaires that had been returned with data missing were excluded from analysis, so that 240 questionnaires were analyzed. Participants' demographic characteristics were evaluated using frequency, percentage, mean, and standard deviation values. The reliability test that was performed to assess the internal consistency of the study tool produced a Cronbach's α of > .70, which confirmed its internal consistency (Noh, 2014).

Validity of the instrument was ensured through EFA and CFA. Item analysis was conducted using the correlations between the total score and the individual factors. For factor extraction, the Kaiser–Meyer–Olkin and Bartlett's sphericity tests were used to determine the number of factors with eigenvalues of ≥ 1.0 in the principal component factor analysis. A cumulative variance of at least 60% was explained by the extracted factors with loadings of > .50. When the number of factors was determined, the model fit of the tool may be confirmed using CFA to show that the significance level of chi-square is $p \geq .05$, the root mean square residual (RMR) is < .08, the standardized root mean square residual (SRMR) is < .05, the root mean square error of approximation (RMSEA) is < .08, the goodness-of-fit index (GFI) is > .90, the normed fit index (NFI) is > .90, the relative fit index is > .90, the incremental fit index (IFI) is > .90, the average variance extracted (AVE) is $\geq .5$, and the composite reliability (CR) is $\geq .7$. In addition, the Pearson's correlation coefficient was used to analyze the correlation between the scale and the patient-perceived quality of care as measured using the PPHEN to verify the convergent validity of the WCPS.

Results

Participant Characteristics

Of the 240 participants, 53.8% were male, 90.9% were middle aged (35–64 years) or older (65 years and over), 65.8% were religious, 84.6% were married, 53.3% had less than a high school level of education, 33.3% were employed, and 79.6% had a previous hospitalization experience. Most (89.2%) had been hospitalized for a period between 2 days and 1 month, and 62.5% were surgery department inpatients (Table 1).

TABLE 1.
Watson Caritas Patient Score, by Participant Characteristics (N = 240)

Characteristic	n	%	WCPS			
			M	SD	t or F	p/Post Hoc
Age (years)					F = 4.40	.013
① 19–34[a]	22	9.2	5.49	1.20		① < ②, ③
② 35–64[b]	107	44.6	6.01	1.24		
③ ≥ 65[b]	111	46.3	6.31	1.28		
Gender					0.65	.519
Male	129	53.8	6.15	1.17		
Female	111	46.2	6.05	1.39		
Religion					−1.42	.156
Yes	158	65.8	6.03	1.36		
No	82	34.2	6.26	1.09		
Marital status					1.95	.052
Married	203	84.6	6.17	1.25		
Single	37	15.4	5.73	1.34		
Education					4.63	< .001
Below high school graduate	128	53.3	6.45	0.96		
Above high school graduate	112	46.7	5.70	1.47		
Occupation					−2.07	.040
Yes	80	33.3	5.87	1.40		
No	160	66.7	6.22	1.19		
Experience of hospitalization					0.97	.335
Yes	191	79.6	6.06	1.32		
No	49	20.4	6.26	1.08		
Hospitalization period (days)					F = 2.07	.133
< 2	113	47.1	6.00	1.35		
2–30	101	42.1	6.30	1.11		
> 30	26	10.8	5.81	1.45		
Hospital ward					0.78	.439
Department of medicine	90	37.5	6.19	1.28		
Department of surgery	150	62.5	6.05	1.27		

Note. WCPS = Watson Caritas Patient Score.

Reliability Test

The item analysis for the reliability test revealed a skewness range of −1.48 to −1.71 and a kurtosis range of 1.34–2.54, indicating regularity (West, Finch, & Curran, 1995). The internal consistency (Cronbach's α) of the five items was .94, indicating that the final tool is reliable.

Validity Verification

Content validity

The content validity of the Korean version of the WCPS was verified by two nursing professors, two ward administrators, and two clinical nurses. The content validity instrument was configured to respond to each item on a 4-point Likert scale ranging from "poor fit" (1) to "excellent fit" (4). The content validity index of the total instrument was assessed by the experts as the proportion of the

five items that scored either 3 or 4. The content validity index of each of the items was 1.0, which means that all of the experts agreed that all of the five items were valid. Therefore, in accordance with usual acceptance criteria (Lee et al., 2009), all five items were included in the final questionnaire.

Exploratory factor analysis

The EFA, analyzed using SPSS 22.0, yielded a Kaiser–Meyer–Olkin index of .89. The Bartlett's sphericity test resulted in $\chi^2 = 1104.27$ and $df = 10$ ($p < .001$). In the EFA, a single factor with an eigenvalue of ≥ 1.0 was extracted from the principal component analysis, with a total explanatory power of 81.36%. The communality ranged from .75 to .87, indicating that all of the questions included satisfied the > .40 criterion (Costello & Osborne, 2005). The factor loading of each item ranged from .86 to .93 (Table 2).

TABLE 2.

Descriptive Statistics, Factor Loading, Reliability, and Correlation Between PPHEN of the Korean Version of WCPS Items (N = 240)

No	WCPS Item	M	SD	Factor Loading	PPHEN r	PPHEN p
1	Deliver my care with loving kindness.	6.15	1.33	.91	.63	< .001
2	Meet my basic human needs with dignity.	6.19	1.29	.90	.62	< .001
3	Have helping and trusting relationships with me.	6.07	1.46	.91	.60	< .001
4	Create a caring environment that helps me heal.	6.01	1.54	.86	.68	< .001
5	Value my personal beliefs and faith, allowing for hope.	6.10	1.45	.93	.70	< .001
Total		6.10	1.28		.72	< .001

Note. Kaiser–Meyer–Olkin values = .89; Bartlett's sphericity test: χ^2 = 1104.27, p < .001; total explanatory power: 81.36%; Cronbach's α = .94. WCPS = Watson Caritas Patient Score; PPHEN = Patient Perception of Hospital Experience with Nursing.

TABLE 3.

Goodness of Fit in the Korean Version of the WCPS Model (N = 240)

Category	χ^2	df	p	RMR	SRMR	RMSEA	GFI	NFI	RFI	IFI	TLI	CFI
Model fit (modified)	3.47	2	.18	.02	.01	.06	.99	.99	.98	.99	.99	.99
Model fit (hypothetical)	35.82	5	< .001	.05	.02	.16	.94	.97	.94	.97	.94	.98
Acceptance value			> .05	< .08	< .05	< .08	> .90	> .90	> .90	> .90	> .90	> .90

Note. WCPS = Watson Caritas Patient Score; RMR = root mean square residual; SRMR = standardized root mean square residual; RMSEA = root mean square error of approximation; GFI = goodness-of-fit index; NFI = normed fit index; RFI = relative fit index; IFI = incremental fit index; TLI = Tucker–Lewis index; CFI = comparative fit index.

Construct validity

The results of the CFA using AMOS 21.0 were χ^2 = 35.82 and p < .001. Because the value of RMSEA was .16, a modification of the model was warranted. Error covariances between Items 1 and 2, Items 2 and 5, and Items 2 and 4 were controlled based on the modification index suggested by the AMOS program, and the goodness of fit of the modified model was determined. The results of χ^2 = 3.47 and p > .05 showed the model to be significant and the overall goodness of fit of the model to be favorable, with RMR = .02 (< .08), SRMR = .01 (< .05), RMSEA = .06 (< .08), and GFI = .99 (> .90). The suitability of this model as a valid instrument was confirmed by all values of the IFIs satisfying the acceptance criteria (Noh, 2014), with NFI = .99 (> .90), relative fit index = .98 (> .90), IFI = .99 (> .90), Tucker–Lewis index = .99 (> .90), and CFI = .99 (> .90; Table 3). When the convergent validity of items is tested, the standardized factor loading for each item should be ≥ .50 (preferably > .70). The loadings for all of the items in the WCPS were > .83. The analysis performed using the equation of Fornell and Larcker (1981) resulted in an AVE of .61 and a CR of .89 (AVE ≥ .50 and CR ≥ .70), indicating that the five items measured the caring concept well (Table 4).

Convergent validity

Convergent validity was shown by a positive correlation between the coefficients for the quality of nursing (PPHEN)

tool and the five items of the WCPS (range: .60–.70, p < .001), with an overall coefficient of .72 (p < .001). This result shows that the same concept is closely measured, which confirms the convergent validity (Table 2).

Discussion

The process of translating the original version of the WCPS prompted several discussions about terms such as "took care

TABLE 4.

Confirmatory Factor Analysis Results of the Korean Version of WCPS (N = 240)

Variable	Number of Items	Standardized Factor Loading	Error Variance	AVE	CR
WCPS	1	.86	.47	.61	.89
	2	.84	.50		
	3	.90	.40		
	4	.84	.69		
	5	.91	.35		
Evaluation criteria		≥ .5		≥ .5	≥ .7

Note. WCPS = Watson Caritas Patient Score; AVE = average variance extracted; CR = composite reliability.

with sincerity," "took care with caritas," and "took kind care with affection" in the context of Item 1: "Deliver my care with loving-kindness." On the basis of the opinion that it would be better to use sentences that allow patients to understand their subjective experiences, the decision was made to use the following expression: "Look after them kindly with compassion." The back-translation process confirmed that this expression reflected the same meaning as the original English version, with the expert group stating that the question provided a valid measure of the concept of caring. Moreover, the participants understood the question without difficulty. Therefore, "look after them kindly with compassion" was deemed as appropriate for inclusion in the Korean version of the WCPS.

The original WCPS consisted of one factor. In this study, a single factor was also used for the Korean version based on an eigenvalue cutoff of ≥ 1.0. Woo (2012) suggested that there is no standard for the number of factors required in valid tools and that at least three observational variables should be used to constitute one potential variable to avoid the identification problem in CFA. The fit of a model in CFA is considered acceptable when RMR is < .08, with a value of ≤ .05 indicating a very suitable model. A value of .05 was obtained in this study, whereas a good fit of .01 was found for the standardized coefficient (SRMR) and the absolute fit index (GFI) was found to be .99 (> .90), which, together, indicated that the overall model was appropriate. Moreover, the IFI, which is an index of how well a research model was measured, was appropriate compared with the null model. In particular, the NFI, which is the most basic index, was .99 (> .90), showing that the research model in the null model improved to 99% and indicating that it is highly relevant. Although the absolute GFI (RMSEA) is best when the value nears zero (good when the index is less than .5 and bad when the index is 1 or greater), a poor goodness of fit with a high RMSEA value will result when the number of variables is small because of the influence of the degree of freedom (Hong, 2000). The goodness-of-fit test of the model in this study resulted in the following: RMSEA = .06 and CFI = .99 (> .90). As CFI is deemed superior to RMSEA for testing the goodness of fit when, as in this study, the number of variables is small (Hong, 2000), the goodness of fit of the model of the WCPS instrument in this study was considered satisfactory.

The result is a model using modified indices that connects Items 1 and 2, 2 and 4, and 2 and 5. In a domestic study, the inpatients asked the nurses to provide a more comfortable environment, kindness in care, and respect for their beliefs. As these requirements reflect the desire of patients to be treated in a dignified manner, they highlight the correlations between the items. In addition, the AVE and CR values, calculated in accordance with Fornell and Larcker (1981), confirmed that the five items measured caring consistently.

On the other hand, the convergent validity of the PPHEN was confirmed through correlations with the WCPS, because the PPHEN was constructed based on the concept of care

and has been used like the WCPS to evaluate the patient-perceived quality of nursing care.

The level of caring measured in this study was 6.10 ± 1.28 ($M \pm SD$), which was similar to the range of 5.7–7.0 found for the original instrument (Brewer & Watson, 2015). Thus, it may be concluded that nurses in the United States and Korea provide human-centered caring. Previous domestic and foreign studies have found differences in how nurses and patients perceive the degree and importance of caring (Kim & Lee, 1999; McCance, Slater, & McCormack, 2009). Because different instruments were used for these measurements, future research should attempt to determine the validity and reliability of the WCPS in clinical applications and use the results as basic data for improving nursing attitudes and perceptions toward patient care.

The caring provided by nurses to patients was found to differ by age, educational level, and occupation. Nearly half (46%) of the participants in this study were aged 65 years or older. The average age of 58.7 years in the study of Brewer and Watson (2015), which used the same instrument, was similar to this study. Whereas the score for perception of care was high in previous studies because of the high proportion of older inpatients, the score for perception of nurses' care among participants aged 35 years or younger in this study was significantly lower than that among the older (65 years and older) group. Similarly, Kim and Lee (1999) reported a low score among participants younger than 30 years old. This appears to be because of the high susceptibility to relationships in this age group, because most subjects in early adulthood are independent from their parents and single. In-depth questions on participant characteristics could not be explored in this study, and Brewer and Watson similarly did not compare the perception of care by age. Therefore, exploring the underlying factors causing young adults to give lower care scores than their older peers and testing the validity of the instrument by age should be pursued in future studies.

Domestic studies of caring have largely relied on qualitative research methods, with quantitative research limited by the lack of appropriate measurement instruments. The results of this study support the Korean version of the WCPS as a valid and easy-to-implement instrument for use in measuring the self-perceived care quality of domestic inpatients. Furthermore, this instrument may help increase research into the care provided by nurses.

Conclusion and Suggestions

This study was designed to develop the Korean version of the WCPS and to verify its validity and reliability. Both the translated single-factor instrument was confirmed as reliable, providing a good fit to the model and showing convergent validity. However, the generalizability of this Korean version of the WCPS is unclear, as it was tested on internal medicine and surgery patients at one general hospital only. A test validation study should be performed to determine the suitability of using the

7-point scoring scheme in this instrument with other patient populations in Korea.

Author Contributions

Study conception and design: SBI
Data collection: All authors
Data analysis and interpretation: All authors
Drafting of the article: MLH
Critical revision of the article: All authors

References

Brewer, B. B., & Watson, J. (2015). Evaluation of authentic human caring professional practices. *The Journal of Nursing Administration, 45*(12), 622–627. https://doi.org/10.1097/NNA.0000000000000275

Costello, A. B., & Osborne, J. W. (2005). Best practices in exploratory factor analysis: Four recommendations for getting the most from your analysis. *Practical Assessment, Research & Evaluation, 10*(7), 1–9.

Dozier, A. M., Kitzman, H. J., Ingersoll, G. L., Holmberg, S., & Schultz, A. W. (2001). Development of an instrument to measure patient perception of the quality of nursing care. *Research in Nursing & Health, 24*(6), 506–517. https://doi.org/10.1002/nur.10007

Edvardsson, D., Watt, E., & Pearce, F. (2017). Patient experiences of caring and person-centredness are associated with perceived nursing care quality. *Journal of Advanced Nursing, 73*(1), 217–227. https://doi.org/10.1111/jan.13105

Fornell, C., & Larcker, D. F. (1981). Evaluating structural equation models with unobservable variables and measurement error. *Journal of Marketing Research, 18*(1), 39–50. https://doi.org/10.2307/3151312

Heo, M. L., & Im, S. B. (2019). Development of the patient caring communication scale. *Journal of Korean Academy of Nursing, 49*(1), 80–91. https://doi.org/10.4040/jkan.2019.49.1.80 (Original work published in Korean)

Hong, S. (2000). The criteria for selecting appropriate fit indices in structural equation modeling and their rationales. *Korean Journal of Clinical Psychology, 19*(1), 161–177. (Original work published in Korean)

Ipek Coban, G., & Kasikci, M. (2010). Reliability and validity of the scale of patient perception of hospital experience with nursing care in a Turkish population. *Journal of Clinical Nursing, 19*(13–14), 1929–1934. https://doi.org/10.1111/j.1365-2702.2009.03125.x

Jung, S. W. (2005). Determinants of patient satisfaction and intent to revisit at national university hospitals in Korea. *Korea Society of Hospital Management, 10*, 1–25. (Original work published in Korean)

Kim, G. S. (2010). *Analysis structural equation modeling.* Seoul, ROK: Hannarae. (Original work published in Korean)

Kim, Y. Y., & Lee, B. S. (1999). Importance of nurses' caring behaviors as perceived by staff nurses and patients. *Journal of Korean Academy of Fundamentals of Nursing, 6*(1), 18–34. (Original work published in Korean)

Lee, B. S. (1996). Concept analysis of caring. *Journal of Korean Academy of Nursing, 26*(2), 337–344. (Original work published in Korean)

Lee, E., Lim, N., Park, H., Lee, I., Kim, J., & Bae, J. (2009). *Nursing study and statistical analysis.* Paju, ROK: Sumoonsa. (Original work published in Korean)

Lee, K. S., Lee, H. J., Cho, K. S., & Seol, D. J. (1998). The satisfaction analysis for patient care service in national university hospitals. *Korea Journal of Hospital Management, 3*, 165–191. (Original work published in Korean)

McCance, T., Slater, P., & McCormack, B. (2009). Using the caring dimensions inventory as an indicator of person-centred nursing. *Journal of Clinical Nursing, 18*(3), 409–417. https://doi.org/10.1111/j.1365-2702.2008.02466.x

McGilton, K. S., Sorin-Peters, R., Rochon, E., Boscart, V., Fox, M., Chu, C. H., & Sidani, S. (2017). The effects of an interprofessional patient-centered communication intervention for patients with communication disorders. *Applied Nursing Research, 39*, 189–194. https://doi.org/10.1016/j.apnr.2017.11.017

Moon, S. (2009). *Basic concepts and applications of structural equation modeling.* Seoul, ROK: Hakjisa. (Original work published in Korean)

Noh, G. (2014). *SPSS & AMOS 21.* Seoul, ROK: Hanbit Academy. (Original work published in Korean)

Paik, H. R., & Kim, K. J. (2014). How to improve patients' satisfaction in healthcare organization?—Healthcare service quality classification using Kano Model. *Korean Journal of Hospital Management, 19*(2), 73–88. (Original work published in Korean)

Park, E. J., & Kim, M. H. (2016). Characteristics of nursing and caring concepts measured in nursing competencies or caring behaviors tools. *Journal of Korean Academy of Nursing Administration, 22*(5), 480–495. https://doi.org/10.11111/jkana.2016.22.5.480 (Original work published in Korean)

Rhodes, M. K., Morris, A. H., & Lazenby, R. B. (2011). Nursing at its best: Competent and caring. *The Online Journal of Issues in Nursing, 16*(2), 10. https://doi.org/10.3912/OJIN.Vol16No02PPT01

Watson, J. (2016). *Caring science-caritas theory practice.* Paper session presented at the Eulji International Nursing Conference "Human Caring: Nursing's Covenant with Humanity". Seoul, ROK.

Watson, J., Brewer, B., & D'Alfonso, J. (2010). *Watson Caritas Patient Survey (WCPS)©.* Boulder, CO: Watson Caring Science Institute.

Watson, J., & Woodward, T. K. (2010). Jean Watson's theory of human caring. In M. E. Parker & M. C. Smith (Eds.), *Nursing theories and nursing practice* (3rd ed.). Philadelphia, PA: F. A. Davis.

West, S. G., Finch, J. F., & Curran, P. J. (1995). Structural equation models with nonnormal variables: Problems and remedies. In R. H. Hoyle (Ed.), *Structural equation modeling: Concepts, issues, and applications* (pp. 56–75). Thousand Oaks, CA: Sage Publications.

Woo, J. P. (2012). *The concept and understanding of structural equation model.* Seoul, ROK: Hannarae Academy. (Original work published in Korean)

World Health Organization. (2017). *Process of translation and adaptation of instruments.* Retrieved from http://www.who.int/substance_abuse/research_tools/translation/en/

24

Psychometric Testing of an Indonesian-Version Diabetes Self-Management Instrument

Henik Tri RAHAYU[1] • Ching-Min CHEN[2*]

ABSTRACT

Background: Self-management is one of the vital elements in diabetes management for adults with Type 2 diabetes mellitus (T2DM). Although the number of people with T2DM in Indonesia has risen, clinical understanding of the problems related to practicing diabetes self-management (DSM) is limited because of the lack of a valid measurement instrument. The 35-item Diabetes Self-Management Instrument (DSMI-35) is one instrument widely used in research to assess DSM-related behavior among patients with diabetes.

Purpose: This study was designed to translate the psychometric properties of the Indonesian version of the DSMI-35 and evaluate the efficacy of this instrument in a sample of Indonesian adults with T2DM.

Methods: Forward and backward translation processes were used to translate the DSMI-35 into Indonesian (IDN-DSMI). Then, the translation equivalence, content validity, face validity, construct validity, and internal consistency were assessed using a sample of 222 Indonesian adults with T2DM from eight public health centers. Confirmatory factor analysis was used to test the data.

Results: The confirmatory factor analysis confirmed that the 35 items all had acceptable goodness of fit. Although the analysis supported removing several of the items, removal of these items was not theoretically justified. The average variance extracted was acceptable, and composite reliability was satisfied. The Cronbach's alpha was .96 for the IDN-DSMI and .84–.93 for the subscales. The significant interitem correlations between some items were consistent with the findings of other previous studies.

Conclusions/Implications for Practice: The IDN-DSMI is a valid and reliable instrument that may be used to measure DSM behavior in Indonesian patients with T2DM in primary healthcare settings.

KEY WORDS:

instrument development and validation, self-management, diabetes, primary healthcare.

Introduction

The number of people with diabetes has been rising rapidly worldwide. In 2019, approximately 463 million adults were living with diabetes, with this number expected to rise to 578 million by 2030 and 700 million by 2045 (International Diabetes Federation, 2019). The rising prevalence of diabetes is associated with the escalating prevalence of obesity, which is a major diabetes risk factor. The global age-standardized prevalence of obesity among adults (aged 18 years and older) has increased 150% since 2016 (World Health Organization, 2020b). Moreover, Indonesia, a developing country in the West Pacific region, had the seventh-largest population of people with diabetes in 2019. Indonesia is expected have the eighth-largest population of people with diabetes in 2045, with the country's 10.7 million people with diabetes in 2019 projected to grow to 13.7 million in 2030 and 16.6 million in 2045 (International Diabetes Federation, 2019).

Diabetes is currently one of the top noncommunicable disease (NCD) causes of death worldwide (World Health Organization, 2020b). In 2016, an estimated 41 million people worldwide (approximately 71% of total deaths) were attributable to NCDs, with approximately 1.6 million directly attributable to diabetes, making diabetes the fourth-largest NCD cause of death after cardiovascular disease, cancer, and chronic respiratory disease (World Health Organization, 2020b). Moreover, diabetes has been associated with a 5% increase in premature mortality. In Indonesia, diabetes is the third-largest direct cause of death after stroke and cardiovascular disease and was also identified as the largest burden disease in 2012 because of its high disability-adjusted life years (DALYs; Kementerian Kesehatan Indonesia, 2015). DALYs is a score equal to the sum of the number of years of life lost because of premature mortality and the number of years of healthy life lost because of disability (World Health Organization, 2020a).

[1]*MSN, Doctoral Student, International Doctoral Program in Nursing, College of Medicine, National Cheng Kung University, Taiwan, ROC, and Lecturer, Department of Nursing, Health Sciences Faculty, University of Muhammadiyah Malang, Malang, Indonesia* • [2]*RN, DNS, Professor, Department of Nursing, Institute of Gerontology, and Institute of Allied Health Sciences, National Cheng Kung University, Taiwan, ROC.*

The high DALYs associated with diabetes is believed to result from severe complications because of poor disease management. The long-term complications of diabetes may lead to heart disease, stroke, kidney disease, blindness, and amputation (Chamberlain et al., 2016). Diabetes and its complication are not only a health problem but also economic, social, and psychological burdens. This disease affects not only the individual but also families, health systems, and the entire country. The global health spending on diabetes treatment and related complication prevention was estimated to be at least USD 760 billion in 2019, which represents about 10% of total health expenditures on adults (International Diabetes Federation, 2019). Although no official information on diabetes expenditures in Indonesia, the International Diabetes Federation reported that total expenditures on diabetes in the Western Pacific region reached USD 162.6 billion in 2019 and are expected to rise to 184.7 billion in 2045 (International Diabetes Federation, 2019). Therefore, promoting disease management to control diabetes is an important strategy for reducing the risk of related complications and the cost for treatments.

Background

Diabetes self-management (DSM) describes how people with diabetes practice self-care. DSM involves a patient's knowledge, attitude, and behavior to both maintain personal health and prevent long-term diabetes complications (International Diabetes Federation, 2012), with knowledge and attitude relating to the activities of daily living that a patient uses to stay healthy (Tol et al., 2011). The key elements of diabetes management are maintaining blood glucose level through dietary management, maintaining good exercise habits, taking prescribed medication, and monitoring blood glucose level to keep this level below 200 mg/dl and glycated hemoglobin A1c (HbA1c) at or below 7 (International Diabetes Federation, 2012). Moreover, on the basis of the American Association of Diabetes Educators, DSM consists of seven domains of self-management behaviors, including healthy eating, controlling blood glucose level, being active, taking medication, maintaining problem-solving abilities, reducing the risk of long-term complications, and having a healthy coping strategy for stress (American Association of Diabetes Educators, 2014). However, most patients with diabetes face obstacles in promoting self-management such as difficulties in coping with diabetes, self-monitoring, and lifestyle changes (Fidan et al., 2020). To evaluate the DSM compliance of patients, a reliable and valid tool to measure the quality of self-management behavior is necessary. However, there remains in Indonesia a widespread lack of information regarding DSM as well as a lack of valid, appropriate tools for assessing DSM status that are adaptable to individual conditions and assess the process rather than the outcome, allowing healthcare providers to identify problems in DSM practices.

Many instruments have been developed to measure DSM efficacy (Lu et al., 2016). Some measure DSM using patients'

compliance or adherence to recommended activities to control blood glucose and prevent complications from diabetes. Some measures, including the Summary of Diabetes Self-Care Activities (Choi et al., 2016; Toobert et al., 2000) and Diabetes Self-Management Questionnaires (Schmitt et al., 2013), are based on the scope of the definition of "self-care" and "self-management" and measure how often adults with diabetes follow each recommended activity associated with controlling blood glucose level and reducing the risk of complications.

However, adults with diabetes have autonomy to manage their diabetes independent from healthcare professionals (Lin et al., 2008), and compelled compliance with a healthcare professional's advice may violate patients' value and autonomy (Anderson et al., 2000; Redman, 2009). To optimize quality of life, DSM should be flexible and adapted to individual conditions (Funnell & Anderson, 2004). Therefore, a preferred definition of DSM is "an active, flexible process in which patients develop strategies for achieving desired goals by regulating their actions, collaborating with their healthcare providers and significant others and performing preventive and therapeutic health-related activities" (Lin et al., 2008, p. 371).

The Diabetes Self-Management Instrument (DSMI), developed by Lin et al. (2008), is the only scale that measures DSM as a process evaluation rather than an outcome. The original instrument was developed in English, translated into Chinese, and then validated in Taiwan. The validation of the Chinese version showed appropriate content validity, internal consistency, and test–retest reliability. Farsi (Persian) and Vietnamese versions of the DSMI have also been translated and validated (Tahmasebi & Noroozi, 2012).

The 35-item, self-report DSMI is designed to assess the frequency with which adults with diabetes performed certain activities during the previous 3-month period using a 4-point Likert scale, with responses ranging from 1 (*never*) to 4 (*always*). The total score for the instrument ranges from 35 to 140, with higher scores representing a higher frequency of self-management activities. The DSMI incorporates the five subscales of self-integration (10 items), self-regulation (nine items), interaction with health professional and significant others (nine items), self-monitoring blood glucose (four items), and adherence to the recommended therapy (three items; Lin et al., 2008).

The validation of the Chinese version of this instrument on 634 adults with Type 2 diabetes mellitus (T2DM) in Taiwan achieved a Cronbach's alpha coefficient of .94 and a test–retest correlation of .73 (Lin et al., 2008). The Iranian version achieved an internal consistency of .91 overall and between .79 and .92 for each subscale as well as a test–retest correlation of .91 (Tol et al., 2011). The Vietnamese version earned an internal consistency of .91 overall and between .81 and .95 for each subscale (Dao-Tran et al., 2017).

Aim

In this study, the original DSMI (35 items) was translated into Indonesian and its psychometric properties were tested to determine the acceptability and appropriateness of applying the translated version (IDN-DSMI) in populations of Indonesian adults with diabetes. It was expected that using the IDN-DSMI would give health professionals in Indonesia a better understanding of how Indonesian adults with diabetes self-manage their health and facilitate the design of appropriate DSM support for patients to reduce the risk of diabetes complications and improve overall health.

The purpose of this study was to conduct a psychometric test of the IDN-DSMI using confirmatory factor analysis (CFA).

Methods

Study Design

This study applied a quantitative study design using a cross-sectional survey. The research reporting guidelines were followed using the TRIPOD Checklist.

Phase 1: Development of the Indonesian version of the Diabetes Self-Management Instrument

First of all, permission to use the original instrument (Lin et al., 2008) was obtained from the original author. The DMSI was then translated into Bahasa (Indonesian) using a forward and backward translation process (Cha et al., 2007) to confirm linguistic equivalence. The English version was translated into Indonesian by two independent bilinguals (Indonesian–English) translators who were nurse lecturers. After the independent, forward English–Indonesian translation was completed, the research team held a consensus meeting with the two translators to establish a single translated version. Subsequently, the back-translated versions were compared with the original instrument by outside experts from the Language Center of Muhammadiyah University of Malang to identify any discrepancies.

After completing the forward and backward translation process, the research team conducted a content validity check of the IND-DSMI. Eight clinical and academic experts in diabetes care in Indonesia were asked to review the content validity of the instrument. An experienced endocrine physician, a medical–surgical nurse specialist, a nurse practitioner, and five lecturers on medical–surgical nursing at a nursing school participated in this content review, rating items on a scale of 1–4 (1 = *not relevant* and 4 = *very relevant*). The experts were further asked regarding the need to modify or eliminate each item. This study earned content validity ratio scores ranging from 0.5 to 1, with a mean score of .93, indicating that most questions are "essential." The reviewer's comments focused primarily on changing word usage to clarify meanings. No reviewer suggested deleting any item. Finally, five patients with diabetes in the Indonesian community were invited to evaluate the face validity of the instrument and to assess from their individual perspectives the clarity of the instrument, ease of item understanding, ease of response, and fit with the purpose of the study (Yasir, 2016).

As mentioned above, adults with diabetes have autonomy to manage their diabetes independent of health professionals (Lin et al., 2008). Thus, although the focus group of patients would have been capable of confirming the cultural adaption and evaluating the content validity, these aspects were not addressed because of time and resource constraints. This condition is recognized as a limitation of this study. However, the original instrument was developed and validated in an Asian country with a culture similar to Indonesia's. Therefore, it hoped that the instrument is also valid for use in Indonesian settings.

Phase 2: Psychometric testing of the Indonesian version of the Diabetes Self-Management Instrument

A cross-sectional survey was used to test the IDN-DSMI to assess its validity and internal consistency.

Setting

Data were collected from July to September 2013 in eight endocrine outpatient departments of public health centers (PHCs) in Malang, Indonesia, using quota sampling methods based on the average daily patient visits to each PHC to calculate the proportion of the sample to be recruited from each PHC. Malang, the second-largest city in East Java, is home to the most people in East Java (3,266,461 people or 8.7% from the total population in East Java; Badan Pusat Statistik, 2010). The sample in this study was recruited from both urban and rural areas. The outpatient department at the PHCs were open 7:30 a.m. to 12:00 p.m. on Mondays through Thursdays, 7:30–10:00 a.m. on Fridays, and 7:30–11:00 a.m. on Saturdays (Department of Health of Malang, 2012).

Participants

Two hundred twenty-two Indonesian adults with T2DM were included in this study. The Rule of 5 from Bryant and Yarnold (1995), used in this study to calculate the sample size, stipulates that the subject-to-variable ratio should not be less than five. The Rule of 200 from Guilford (1954) was also used, which suggests that N should be at least 200 cases (Garson, 2008; Shah, 2012). Three inclusion criteria were used to select samples, including being $\geq$ 20 years old, having a confirmed diagnosis of T2DM, and being willing to participate. Those unable to read and write Indonesian and those with severe diabetes complications such as blindness, amputation, and renal failure were excluded.

Procedure

Potential participants were identified by doctors and nurses working in the PHCs and provided with study information sheets and consent forms. When the prospective participant clearly understood the study and agreed to participate, he or she signed the consent form. Data were collected by the first author and the research assistants.

Data Analysis

On the basis of the results of psychometric testing in the original Taiwanese study (Lin et al., 2008), a CFA using maximum likelihood estimation was performed to test the consistency of the factor structure with the original version. CFA is used to examine the extent to which, a priori, the theoretical model of factor loadings provides an adequate fit for the actual data (Brown & Moore, 2012; Fabrigar et al., 1999). Descriptive analysis and CFA were performed using IBM SPSS AMOS Version 23 (IBM, Inc., Armonk, NY, USA) software. In the CFA, a good-fitting model is deemed to be one that has a weighted chi-square $(x^2)/df < 3$ (Bollen, 1990; MacCallum et al., 1996), a cumulative fit index (CFI) > .90 (Kline, 2005), and a root of mean square error of approximation (RMSEA) < .06 (Browne &Cudeck, 1992; Hooper et al., 2008), with $z = 0.30$ used as a cutoff for items loading onto a factor (Watson & Thompson, 2006). A model was considered to have an adequate fit if two of the above three criteria were met and if the third criterion had an acceptable but not good fit (e.g., RMSEA < .80; Browne & Cudeck, 1992; Hooper et al., 2008). The average variance extracted (AVE) and composite reliability (CR) were calculated to evaluate the construct validity, with the AVE expected to score $\geq .5$ and CR expected to score > .7 (Fornell & Larcker, 1981). For reliability testing, the instrument was considered to have acceptable internal reliability when Cronbach's alpha was $\geq .70$ for the overall scale and all of the subscales (Pallant, 2010).

Item analysis was performed using SPSS 23.0 (IBM, Inc., Armonk, NY, USA) to determine the continued inclusion or removal of individual items in the instrument. Items that met any two of following criteria were eliminated: (a) The means of the items were either extreme or the variance was zero, (b) items with skewness > 3 or kurtosis > 10, (c) low item discrimination ($SD < 0.75$), (d) the corrected item–total correlation was < 0.3, (e) the Cronbach's alpha of the total scale increased when an item was dropped, and (f) factor loading was < .5 (Lee et al., 2016).

Ethical Approval

The study was approved by the Health Research Ethics of the National Institute of Health Research and Development, Indonesia Ministry of Health (Reference No. LB.02.01/5.2/KE.513/2013). All of the participants provided written informed consent.

Results

Participant Characteristics

Two hundred fifty-six participants were eligible for participation. Ten refused because of lack of sufficient spare time, and 24 declined because of lack of interest. The ages of the remaining 222 participants ranged from 25 to 81 years (mean = 55.2, $SD = 10.8$). Men and women were equally represented, with women (50.9%) holding a slight majority. Most participants were married (87%), nearly one third (29.3%) were university educated, one quarter (24.3%) were unemployed, and most (52.3%) earned a low monthly income (< 74.6 USD). The average duration of having diabetes was 4.3 ± 4.4 years, ranging from 0.02 to 25 years, and most (81.5%) received oral drug treatment. Only 4.5% received regular insulin injections.

Factorial Construct Validity

The results of the item analysis are presented in Table 1. No items were deleted based on the item analysis. CFA was used to test construct validity (Watson & Thompson, 2006). The original model for the IDN-DSMI (five domains with 35 items) was identified as an inferior good-fitting model based on two of three criteria $((x^2)/df = 3.2$, CFI = .770) and an adequate fit using the remaining fit statistic (RMSEA = .101; Figure 1). The raw chi-square was 1777.97 ($df = 550$, $p < .01$). Although the CRs of all the factors were satisfactory (> .7), the AVE of this model was unacceptable (the AVEs of two factors were < .5). Thus, this model was rejected, and further modifications were made.

The initial modification, which added the covariance correlations, improved the goodness of fit $((x^2)/df = 2.727$, CFI = .827, RMSEA = .088), although the AVE remained unchanged (Figure 2). Further sequential modification considering the modification indices, item loading, and residual analysis suggested deleting at least 11 items to achieve a quite good-fitting model $((x^2)/df = 2.38$, CFI = .911, RMSEA = .079) with acceptable AVE and CR (the AVEs of the constructs were all > .5, and the CRs of the constructs were all > .7). From the 11 items suggested for deletion, five were from the self-integration domain and four were from the self-regulation domain. In the self-integration domain, the items suggested for deletion included questions on managing diabetes in daily life such as "daily lifestyle is healthier than before because of having diabetes," "successfully merged diabetes into daily life," "adjust diabetes routine to fit a new situation," "exercise to control blood glucose," and "keep weigh within the recommended range." In the self-regulation domain, the items suggested for deletion included "pay attention to signals of the body related to blood glucose level," "monitor progress toward desired goals by keeping track of blood glucose levels and A1c," "decide action based on experience," and "know how to treat if blood glucose levels become low." Besides, the two items "comfortable asking other people with diabetes for tips about managing diabetes" and "check blood glucose to help make self-care decisions" were also considered for deletion based on the analysis. However, every modification resulted in an unstable fit. In addition, the items suggested for deletion in the analysis were all considered key points of DSM. Thus, their deletion to achieve a good-fitting model did not make theoretical sense. MacCallum et al. (1992) warned that "when an initial model fits well, it is probably unwise to modify it to achieve an even better fit because modifications may simply be benefitting small, idiosyncratic characteristics of the sample" (p. 501). Besides, using the initial construct must achieve good

Table 1

Results of Item Analysis

No. Item	Item	Mean	SD < 0.75	Kurtosis > 10	Skewness > 3	Corrected Item–Total Correlation	Cronbach's α of the Total Scale Increased When an Item Was Deleted	Factor Loading < .5
Self-integration								
1	Considering the effect on my blood sugars when choosing foods and portions to eat.	2.634	0.979	−1.004	0.060	.609	.958	.665
2	Managing diabetes and participating in social activity.	2.778	1.015	−0.953	−0.321	.532	.958	.569
3	Managing food portions and choices when eating out.	2.781	1.024	−1.050	−0.263	.664	.957	.737
4	Managing diabetes as way to stay healthy	2.963	1.029	−0.881	−0.548	.594	.958	.687
6	Daily life style is healthier than before because of having diabetes.	2.635	0.997	−0.912	−0.221	.536	.958	.598
7	Successfully merged diabetes into daily life.	2.588	1.029	−1.051	−0.106	.577	.958	.615
18	Adjust diabetes routine to fit new situations (such as being away from home, changing my schedule, and celebration).	2.514	1.056	−1.127	−0.060	.551	.958	.561
29	Manage food choices to help control blood glucose.	3.066	0.938	−0.516	−0.663	.719	.957	.733
31	Exercise enough to help control blood glucose and weight.	2.703	0.998	−0.957	−0.195	.377	.959	.406 [a]
32	Keep weight within the range set up by my healthcare provider and me.	2.785	0.989	−0.791	−0.392	.517	.958	.540
Self-regulation								
8	Pay attention to body signals related to blood glucose level.	2.757	1.008	−1.027	−0.219	.647	.958	.690
9	Pay attention to situations in daily life that may cause blood glucose levels to change.	2.864	0.999	−0.773	−0.481	.670	.957	.723
10	Recognize which signs and symptoms tell the most about blood glucose level.	2.837	1.014	−0.749	−0.521	.611	.958	.677
11	Figure out the reasons for changes in blood glucose levels.	2.620	0.980	−0.824	−0.267	.606	.958	.696
12	Compare the differences between current blood sugar levels and target blood glucose levels.	2.543	1.043	−1.097	−0.032	.603	.958	.703
13	Monitor progress toward desired goals by keeping track of blood glucose levels and A1c.	2.428	1.139	−1.359	0.034	.485	.959	.560
14	Take action based on body signals such as thirst, losing my temper, and feeling anxious.	2.597	0.971	−0.859	−0.130	.528	.958	.595
16	Making decision based on experience	2.704	1.018	−0.996	−0.228	.637	.958	.641
34	Know how to treat if get a low blood glucose	2.917	1.015	−0.806	−0.530	.626	.958	.585
Interaction with health professionals and significant others								
5	Comfortable asking other for tips about managing diabetes.	2.605	0.958	−0.826	−0.131	.610	.958	.524

(continues)

Table 1

Results of Item Analysis, Continued

No. Item	Item	Mean	SD < 0.75	Kurtosis > 10	Skewness > 3	Corrected Item–Total Correlation	Cronbach's α of the Total Scale Increased When an Item Was Deleted	Factor Loading < .5
20	Comfortable asking healthcare provider questions about treatment plan.	3.040	0.944	−0.349	−0.727	.710	.957	.858
21	Work with healthcare providers to identify the possible causes when diabetes control is poor.	2.954	0.944	−0.444	−0.621	.682	.957	.824
22	Comfortable telling healthcare provider how much flexibility in treatment plan.	2.997	0.985	−0.548	−0.676	.711	.957	.853
23	Comfortable telling healthcare provider about changes I would like to make in treatment plan.	2.919	0.981	−0.653	−0.557	.697	.957	.844
24	Tell others about the situations in which need their help for controlling my diabetes.	2.847	0.945	−0.602	−0.462	.614	.958	.628
25	Comfortable discussing the results of out-of-range blood glucose tests with my healthcare providers.	3.063	0.936	−0.354	−0.728	.756	.957	.889
26	Ask others to help with high blood glucose reaction if needed.	2.789	0.987	−0.805	−0.383	.583	.958	.646
27	Comfortable asking healthcare provider about resources that could help manage diabetes.	3.043	0.957	−0.506	−0.685	.744	.957	.827
Self-monitoring blood glucose								
15	Check blood glucose levels when feel as though blood glucose is too low.	2.742	1.077	−1.019	−0.424	.581	.958	.703
17	Check blood glucose when feeling unwell.	2.777	1.044	−1.036	−0.341	.642	.958	.759
19	Check blood glucose level when feeling as though blood glucose is too high.	3.019	0.958	−0.583	−0.627	.760	.957	.866
28	Check blood glucose to help make self-care decisions (e.g., medications, diet, exercise).	3.004	0.924	−0.506	−0.724	.671	.957	.710
Adherence to recommended therapy								
30	Take diabetes medications at the times prescribed.	3.377	0.904	1.115	−1.432	.673	.957	.830
33	See diabetes provider every 1–3 months.	3.119	0.997	−0.356	−0.869	.601	.958	.719
35	Take the amount of diabetes medication that has been prescribed.	3.326	0.860	0.856	−1.242	.650	.958	.875

[a]Represents modulus of skewness > 3, modulus of kurtosis > 10, SD < 0.75, item–total correlation < 0.3, and factor loading < .5; Cronbach's alpha increased when item dropped.
[b]Represents the item deleted after item analysis (there were no items deleted from the analysis).

reliability (the Cronbach's alpha of each scale ranged from .84 to .93). Therefore, the final IDN-DSMI retained all 35 items in the original model.

Internal Consistency Reliability

The Cronbach's alpha of the final model was .96. The level of internal consistency for each subscale was .86 for self-integration, .87 for self-regulation, .93 for interactions

with health professionals and significant others, .86 for self-monitoring blood glucose, and .84 for adherence to recommended therapy (Table 2).

Item Correlations

The examination of item-to-item correlations highlighted that some items were highly correlated ($r \geq .70$; full item correlation table shown in Table 3). Furthermore, strong interitem

Figure 1

The Indonesian Version of the 35-Item Diabetes Self-Management Instrument Based on the Original Model With Factor Loadings and Interfactor Correlations (N = 222)

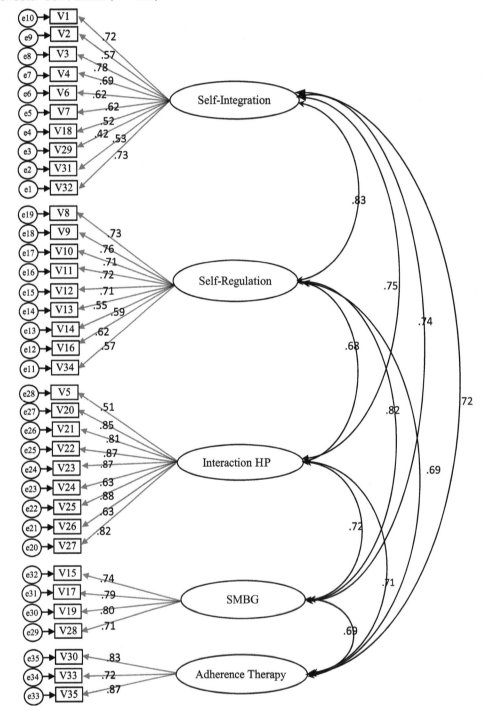

Note. HP = health professional; SMBG = self-monitoring blood glucose. Chi-square = 1777.97 (*df* = 550, *p* < .01), χ^2/df = 3.2; *CFI* = .770, *RSMEA* = .101.

correlations were found among Items 20–23 and 25 and among Items 23, 25, and 27, with all of the items in the domain of "interaction with health professionals and significant others" and Items 30 and 35 in the domain of "adherence to recommended therapy." It also indicated that some items may be redundant.

Discussion

The purpose of this study was to evaluate the validity and reliability of the IDN-DSMI. CFA was used to determine whether the original model may be applied on the IDN-DSMI model as well.

On the basis of a thorough investigation of the literature, this article is believed to be the first study to develop an Indonesian version of the DSMI and to examine its psychometric properties in adults with T2DM in Indonesia. Our findings suggested that IDN-DSMI attained good validity and reliability. The CFA supported acceptable goodness of fit for all of the 35 items, which cover the same five domains as the English version. Furthermore, these findings are consistent with the CFA results conducted in other countries (Taiwan, Iran, and Vietnam; Dao-Tran et al., 2017; Lin et al., 2008; Tol et al., 2011).

Figure 2

Final Model of the Indonesian Version of the 35-item Diabetes Self-Management Instrument with Factor Loadings, Interfactor Correlations, and Covariance Correlations (N = 222)

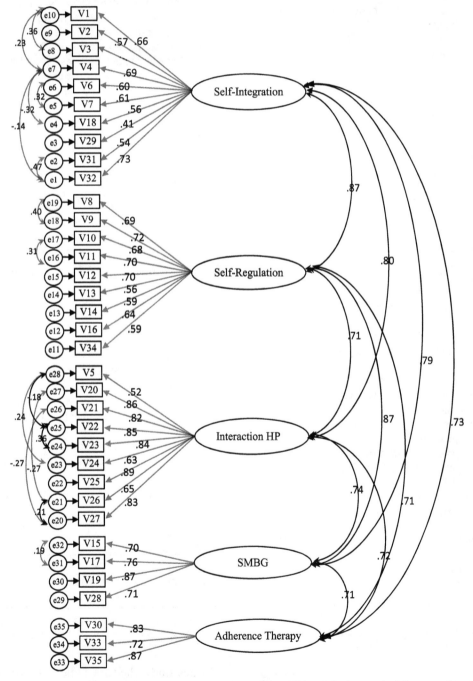

Note. HP = health professional; SMBG = self-monitoring blood glucose. Chi-square = 1458.834 (*df* = 535, *p* < .01), χ^2/df = 2.727; *CFI* = .827, *RSMEA* = .088.

Table 2

Factor Loading of IND-DSMI Final Model: AVE, CR, and Cronbach's Alpha

No. Item	Factor	Factor Loading
Factor 1: self-integration (AVE = .38, CR = .86, Cronbach's α = .86)		
1	I consider the effect on my blood sugars when choosing foods and portions to eat.	.665
2	I can participate in the social activities and still manage my diabetes.	.569
3	I know how to manage food portions and choices when I eat out.	.737
4	I regard my diabetes management as a way to stay healthy overall.	.687
6	My daily life style is healthier than before because of having diabetes.	.598
7	I have successfully merged diabetes into my daily life.	.615
18	I can adjust my diabetes routine to fit new situations (such as being away from home, changing my schedule, and celebration).	.561
29	I manage my food choices to help control my blood glucose.	.733
31	I exercise enough to help control my blood glucose and my weight.	.406
32	I keep my weight within the range set up by healthcare provider and me.	.540
Factor 2: self-regulation (AVE = .43, CR = .87, Cronbach's α = .87)		
8	I pay attention to signals my body gives me related to my blood glucose level.	.690
9	I pay attention to situations in my daily life that might cause my blood glucose levels to change.	.723
10	I can recognize which signs and symptoms tell me the most about my blood glucose level.	.677
11	I can usually figure out the reasons for changes in my blood glucose levels.	.696
12	I compare the differences between my current blood sugar levels and my target blood glucose levels.	.703
13	I monitor my progress toward my desired goals by keeping track of blood glucose levels and A1c.	.560
14	I take action based on body signals such as thirst, losing my temper, and feeling anxious.	.595
16	I decide what action to take based on the results of my previous actions.	.641
34	If I get a low blood glucose reaction I know how to treat it.	.585
Factor 3: interaction with health professionals and significant others (AVE = .60, CR = .93, Cronbach's α = .93)		
5	I am comfortable asking other people with diabetes for tips about managing diabetes.	.524

(continues)

Table 2

Factor Loading of IND-DSMI Final Model: AVE, CR, and Cronbach's Alpha, Continued

No. Item	Factor	Factor Loading
20	I am comfortable asking my healthcare provider questions about my treatment plan.	.858
21	I work with my healthcare providers to identify the possible causes when my diabetes control is poor.	.824
22	I am comfortable telling my healthcare provider how much flexibility I want in my treatment plan.	.853
23	I am comfortable telling my healthcare provider about changes I would like to make in my treatment plan	.844
24	I tell others (e.g., my friends, my family) about the situations in which I need their help for controlling my diabetes.	.628
25	I am comfortable discussing the results of out-of-range blood glucose tests with my healthcare providers.	.889
26	I ask others (e.g., my friends, my family) to help me with my high blood glucose re action if needed.	.646
27	I am comfortable asking my healthcare provider about resources that could help me manage my diabetes.	.827
Factor 4: self-monitoring blood glucose (AVE = .58, CR = .83, Cronbach's α = .86)		
15	When I feel as though my blood glucose is too low, I check my blood glucose levels as soon as possible.	.703
17	When I feel unwell but I am not sure if the cause is either high or low blood glucose, I check my blood glucose as soon as possible.	.759
19	When I feel as though my blood glucose is too high, I check my blood glucose levels as soon as possible.	.866
28	I check my blood glucose to help me make self-care decisions (e.g., medications, diet, exercise).	.710
Factor 5: adherence to recommended therapy (AVE = .66, CR = .85, Cronbach's α = .84)		
30	I take my diabetes medications at the times prescribed.	.830
33	I see my diabetes provider every 1–3 months.	.719
35	I take the amount diabetes medication that has been prescribed for me.	.875

Note. Cronbach's α of all scales = .96. IND-DSMI = Indonesian-Version Diabetes Self-Management Instrument; AVE = average variance extracted; CR = composite reliability.

In this study, the CFA indicated a need to remove some items. However, doing so would not make sense theoretically

Table 3

Interitem Correlation Matrix of Indonesian-Version Diabetes Self-Management Instrument

No. Item	V1	V2	V3	V4	V9	V10	V11	V12	V14	V15	V17	V19
V1	1.000	.406	.678	.609	.439	.259	.289	.364	.145	.337	.451	.446
V2	.406	1.000	.505	.395	.413	.305	.376	.390	.136	.282	.329	.400
V3	.678	.505	1.000	.598	.494	.403	.398	.474	.299	.316	.396	.496
V4	.609	.395	.598	1.000	.367	.292	.341	.410	.273	.254	.345	.420
V9	.439	.413	.494	.367	1.000	.577	.508	.519	.387	.386	.445	.572
V10	.259	.305	.403	.292	.577	1.000	.634	.487	.541	.424	.403	.494
V11	.289	.376	.398	.341	.508	.634	1.000	.584	.500	.453	.429	.495
V12	.364	.390	.474	.410	.519	.487	.584	1.000	.378	.438	.453	.516
V14	.145	.136	.299	.273	.387	.541	.500	.378	1.000	.487	.384	.511
V15	.337	.282	.316	.254	.386	.424	.453	.438	.487	1.000	.666	.618
V17	.451	.329	.396	.345	.445	.403	.429	.453	.384	.666	1.000	.686
V19	.446	.400	.496	.420	.572	.494	.495	.516	.511	.618	.686	1.000
V20	.462	.458	.461	.477	.412	.364	.310	.317	.269	.327	.474	.564
V21	.414	.339	.395	.468	.422	.409	.304	.349	.318	.297	.422	.482
V22	.431	.432	.432	.402	.376	.400	.392	.307	.336	.334	.419	.556
V23	.443	.382	.390	.469	.406	.345	.329	.324	.364	.352	.358	.509
V24	.374	.357	.335	.346	.438	.329	.325	.268	.327	.368	.420	.553
V25	.480	.452	.499	.501	.453	.389	.361	.344	.335	.380	.488	.523
V26	.176	.278	.288	.263	.342	.383	.364	.292	.432	.399	.376	.431
V27	.344	.463	.437	.358	.447	.450	.425	.379	.407	.476	.418	.557
V29	.539	.427	.546	.469	.467	.328	.449	.461	.295	.544	.564	.585
V30	.455	.365	.394	.457	.398	.414	.389	.401	.347	.410	.501	.540
V33	.464	.461	.445	.314	.430	.317	.270	.345	.279	.315	.406	.543
V35	.420	.368	.437	.443	.432	.437	.356	.363	.359	.354	.420	.527

Note. Bold values indicate that value were above .7 (high inter-items correlation).

and would probably be unwise to make modifications only to achieve better statistical results (MacCallum et al., 1992; Schreiber et al., 2006). Therefore, the final version of the IDN-DSMI retains the same set of items as in the original because the reliability of the original instrument was shown to be excellent. The items with lower loadings and higher residuals may be more sensitive to differences in cultural, education, and social variables across country settings. Compared with countries such as Taiwan and Vietnam, Indonesia has fewer resources and facilitation assistance available to support DSM. Moreover, the health education system in clinical settings, particularly in the primary health services, remains limited in Indonesia, which might be less optimal for the patients. In addition, sampling bias (participants were only recruited from public health services) may have biased the results. In addition, demographic characteristics such as age, level of education, family income, and occupation may have influenced the findings. Although some of the participants had a university degree, the proportion of participants with a less-than-university-degree education was much higher. Participants with lower levels of education tend to prefer that information be

presented simply and in a manner that can be easily understood (Baker et al., 2011; Nutbeam, 2008).

In our findings, self-integration was the domain with most items designated for removal. Three of these, including "daily lifestyle is healthier than before because of having diabetes," "successfully merged diabetes into daily life," and "adjust diabetes routine to fit a new situation," conveyed similar contents and may be redundant. In addition, two items, including "exercise to control blood glucose" and "keep body weight within the recommended range," may relate to Indonesians with low self-awareness to do exercise and keep a healthy body weight. Thus, these two items had the lowest factor loading. In the self-regulation domain, the items designated for removal were related to decision making, which may be influenced by the level of knowledge, such as "pay attention to signals of the body related to blood glucose level," "decide action based on experience," and "know how to treat low blood glucose." The item "monitor progress toward desired goals by keeping track of blood glucose levels and A1c" was also designated for removal, perhaps because participants were unfamiliar with using A1c as a monitoring

V20	V21	V22	V23	V24	V25	V26	V27	V29	V30	V33	V35
.462	.414	.431	.443	.374	.480	.176	.344	.539	.455	.464	.420
.458	.339	.432	.382	.357	.452	.278	.463	.427	.365	.461	.368
.461	.395	.432	.390	.335	.499	.288	.437	.546	.394	.445	.437
.477	.468	.402	.469	.346	.501	.263	.358	.469	.457	.314	.443
.412	.422	.376	.406	.438	.453	.342	.447	.467	.398	.430	.432
.364	.409	.400	.345	.329	.389	.383	.450	.328	.414	.317	.437
.310	.304	.392	.329	.325	.361	.364	.425	.449	.389	.270	.356
.317	.349	.307	.324	.268	.344	.292	.379	.461	.401	.345	.363
.269	.318	.336	.364	.327	.335	.432	.407	.295	.347	.279	.359
.327	.297	.334	.352	.368	.380	.399	.476	.544	.410	.315	.354
.474	.422	.419	.358	.420	.488	.376	.418	.564	.501	.406	.420
.564	.482	.556	.509	.553	.523	.431	.557	.585	.540	.543	.527
1.000	**.719**	**.751**	**.759**	.555	**.778**	.418	.650	.530	.571	.497	.492
.719	1.000	.737	.714	.516	**.721**	.498	.588	.433	.473	.443	.497
.751	.737	1.000	.827	.510	**.743**	.527	.681	.474	.467	.452	.461
.759	**.714**	**.827**	1.000	.559	**.729**	.504	.717	.453	.473	.395	.440
.555	.516	.510	.559	1.000	.523	.469	.479	.420	.384	.419	.358
.778	**.721**	**.743**	**.729**	.523	1.000	.579	.768	.561	.594	.488	.568
.418	.498	.527	.504	.469	.579	1.000	.683	.398	.383	.369	.403
.650	.588	.681	**.717**	.479	**.768**	.683	1.000	.547	.500	.517	.562
.530	.433	.474	.453	.420	.561	.398	.547	1.000	.600	.459	.506
.571	.473	.467	.473	.384	.594	.383	.500	.600	1.000	.533	**.738**
.497	.443	.452	.395	.419	.488	.369	.517	.459	.533	1.000	.653
.492	.497	.461	.440	.358	.568	.403	.562	.506	**.738**	.653	1.000

parameter of blood glucose level. Diabetes testing in this study was conducted primarily in PHC settings, which did not have the facilities necessary to measure HbA1c. Although HbA1c is one of the international standards for measuring DSM, most healthcare facilities in Indonesia, especially primary care settings, do not have the tools necessary to measure this variable. Thus, traditional tools such as the blood glucose stick are still widely used to monitor blood glucose levels.

The IDN-DSMI achieved the preferred internal consistency (α = .96), which is comparable with the instrument validations conducted in Taiwan (α = .94), Iran (α = .91), and Vietnam (α = .92; Dao-Tran et al., 2017; Lin et al., 2008; Tol et al., 2011). This evaluation suggests that IDN-DSMI is a reliable tool for measuring the concept of DSM among Indonesians with diabetes. However, a Cronbach's alpha of .90 or higher indicates the possibility of unnecessary items (Tavakol & Dennick, 2011). Besides, the high item-to-item correlation suggests that most of the questions overlap. Thus, further study may beneficial to investigate the potential for developing a shorter version of the IDN-DSMI.

This study also indicates that the problem of poor-fitting model may relate to limitations inherent to the healthcare system, particularly primary healthcare, and infrastructure in Indonesia. Promoting the health education competence of PHC medical personnel is essential to supporting patients with diabetes. Providing psychosocially based educational interventions and addressing cultural issues that may improve patients' self-care behavior are also essential (Tan et al., 2018). Moreover, providing an empowerment program to people with diabetes may be beneficial to improving DSM (Chen et al., 2017).

Limitations

First, the instrument was validated in adults with T2DM in the outpatient department of PHCs in Malang City, Indonesia, only. Therefore, this study may not be generalizable to other populations. Second, the demographic characteristics of the participants, particularly in terms of level of education, was quite extreme (nearly three quarters with less than a university degree). Thus, future investigations should better reflect the demographic characteristics of the general population by sampling a broader population of patients.

Conclusions

The IDN-DSMI is a valid and reliable instrument for measuring DSM behavior in the Indonesian community, especially among patients in primary healthcare. Cultural factors and facilities supporting healthcare services may cause problems of poor fit model. The findings highlight the importance of promoting the health education system and improving infrastructures to promote better DSM by patients with diabetes.

Relevance to Clinical Practice

The IDN-DSMI is a new tool for assessing the self-management behavior of patients with diabetes. This tool may be used by healthcare providers to identify patient problems relating to DSM.

Acknowledgments

This study was supported by the Indonesia Endowment Fund for Education. We would like to thank the patients with diabetes at the PHCs who participated in this study, the research assistants who helped collect the data, and the nursing staffs who facilitated the data collection process.

Author Contributions

Study conception and design: HTR, CMC
Data collection: HTR
Data analysis and interpretation: HTR
Drafting of the article: HTR
Critical revision of the article: CMC

References

American Association of Diabetes Educators. (2014). *AADE 7™ self-care behaviors: American Association of Diabetes Educators (AADE) position statement*. https://www.diabeteseducator.org/docs/default-source/practice/practice-resources/position-statements/aade7-self-care-behaviors-position-statement.pdf?sfvrsn=6

Anderson, R. M., Funnell, M. M., Fitzgerald, J. T., & Marrero, D. G. (2000). The diabetes empowerment scale: A measure of psychosocial self-efficacy. *Diabetes Care, 23*(6), 739–743. https://doi.org/10.2337/diacare.23.6.739

Badan Pusat Statistik. (2010). *Regulation of the Head of the Central Statistics Agency No. 37 of 2010 concerning Urban and Rural Classifications in Indonesia*. http://www.datastatistik-indonesia.com (Original work published in Bahasa Indonesia)

Baker, D. W., DeWalt, D. A., Schillinger, D., Hawk, V., Ruo, B., Bibbins-Domingo, K., Weinberger, M., Macabasco-O'Connell, A., & Pignone, M. (2011). "Teach to goal": Theory and design principles of an intervention to improve heart failure self-management skills of patients with low health literacy. *Journal of Health Communication, 16*(3, Suppl.), 73–88. https://doi.org/10.1080/10810730.2011.604379

Bollen, K. A. (1990). Overall fit in covariance structure models: Two types of sample size effects. *Journal Psychological Bulletin, 107*(2), 256–259. https://doi.org/10.1037/0033-2909.107.2.256

Brown, T. A., & Moore, M. T. (2012). Confirmatory factor analysis. In R. H., Hoyle (Ed.), *Journal handbook of structural equation modeling* (pp. 361–379). Guilford Press.

Browne, M. W., & Cudeck, R. (1992). Alternative ways of assessing model fit. *Sociological Methods & Research, 21*(2), 230–258. https://doi.org/10.1177/0049124192021002005

Bryant, F. B., & Yarnold, P. R. (1995). Principal-components analysis and exploratory and confirmatory factor analysis. In L. G., Grimm & P. R., Yarnold (Eds.), *Reading and understanding multivariate statistics* (pp. 99–136). American Psychological Association.

Cha, E. S., Kim, K. H., & Erlen, J. A. (2007). Translation of scales in cross-cultural research: Issues and techniques. *Journal of Advanced Nursing, 58*(4), 386–395. https://doi.org/10.1111/j.1365-2648.2007.04242.x

Chamberlain, J. J., Rhinehart, A. S., Shaefer, C. F. Jr., & Neuman, A. (2016). Diagnosis and management of diabetes: Synopsis of the 2016 American Diabetes Association standards of medical care in diabetes. *Annals of Internal Medicine, 164*(8), 542–552. https://doi.org/10.7326/M15-3016

Chen, M.-F., Hung, S.-L., & Chen, S.-L. (2017). Empowerment program for people with prediabetes: A randomized controlled trial. *The Journal of Nursing Research, 25*(2), 99–111. https://doi.org/10.1097/jnr.0000000000000193

Choi, T. S. T., Davidson, Z. E., Walker, K. Z., Lee, J. H., & Palermo, C. (2016). Diabetes education for Chinese adults with type 2 diabetes: A systematic review and meta-analysis of the effect on glycemic control. *Diabetes Research and Clinical Practice, 116*, 218–229. https://doi.org/10.1016/j.diabres.2016.04.001

Dao-Tran, T. H., Anderson, D. J., Chang, A. M., Seib, C., & Hurst, C. (2017). Vietnamese version of Diabetes Self-Management Instrument: Development and psychometric testing. *Research in Nursing & Health, 40*(2), 177–184. https://doi.org/10.1002/nur.21777

Department of Health of Malang. (2012). *Opening hours of public services at the health center in the city of Malang*. https://puskgribig.malangkota.go.id/jam-pelayanan/ (Original work published in Bahasa Indonesia)

Fabrigar, L. R., Wegener, D. T., MacCallum, R. C., & Strahan, E. J. (1999). Evaluating the use of exploratory factor analysis in psychological research. *Psychological Methods, 4*(3), 272–299. https://doi.org/10.1037/1082-989X.4.3.272

Fidan, Ö., Takmak, S., Zeyrek, A. S., & Kartal, A. (2020). Patients with type 2 diabetes mellitus: Obstacles in coping. *The Journal of Nursing Research, 28*(4), Article e105. https://doi.org/10.1097/jnr.0000000000000379

Fornell, C., & Larcker, D. F. (1981). Evaluating structural equation models with unobservable variables and measurement error. *Journal of Marketing Research, 18*(1), 39–50. https://doi.org/10.1177/002224378101800104

Funnell, M. M., & Anderson, R. M. (2004). Empowerment and self-management of diabetes. *Clinical Diabetes, 22*(3), 123–127. https://doi.org/10.2337/diaclin.22.3.123

Garson, D. G. (2008). *Factor analysis: Statnotes.* North Carolina State University Public Administration Program. https://www.encorewiki.org/download/attachments/25657/Factor%20Analysis_%20Statnotes%20from%20North%20Carolina%20State%20University.pdf?api=v2

Guilford, J. P. (1954). *Psychometric methods* (2nd ed.). McGraw-Hill.

Hooper, D., Coughlan, J., & Mullen, M. R. (2008). Structural equation modelling: Guidelines for determining model fit. *The Electronic Journal of Business Research Methods, 6*(1), 53–60.

International Diabetes Federation. (2012). *Clinical guideline task force: Global guideline for type 2 diabetes.* https://www.iapb.org/wp-content/uploads/Global-Guideline-for-Type-2-Diabetes-IDF-2012.pdf

International Diabetes Federation. (2019). *IDF diabetes atlas* (9th ed.). https://www.diabetesatlas.org/en/resources/

Kementerian Kesehatan Indonesia. (2015). Morbidity and multi-morbidity in the elderly group in Indonesia. *The Indonesia Journal of Biotechnology Medicine, 4*(2), 77–88. https://media.neliti.com/media/publications/76059-ID-morbiditas-dan-multi-morbiditas-pada-kel.pdf (Original work published in Indonesian)

Kline, T. (2005). *Psychological testing: A practical approach to design and evaluation.* SAGE Publication.

Lee, C. L., Lin, C. C., & Anderson, R. (2016). Psychometric evaluation of the Diabetes Self-Management Instrument Short Form (DSMI-20). *Applied Nursing Research, 29,* 83–88. https://doi.org/10.1016/j.apnr.2015.04.013

Lin, C. C., Anderson, R. M., Chang, C. S., Hagerty, B. M., & Loveland-Cherry, C. J. (2008). Development and testing of the Diabetes Self-Management Instrument: A confirmatory analysis. *Research in Nursing & Health, 31*(4), 370–380. https://doi.org/10.1002/nur.20258

Lu, Y., Xu, J., Zhao, W., & Han, H. R. (2016). Measuring self-care in persons with type 2 diabetes: A systematic review. *Evaluation & the Health Professions, 39*(2), 131–184. https://doi.org/10.1177/0163278715588927

MacCallum, R. C., Browne, M. W., & Sugawara, H. M. (1996). Power analysis and determination of sample size for covariance structure modeling. *Journal Psychological methods, 1*(2), 130–149. https://doi.org/10.1037/1082-989X.1.2.130

MacCallum, R. C., Roznowski, M., & Necowitz, L. B. (1992). Model modifications in covariance structure analysis: The problem of capitalization on chance. *Psychological Bulletin, 111*(3), 490–504.

Nutbeam, D. (2008). The evolving concept of health literacy. *Social Science & Medicine, 67*(12), 2072–2078. https://doi.org/10.1016/j.socscimed.2008.09.050

Pallant, J. (2010). *SPSS survival manual: A step by step guide to data analysis using SPSS* (4th ed.). Open University Press.

Redman, B. K. (2009). Patient adherence or patient self-management in transplantation: An ethical analysis. *Progress in Transplantation, 19*(1), 90–94. https://doi.org/10.1177/152692480901900113

Schmitt, A., Gahr, A., Hermanns, N., Kulzer, B., Huber, J., & Haak, T. (2013). The Diabetes Self-Management Questionnaire (DSMQ): Development and evaluation of an instrument to assess diabetes self-care activities associated with glycaemic control. *Health and Quality Life Outcomes, 11*(1), Article No. 138. https://doi.org/10.1186/1477-7525-11-138

Schreiber, J. B., Stage, F. K., Nora, A., Barlow, E. A., & King, J. (2006). Reporting structural equation modeling and confirmatory factor analysis results: A review. *The Journal of Educational Research, 99*(6), 323–337. https://doi.org/10.3200/JOER.99.6.323-338

Shah, R. B. (2012). A multivariate analysis technique: Structural equation modeling. *Asian Journal of Multidimensional Research, 1*(4), 73–81.

Tahmasebi, R., & Noroozi, A. (2012). Cross-cultural validation of the diabetes self-management scale in Iranian patients. *HealthMED, 6*(8), 2635–2641.

Tan, C. C. L., Cheng, K. K. F., Sum, C. F., Shew, J. S. H., Holydard, E., & Wang, W. (2018). Perceptions of diabetes self-care management among older Singaporeans with type 2 diabetes: A qualitative study. *The Journal of Nursing Research, 26*(4), 242–249. https://doi.org/10.1097/jnr.0000000000000226

Tavakol, M., & Dennick, R. (2011). Making sense of Cronbach's alpha. *International Journal of Medical Education, 2,* 53–55. https://doi.org/10.5116/ijme.4dfb.8dfd

Tol, A., Mohajeri Tehrani, M. R., Mahmoodi, G., Alhani, F., Shojaeezadeh, D., Eslami, A., & Sharifirad, G. (2011). Development of a valid and reliable Diabetes Self-Management Instrument: An Iranian version. *Journal of Diabetes and Metabolic Disorders, 10,* 1–6. http://jdmd.tums.ac.ir/index.php/jdmd/article/view/289

Toobert, D. J., Hampson, S. E., & Glasgow, R. E. (2000). The summary of diabetes self-care activities measure: Results from 7 studies and a revised scale. *Diabetes Care, 23*(7), 943–950. https://doi.org/10.2337/diacare.23.7.943

Watson, R., & Thompson, D. R. (2006). Use of factor analysis in journal of advanced nursing: Literature review. *Journal of Advanced Nursing, 55*(3), 330–341. https://doi.org/10.1111/j.1365-2648.2006.03915.x

World Health Organization. (2020a). *Health statistics and information systems: Metrics: Disability-adjusted life year (DALY).* Retrieved June 27, 2020, from https://www.who.int/healthinfo/global_burden_disease/metrics_daly/en/

World Health Organization. (2020b). *World health statistic 2020: Monitoring health for the SDGs.* https://www.who.int/gho/publications/world_health_statistics/2020/en/

Yasir, A. S. M. (2016). Cross cultural adaptation & psychometric validation of instruments: Step-wise description. *International Journal of Psychiatry, 1*(1), 1–4. https://www.opastonline.com/wp-content/uploads/2016/07/cross-cultural-adaptation-psychometric-validation-of-instruments-step-wise-description-ijp-16-001.pdf

25

Knowledge and Attitudes Regarding Organ Transplantation Among Cyprus Residents

Evanthia ASIMAKOPOULOU[1]* • Vaso STYLIANOU[2] • Ioannis DIMITRAKOPOULOS[3] •
Alexandros ARGYRIADIS[4] • Panagiota BELLOU–MYLONA[5]

ABSTRACT

Background: Organ transplantation was one of the greatest achievements of medical science during the 20th century. Knowledge, education, and culture all play prominent roles in transplantation because of the complexity of the process from donation to transplantation.

Purpose: The aim of this research was to determine and analyze the knowledge and attitudes about organ donation and transplantation among the general population in Limassol, Cyprus.

Methods: A quantitative research approach was followed, and a questionnaire consisting of closed-ended questions was completed by adults from the general population in Limassol.

Results: One thousand two hundred adults out of the 1,346 adults who were contacted responded to the survey (response rate: 89%) and were included as participants. Of the participants, 93.4% ($p < .05$) considered organ donation to be lifesaving, 57% expressed interest (and 39.8% expressed disinterest) in becoming organ donors, 80.6% ($p < .05$) expressed awareness of there being a waiting list for people in need of organ transplantation, 50.4% agreed that brain death must be confirmed before organ removal for transplantation, and 47% recalled having been informed about organ donation through the media, with 31.5% stating that they had never been informed about organ donation.

Conclusions: The participants demonstrated limited awareness regarding the organ donation system in Cyprus. Furthermore, a significant percentage stated that they lacked a source for obtaining related information. The Cypriot society should be informed and encouraged to participate in organ donation to increase the rate of organ transplantation.

KEY WORDS:
attitudes, Cyprus, knowledge levels, organ donation, transplantation.

Introduction

Transplantation, one of the most progressive areas in the healthcare sciences, has moved from experimental trials to acceptable therapies and is being used to treat many severe health problems (Shafran et al., 2014). Organ donation is a voluntary process that leads to the transfer of life to a person who needs a healthy organ to live or to improve their quality of life (Chen et al., 2007). This action has no financial benefit and thus represents a purely a humanitarian effort (Voo, 2015).

According to Caplan (2009), about a dozen people in the United States waiting for organ transplants die each day. Many deaths may be prevented if more organs are available. This pressure is getting worse because waiting lists are growing faster than the supply of organs. Therefore, healthcare professionals must consider new options for including more people in organ donation programs, and transplantation centers may need to reconsider their waiting list criteria and priorities (Caplan, 2009; Shafran et al., 2014). The decisions related to organ transplantation involve a myriad of difficult ethical and legal issues.

The first organ transplant attempts in Cyprus were made in 1986 from living kidney donors. Since then, only kidney transplants have been performed in Cyprus, while patients who need other organs have been required to list abroad (Kyriakides et al., 2002). There is an intensive need to expand the transplant methods used in Cyprus and to include many other organs in the process. Moreover, there is a lack of transplant coordinators and education for healthcare professionals in Cyprus.

Transplantation, which is the implantation of a tissue, cell, or organ (called a graft), is often the only effective treatment for organ failure (Cho et al., 2018). The process of transplanting organs from donors to patients is governed by strict rules and regulations (Prabhu, 2019). A transplant from a living donor has many advantages, as it is a planned operation in which the person is hemodynamically stable and well oxygenated (Tong et al., 2013). However, donors

[1] PhD, RN, Lecturer, School of Health Sciences, Frederick University, Nicosia, Cyprus • [2] PhD(c), RN, Staff Nurse, School of Health Sciences, Frederick University, Nicosia, Cyprus • [3] MSc, RN, Special Teaching Staff, School of Health Sciences, Frederick University, Nicosia, Cyprus • [4] PhD, RN, Assistant Professor, School of Health Sciences and School of Education and Social Sciences, Frederick University, Nicosia, Cyprus • [5] PhD, Professor, School of Health Sciences, Frederick University, Nicosia, Cyprus.

who have experienced brain death and are hospitalized in intensive care units are the primary source of transplants, which requires tests and checks by doctors in different specialties at different times to confirm the time of brain death, qualify the donation, and confirm compatibility (Chinen & Buckley, 2010). The total process is very complicated and time sensitive. Transport and storage conditions for donated organs must follow applicable European directives. In addition, European Union member states must ensure that transplantation takes place in or under the supervision of transplantation centers that comply with the rules of the European Union (Bouwman et al., 2013).

Social media networks are an important factor driving changing views and attitudes toward organ transplantations. Social networks may positively affect public opinion through information campaigns about organ donation (Cameron et al., 2013; Jiang et al., 2019). On the other hand, misinformation about transplants, which confuses public opinion and leads to distrust in the medical community, is considered an underlying cause of low organ donor registration rates (Cameron et al., 2013). Religion is also an important factor that influences personal decision-making regarding becoming an organ donor. If a patient has an irreversible medical condition and observes all legal protocols, churches are generally in favor of organ donation (Bruzzone, 2008).

Donation decisions are influenced by religious, cultural, altruistic, and knowledge-based beliefs (Ríos et al., 2018). In addition, family, school, and the state affect related directions and policies on this issue. School courses, government campaigns, and social media have all been used to promote organ donation awareness and registration.

Because of the intense interest in transplantation and of Cyprus' high position on the European transplantation charts (Kyriakides et al., 2002) in terms of living donors, this study was conducted to assess the attitudes and knowledge of Limassol residents about organ transplantation.

Methods

The survey, conducted in Limassol, Cyprus, adopted a quantitative approach because of the main aim of this study. The research tool used was the questionnaire, and the distribution of the questionnaires took place in public areas where people were waiting to access public services. The sample used in the analysis included 1,200 adult men and women of all education levels. Data collection lasted 4 months, from June 2017 to September 2017.

The sampling method used was convenience sampling. Despite the risks, this method is very useful for investigating phenomena because of its low cost, deep access to information, and the relatively brief time required to collect data (Gravetter & Forzano, 2011).

The items on the questionnaire were drafted after a thorough literature review and were checked by two relevant experts for appropriateness (Bedi et al., 2015; Burra et al., 2005; Tsavdaroglou et al., 2013). The questionnaire was then pilot tested on a sample of 10 individuals for ease of comprehension and item appropriateness. These 10 individuals were not included in the main study. The original questionnaire consisted of a smaller number of questions. After the pilot study, adjustments were made to address several difficulties noted regarding terminology. The questionnaire was divided into four sections: sociodemographic details, awareness regarding donation, experience with organ donation, and intentions regarding donation. Each participant was given 10 minutes to complete the questionnaire, and informed consent was obtained from all participants beforehand.

Each correct answer was assigned a score of 1, and each wrong or equivocal (i.e., I do not know) answer was assigned a score of 0. Next, a total score for each participant was calculated, divided by the total number of questions ($n = 12$), and then multiplied by 100 to extract a percentage scale (0–100). A larger percentage scale value indicated better knowledge, with a minimum scale value of 60% used to distinguish between "inadequate" and "adequate" knowledge categories, having responded correctly to most of the questions (at least 6 out of 10; Albert et al., 2002; Sánchez-Mendiola et al., 2012; Testa et al., 2018).

Data analysis for this study was conducted using IBM SPSS Version 21.0 (IBM, Inc., Armonk, NY, USA). The reliability coefficients and Cronbach's internal consistency of the attitudes scale were assessed. The knowledge score, frequency distributions of the participants' characteristics, estimated relative frequencies, and 95.0% confidence intervals were calculated, and a chi-square test was used in categorical data. Differences in knowledge scale attributable to sociodemographic characteristics and heterogeneity were tested using the variance analysis method and the Levene method, respectively. The difference between high and low knowledge scale attributable to sociodemographic characteristics was checked by a chi-square test, and the acceptable level of significance was set at .05 (Linardakis & Dellaportas, 2003).

The National Bioethics Committee of Cyprus and the Data Protection Office approved the study (Protocol No. EEBK ΕΠ2014.01.105).

Results

Less than two thirds (59.7%; highest notable frequency, $p < .05$) responded correctly to the questionnaire statement that someone must be completely healthy to be an organ donor, 80.6% responded that there is a waiting list for recipients, 50.4% responded that brain death must be confirmed before organ removal, 67.2% (highest notable frequency, $p < .05$) responded that all donors are tested for transmittable diseases, 69.1% responded that you may change your mind after registering as a donor, 45.5% responded that anyone may become a donor regardless of their age, 42.3% responded that individuals may designate who their organs will be given to in case of brain death, and 93.4% (highest notable frequency, $p < .05$) responded that organ donation saves lives. Less than half (45.1%; highest notable frequency,

$p < .05$) responded that they were not aware of the view of the church toward organ donation; 19.2% (lowest notable frequency, $p < .05$) did not know whether, in case of brain death, the next of kin could make the decision regarding donation; and 27.8% (lowest notable frequency, $p < .05$) did not know if brain death was reversible (Table 1).

The highest percentage of participants who had been informed about organ donation by a doctor were those with a primary level of education (24%), whereas only 9.1% of those had university education. A large percentage of participants at all levels of education indicated having never received information on organ donation, with the highest percentages being 35.4% and 30.7%, respectively, for participants educated to the high school and university levels (Table 2).

Over half, 61.8% and 52.9% (highest notable frequency, $p < .05$), respectively, responded negatively about knowing a family member or a close acquaintance needing a transplant or previously declaring an interest in becoming a donor and whether the people in their environment held negative attitudes toward donation. A high percentage (50.8%; highest notable frequency, $p < .05$) responded that they did not know if anyone in their family or close environment had shown interest in becoming an organ donor, whereas 57.0% stated that they would become a donor and 39.8% responded that they would not become a donor (highest notable frequency, $p < .05$). Slightly over half (52.3%; highest notable frequency, $p < .05$) agreed strongly that the reason they would like to become a donor is because they desired to help their fellow man. Respective percentages of 39.5%, 34.5%, and 44.7% (highest notable frequency, $p < .05$) completely disagreed, which could be affected or sensitized by a family member or a friend who was either a donor or needed a transplant and become a donor only for someone dear to them.

Respective percentages of 40.3%, 41.1%, and 37.7% (highest notable frequency, $p < .05$) answered affirmatively to being afraid, to not trusting the unions and the doctors about how they will be treated knowing that they are donors, and to being unsure whether their transplanted organs would be used properly. Respective percentages of 37.1% and 44.9% (highest notable frequency, $p < .05$) agreed about not being interested in organ donation and on not being sufficiently aware of the issue of organ donation. More than 4 of 10 participants (42.1%; highest notable frequency, $p < .05$) questioned brain death and agreed that there was still hope for life until the last breath. However, 44.2% (highest notable frequency, $p < .05$) accepted brain death as physical death (Table 3). Respective percentages of 32.0%, 37.3%, and 32.7% (highest notable frequency, $p < .05$) agreed that they were positively affected by mass media, the title of organ donor gives a sense of satisfaction and pride, and organ donation offers a way to live on after death (Table 3).

A higher percentage of women participants were motivated by altruistic motives than their male counterparts. Desire to limit organ donations only to close friends or family fell with rising education level (highest notable relation, $p < .05$). The percentage of those expressing willingness to

Table 1

Awareness Score According to the Correct Answers Given in the 12 Questions Regarding Organ Donation in Correspondence to the Demographic Details of the Participants

Characteristic	Awareness Score					p
	n	M	SD	p	Score ≥ 60 (%)	
Total	1,200	52.3	17.7	—	28.5	—
Gender				.876		.053
Male	519	52.4	19.1		31.4	
Female	681	52.3	16.5		26.3	
Age (years)				.040*		.014*
18–29	392	51.3	17.7		26.3	
30–39	403	51.4	16.9		25.3	
40–49	196	54.5	17.9		34.7	
50–59	156	53.2	18.9		31.4	
≥ 60	53	56.0	17.9		37.7	
Education				.280		.461
Up to primary school	25	54.3	23.3		32.0	
Secondary school	45	55.7	18.6		35.6	
High school	353	51.6	17.2		25.5	
Technological institute	148	50.0	18.9		25.7	
University	629	52.9	17.3		30.2	

*$p < .05$.

Table 2

Frequencies of Stated Sources of Information Regarding Organ Donation, by Level of Education

Source of Information[a]	Education Level (%)					p
	Up to Primary School	Secondary School	High School	Tech. Institute	University	
Doctor	24.0	20.0	10.5	15.5	9.1	.015*
Family	16.0	11.1	17.6	17.3	13.5	.131
Close contacts	32.0	26.7	30.0	30.4	31.2	.638
Mass media	60.0	44.4	45.6	43.2	48.5	.716
Medical journals	20.0	17.8	15.0	12.8	15.1	.670
Conventions—events	4.0	4.4	2.0	4.7	3.3	.592
University	0.0	0.0	0.0	2.0	1.0	.107
Movies	0.0	0.0	0.3	0.0	0.8	.188
No one (no source)	24.0	28.9	35.4	27.7	30.7	.525

[a]Multiple choice.
*$p < .05$.

Table 3

Agreeability Degree Frequencies From the Participants Who Did Not Express/Expressed Willingness to Become a Donor (y = 474) in Questions About Personal Views Regarding Organ Donation

Question	Completely Disagree	Disagree	Agree	Completely Agree	I Do Not Know
	%	%	%	%	%
Unwilling					
1. I'm afraid.	13.6	23.9	40.3*	13.8	8.4
2. I do not trust the unions to provide needed treatments to registered donors.	8.8	24.5	41.1*	15.9	9.6
3. I do not trust doctors and the way that I would be treated during hospitalization as a registered donor.	11.1	27.3	37.9*	16.8	6.9
4. I do not believe that the transplant would be used correctly.	11.7	29.6	37.7*	14.3	6.7
5. I find it irrelevant and am not really concerned about the matter.	26.8	44.2*	13.4	5.9	9.6
6. I disregard the matter and have not given it any serious thought.	15.3	24.9	37.1*	18.0	4.6
7. I'm still not aware or decided regarding organ donation.	13.4	19.7	44.9*	17.4	4.6
8. I question brain death, since there is still hope for life until the last breath.	7.5	20.8	42.1*	28.3	1.3
Willing					
1. I really want to help a fellow person.	2.3	2.3	41.5	52.3*	1.5
2. By donating an organ, you are saving a life, which is something that agrees with my religious beliefs.	7.5	7.6	38.0	38.9	8.0
3. I have been affected by a family member or a friend that is a donor.	39.5*	28.9	14.6	7.7	9.2
4. I have been sensitized by a family member or friend that needed a transplant.	34.5*	24.6	19.7	13.9	7.3
5. I would only become a donor for someone dear to me.	44.7*	30.1	12.6	7.7	4.8
6. The mass media has had a positive effect on me about becoming a donor.	24.6	21.9	32.0*	12.3	9.2
7. The title of organ donor gives me a sense of satisfaction and pride.	16.5	13.9	37.3*	27.6	4.7
8. By becoming an organ donor I feel that a piece of me will live on after my death.	19.0	14.8	32.7*	25.9	7.6

*$p < .05$.

become a donor and disagreeing about being sensitized by a family member or a close friend who needed a transplant rose with the education level of the participant. Women participants disagreed more than their male counterparts about being unconcerned or only mildly concerned regarding the subject of donation (highest notable relation, $p < .05$). Among those who expressed unwillingness to become a donor, older age was associated negatively with the interest in organ donation and accepting brain death as physical death (highest notable relation, $p < .05$). Among those participants who did not express willingness to become a donor, awareness level was positively associated with disagreeing about being afraid, finding the subject of organs irrelevant, and being unconcerned about organ donation.

Discussion

The literature on the knowledge and attitudes of Cypriots regarding organ transplantation–donation is very limited. After evaluating the awareness of the participants, some important results were found in this study. A high percentage answered positively to the questions that someone must be completely healthy to become a donor and that there is a waiting list for perspective donors.

A very high percentage of the participants (93.4%) agreed that organ donation saves lives. In a similar survey in Greece (Tsavdaroglou et al., 2013), 90.5% of nursing students considered that organ donation saves lives. In a survey in Pakistan (Ali et al., 2013), 81.6% of medical students agreed that it was ethically correct to donate an organ. In another survey in Saudi Arabia (Mohamed & Guella, 2013), over 90% of a random general-population sample were aware of organ transplantation donation. Moreover, a survey conducted in an African American community in Buffalo, New York, showed high organ donation awareness, with 88% of the participants being familiar with organ donation, 36% indicating they would not donate organs, 31% indicating that they would donate, and 33% indicating being unsure (Minniefield & Muti, 2002). Similar results were also found in young British adults, who showed positive attitudes toward donation (90% are in favor of organ donation) and 63.9% and 78.2% expressing respective willingness to donate and to receive organs (Coad et al., 2013). Moreover, 72% of nonmedical hospital staffs expressed being in favor of donating organs after death in Spain and Latin American. This percentage varies greatly by country, with 98% of Cuban, 80% of Mexican, 66% of Costa Rican, and 52% of Spanish respondents responding favorably (Ríos et al., 2013).

With regard to experiences with organ donation, high percentages in this study answered that family members or close acquaintances had never needed a transplant and had never officially declared wanting to be a donor. A similar percentage expressed not knowing if any close acquaintance wanted to become a donor. However, a high percentage answered negatively to the question whether their close acquaintances held negative attitudes toward organ donation.

In this study, 57.0% agreed to become an organ donor, whereas 39.0% declined. In a similar survey in Greece (Theodorakopoulou & Bakalis, 2010), 62.0% and 68.0% of nurses and nursing students, respectively, responded they would become organ donors. In the Buffalo, New York, study (Minniefield & Muti, 2002), 33% respondents indicated that they would donate their organs, 36% said no, and 33% were unsure. In Brazil (Peron et al., 2004), 68.2% of university health students expressed willingness to be organ donors. On the other hand, more than 90% of medical students in Italy showed strongly positive attitudes; most of these were prepared to donate their organs after death, and 63% had already signed a donor card (Burra et al., 2005).

The main reasons for participants in this study not intending to be organ donors included fear (40.3%), distrust in organizations (41.1%), distrust in doctors during hospitalization (37.9%), and hope for life until their last breath (42.1%). In a survey in Greece (Theodorakopoulou & Bakalis, 2010), 32% of nurses and 17% nursing students expressed distrust in the transplantation selection process. In Saudi Arabia (Mohamed & Guella, 2013), 15.2% expressed fear of the operation, and in Brazil (Peron et al., 2004), almost 79.4% of the student participants did not believe that the waiting list for transplants was followed.

In a survey of the adult population in Pakistan regarding the allowance of organ donation by religion, "yes," "no," and "do not know" earned roughly equal percentages (Saleem et al., 2009). In that survey, religion was the leading reason (45.4%) expressed that organ donation should not be promoted. A meta-analysis in 2013 (Tong et al., 2013) showed that most were in favor of living-directed donation (85.5%), with the barriers identified including fear of surgery and health risks, lack of knowledge, respect for cultural norms, financial loss, distrust in hospitals, and avoiding recipient indebtedness. In addition, 32% of the sample in the survey in Buffalo, New York, stated that they did not trust doctors, and most of the young adult respondents were afraid they would not receive proper medical attention if they were registered as organ donors (Minniefield & Muti, 2002). Finally, the main reason among nursing students for hesitating to donate organs was fear of the commercialization of organ donation (Tsavdaroglou et al., 2013).

In term of religion, a high percentage in this study seemed not to know the church's position toward donation, whereas a small percentage reflected a belief that the church forbids organ donation. This study found that a large percentage (45.1%) does not know the position of the church. From a religious point of view, 68.6% of Saudi Arabians consider it legal to donate organs and 26.2% do not (Mohamed & Guella, 2013). The African American respondents most often cited religious reasons for not donating (Minniefield & Muti, 2002).

A high percentage of participants identified the mass media as their main source of information, whereas a smaller percentage identified their close acquaintances, medical journals, and their doctor as their primary source. A significant percentage stated that they had no source of related information. This raises concerns regarding how accurately the public is being informed. In this study, 47.1% were informed by the media, 30.6% were informed by friends, and 17.6% were informed by family. Notably, a large percentage (31.5%) indicated being informed by no one. Similarly, in a study in Pakistan (Ali et al., 2013), most of the students (64.6%) were made aware of organ donation through print and electronic media, whereas only 27.8% were made aware by their healthcare providers. These results suggest that nonphysicians are frequently overlooked and are not provided with the necessary information to help them better understand the organ donation and transplantation process (Zambudio et al., 2012).

A very small percentage in this study answered that there are no regulations governing organ donation. One out of 10 (9.8%) expressed the belief that no regulations existed, whereas 45.8% were unaware whether there was related regulations in Cyprus. A study in Greece (Theodorakopoulou & Bakalis, 2010) found that 82% of nursing students and 62.5% of the nurses were unaware of related regulations. In an international study (Ramadurg & Gupta, 2014), it was found that awareness of regulations governing transplantation among medical students was poor (44.3% were unaware regarding the existence of related laws).

In cases of brain death, with regard to whether relatives could decide about organ donation regardless of the patient's declared intent while alive, 43% of the participants in this study disagreed and 19.2% did not know. However, in another study, 61.2% of subjects expressed that relatives could donate a patient's organs after brain death (Mohamed & Guella, 2013). Family members continue to play a prominent role in donation decisions at time of death, as many participants relied on their family to make end-of-life care decisions for them in the absence of a written advance directive (Ríos et al., 2019; Rodrigue et al., 2006).

A high percentage in this study expressed awareness that the donor must be declared brain dead in order for an organ to be removed. However, relatively high percentages of the respondents seemed not to know that brain death was irreversible, with 37.3% believing brain death to be reversible and 27.8% being unsure.

In responding to the statement that a person could predetermine where their organs would be given, 44.7% of the sample disagreed and only 12.6% agreed. In this study, a high percentage believed that anyone could donate organs no matter their age. A similar general-population survey in Pakistan (Saleem et al., 2009) found that half (51.1%) would donate their organs to a family member. In a cohort study of Latin Americans living in the United States, respondents who were in favor of donating a family member's organs were more in favor of donating their own organs, whereas those who had previously discussed the subject of organ donation in their family circle held a more favorable attitude (Ríos et al., 2017). In a study of university students in China, 62.4% respondents indicated that designated relatives were their most probable recipients (Zhang et al., 2007).

Although this study achieved its aims, there are some limitations. The survey was conducted only in Limassol and not in the other cities of Cyprus. Therefore, to generalize the results, the study should involve participants from different areas of the country. Also, the results may have been affected by cultural bias, as the origin and cultural background of the participants were not considered.

Conclusions

In conclusion, a high percentage of participants expressed a desire to become a donor, whereas a very small percentage expressed that they did not know. Those who expressed willingness to become an organ donor agreed that a main reason for doing so was to help their fellow man. Furthermore, high percentages of donors were found among those who were affected by mass media, those who felt the title of donor conferred a sense of satisfaction/pride, and those who felt that donating would allow a part of their being to live on after their death. A high percentage of those unwilling to become organ donors stated fear as their main reason, with distrust of doctors and concern that they would not receive necessary treatment as registered donors also noted as important reasons.

The results support that Cypriots have a relatively high level of awareness regarding organ donation. As transplant waiting lists have increased exponentially worldwide during recent decades, there is a need to develop community programs to further raise public awareness about organ and tissue donation in Cyprus. Public education, mainly through the media, nongovernmental organizations, and lectures by experts, has been the main strategy to change social attitudes toward organ donation and transplantation.

Acknowledgment

The authors would like to thank all of those who participated in this study.

Author Contributions

Study conception and design: EA, VS
Data collection: VS, ID
Data analysis and interpretation: EA, ID, AA
Drafting of the article: EA, AA
Critical revision of the article: PBM

References

Albert, N. M., Collier, S., Sumodi, V., Wilkinson, S., Hammel, J. P., Vopat, L., Willis, C., & Bittel, B. (2002). Nurses' knowledge of heart failure education principles. *Heart & Lung, 31*(2), 102–112. https://doi.org/10.1067/mhl.2002.122837

Ali, N. F., Qureshi, A., Jilani, B. N., & Zehra, N. (2013). Knowledge and ethical perception regarding organ donation among medical students. *BMC Medical Ethics, 14,* Article 38. https://doi.org/10.1186/1472-6939-14-38

Bedi, K. K., Hakeem, A. R., Dave, R., Lewington, A., Sanfey, H., & Ahmad, N. (2015). Survey of the knowledge, perception, and attitude of medical students at the University of Leeds toward organ donation and transplantation. *Transplantation Proceedings, 47*(2), 247–260. https://doi.org/10.1016/j.transproceed.2014.11.033

Bouwman, R., Lie, J., Bomhoff, M., & Friele, R. D. (2013). *Study on the set-up of organ donation and transplantation in the EU Member States, uptake and impact of the EU Action Plan on Organ Donation and Transplantation (2009–2015): ACTOR study.* NIVEL. https://ec.europa.eu/health/sites/health/files/blood_tissues_organs/docs/organs_actor_study_2013_en.pdf

Bruzzone, P. (2008). Religious aspects of organ transplantation. *Transplantation Proceedings, 40*(4), 1064–1067. https://doi.org/10.1016/j.transproceed.2008.03.049

Burra, P., De Bona, M., Canova, D., D'Aloiso, M. C., Germani, G., Rumiati, R., Ermani, M., & Ancona, E. (2005). Changing attitude to organ donation and transplantation in university students during the years of medical school in Italy. *Transplantation Proceedings, 37*(2), 547–550. https://doi.org/10.1016/j.transproceed.2004.12.255

Cameron, A. M., Massie, A. B., Alexander, C. E., Stewart, B., Montgomery, R. A., Benavides, N. R., Fleming, G. D., & Segev, D. L. (2013). Social media and organ donor registration: The Facebook effect. *American Journal of Transplantation, 13,* 2059–2065. https://doi.org/10.1111/ajt.12312

Caplan, L. A. (2009). *The Penn Center guide to bioethics.* Springer.

Chen, W.-C., Chen, C.-H., Lee, P.-C., & Wang, W.-L. (2007). Quality of life, symptom distress, and social support among renal transplant recipients in southern Taiwan: A correlational study. *The Journal of Nursing Research, 15*(4), 319–329. https://doi.org/10.1097/01.JNR.0000387628.33425.34

Chinen, J., & Buckley, R. H. (2010). Transplantation immunology: Solid organ and bone marrow. *The Journal of Allergy and Clinical Immunology, 125*(2, Suppl.), S324–S325. https://doi.org/10.1016/j.jaci.2009.11.014

Cho, S., Mohan, S., Husain, S. A., & Natarajan, K. (2018). Expanding transplant outcomes research opportunities through the use of a common data model. *American Journal of Transplantation, 18*(6), 1321–1327. https://doi.org/10.1111/ajt.14892

Coad, L., Carter, N., & Ling, J. (2013). Attitudes of young adults from the UK towards organ donation and transplantation. *Transplantation Research, 2*(1), Article No. 9. https://doi.org/10.1186/2047-1440-2-9

Gravetter, F. J., & Forzano, L.-A. B. (2011). *Research methods for the behavioural sciences* (4th ed.). Wadsworth Publishing.

Jiang, X., Jiang, W., Cai, J., Su, Q., Zhou, Z., He, L., & Lai, K. (2019). Characterizing media content and effects of organ donation on a social media platform: Content analysis. *Journal of Medical Internet Research, 21*(3), Article e13058. https://doi.org/10.2196/13058

Kyriakides, G., Pouloukas, S., Hadjigavriel, M., & Nicolaidou, A. (2002). Living unrelated renal transplants in Cyprus. *Transplantation Proceedings, 34*(8), 3104–3105. https://doi.org/10.1016/S0041-1345(02)03600-X

Linardakis, M., & Dellaportas, P. (2003). Assessment of Athens's metro passenger behaviour via a multiranked probit model. *Journal of the Royal Statistical Society, 52,* 185–200. https://doi.org/10.1111/1467-9876.00397

Minniefield, W. J., & Muti, P. (2002). Organ donation survey results of a Buffalo, New York, African American community. *Journal of the National Medical Association, 94*(11), 979–986.

Mohamed, E., & Guella, A. (2013). Public awareness survey about organ donation and transplantation. *Transplantation Proceedings, 45*(10), 3469–3471. https://doi.org/10.1016/j.transproceed.2013.08.095

Peron, A. L., Rodrigues, A. B., Leite, D. A., Lopes, J. L., Ceschim, P. C., Alter, R., Roza, B. A., Pestana, J. O., & Schirmer, J. (2004). Organ donation and transplantation in Brazil: University students' awareness and opinions. *Transplantation Proceedings, 36,* 811–813. https://doi.org/10.1016/j.transproceed.2004.04.040

Prabhu, P. K. (2019). Is presumed consent an ethically acceptable way of obtaining organs for transplant? *Journal of the Intensive Care Society, 20*(2), 92–97. https://doi.org/10.1177/1751143718777171

Ramadurg, U. Y., & Gupta, A. (2014). Impact of an educational intervention on increasing the knowledge and changing the attitude and beliefs towards organ donation among medical students. *Journal of Clinical and Diagnostic Research, 8*(5), JC05–JC07. https://doi.org/10.7860/JCDR/2014/6594.4347

Ríos, A., López-Navas, A., Ayala-García, M. A., Sebastian, M. J., Abdo-Cuza, A., Alán, J., Martínez-Alarcón, L., Ramírez-Barba, E. J., Muñoz-Jiménez, G., Palacios, G., Suárez-López, J., Castellanos, R., González-Yebra, B., Martínez-Navarro, M. Á., Díaz-Chávez, E., Nieto, A., Ramírez, P., & Parrilla, P. (2013). Attitudes of non-medical staff in hospitals in Spain, Mexico, Cuba and Costa Rica towards organ donation. *Nefrología, 33*(5), 699–708. https://doi.org/10.3265/Nefrologia.pre2013.Jun.11296

Ríos, A., López-Navas, A. I., De-Francisco, C., Sánchez, Á., Hernández, A. M., Ramírez, P., & Parrilla, P. (2018). Psychometric characteristics of the attitude questionnaire toward the donation of organs for transplant (PCID-DTO-RIOS). *Transplantation Proceedings, 50*(2), 345–349. https://doi.org/10.1016/j.transproceed.2017.11.063

Ríos, A., López-Navas, A. I., García, J. A., Garrido, G., Ayala-García, M. A., Sebastian, M. J., Hernandez, A. M., Ramírez, P., & Parrilla, P. (2017). The attitude of Latin American immigrants in Florida (USA) towards deceased organ donation— A cross-section cohort study. *Transplant International, 30*(10), 1020–1031. https://doi.org/10.1111/tri.12997

Ríos, A., López-Navas, A. I., Garrido, G., Ayala-García, M. A., Sebastián, M. J., Hernández, A. M., Ramírez, P., & Parrilla, P. (2019). The knowledge of the brain death concept among Latin Americans residing in Florida (USA). *Experimental and Clinical Transplantation, 17*(2), 147–154. https://doi.org/10.6002/ect.2017.0254

Rodrigue, J. R., Cornell, D. L., & Howard, R. J. (2006). Organ donation decision: Comparison of donor and nondonor families. *American Journal of Transplantation, 6*(1), 190–198. https://doi.org/10.1111/j.1600-6143.2005.01130.x

Saleem, T., Ishaque, S., Habib, N., Hussain, S. S., Jawed, A., Khan, A. A., Ahmad, M. I., Iftikhar, M. O., Mughal, H. P., & Jehan, I. (2009). Knowledge, attitudes and practices survey on organ donation among a selected adult population of Pakistan. *BMC Medical Ethics, 10*, Article 5. https://doi.org/10.1186/1472-6939-10-5

Sánchez-Mendiola, M., Kieffer-Escobar, L. F., Marín-Beltrán, S., Downing, S. M., & Schwartz, A. (2012). Teaching of evidence-based medicine to medical students in Mexico: A randomized controlled trial. *BMC Medical Education, 12*, Article 107. https://doi.org/10.1186/1472-6920-12-107

Shafran, D., Kodish, E., & Tzakis, A. (2014). Organ shortage: The greatest challenge facing transplant medicine. *World Journal of Surgery, 38*, 1650–1657. https://doi.org/10.1007/s00268-014-2639-3

Testa, S., Toscano, A., & Rosato, R. (2018). Distractor efficiency in an item pool for a statistics classroom exam: Assessing its relation with item cognitive level classified according to Bloom's taxonomy. *Frontiers in Psychology, 9*, Article 1585. https://doi.org/10.3389/fpsyg.2018.01585

Theodorakopoulou, G., & Bakalis, N. (2010). The attitude of nursing students and nurses about transplantations. *Hellenic Journal of Nursing Science, 4*, 104–109. (Original work published in Greek)

Tong, A., Chapman, J. R., Wong, G., Josephson, M. A., & Craig, J. C. (2013). Public awareness and attitudes to living organ donation: Systematic review and integrative synthesis. *Transplantation, 96*(5), 429–437. https://doi.org/10.1097/TP.0b013e31829282ac

Tsavdaroglou, T., Paleolouga, C., Droulia, P., Fotos, N., & Brokalaki, I. (2013). Attitude and knowledge of nursing students towards donation and transplantation of organs and tissues. *Hellenic Journal of Nursing, 52*, 215–222. (Original work published in Greek)

Voo, T. C. (2015). Altruism and reward: Motivational compatibility in deceased organ donation. *Bioethics, 29*, 190–202. https://doi.org/10.1111/bioe.12078

Zambudio, A. R., López-Navas, A., Ayala-García, M., José Sebastián, M., Abdo-Cuza, A., Alán, J., Martínez-Alarcón, L., Ramírez, E. J., Muñoz, G., Palacios, G., Suárez-López, J., Castellanos, R., González, B., Martínez, M. A., Díaz, E., Ramírez, P., & Parrilla, P. (2012). Level of awareness of personnel in hospital services related to the donation process: A Spanish and Latin American multicenter study. *The Journal of Heart and Lung Transplantation, 31*(8), 850–857. https://doi.org/10.1016/j.healun.2012.03.011

Zhang, L., Li, Y., Zhou, J., Miao, X., Wang, G., Li, D., Nielson, K., Long, Y., & Li, J. (2007). Knowledge and willingness toward living organ donation: A survey of three universities in Changsha, Hunan Province, China. *Transplantation Proceedings, 39*, 1303–1309. https://doi.org/10.1016/j.transproceed.2007.02.096

Permissions

List of Contributors

Jiwon LEE, Ari LEE and Hanul LEE
College of Nursing, The Catholic University of Korea, Seoul, Republic of Korea

Younghye PARK
Seoul St. Mary's Hospital, College of Medicine, The Catholic University of Korea, Seoul, Republic of Korea

Kyounjoo LIM
Department of Nursing, Kyungbuk College, Yeongju-si, Republic of Korea

Jong-Eun LEE
College of Nursing, The Catholic University of Korea, Seoul, Republic of Korea

Julián RODRÍGUEZ-ALMAGRO and David RODRÍGUEZ-ALMAGRO
Department of Emergency, University General Hospital of Ciudad Real, Ciudad Real, Spain

MCarmen SOLANO-RUIZ and José SILES-GONZÁLEZ
Department of Nursing, School of Health Sciences, University of Alicante, Alicante, Spain

Antonio HERNÁNDEZ-MARTINEZ
Nurse Midwife Teaching Unit, General Hospital Mancha-Centro, Alcázar de San Juan, Ciudad Real, Spain

Özlem FİDAN, Arife Şanlialp ZEYREK and Şenay TAKMAK
Institute of Health Sciences, Pamukkale University, Denizli, Turkey

Asiye KARTAL
Faculty of Health Sciences, Department of Nursing, Pamukkale University, Denizli, Turkey

Mei-Chen SU
School of Nursing, National Taipei University of Nursing and Health Sciences, Taipei City, Taiwan

An-Shine CHAO
Department of Obstetrics and Gynecology, New Taipei Municipal TuCheng Hospital, New Taipei City, Taiwan

Min-Yu CHANG
Department of Nursing, New Taipei Municipal TuCheng Hospital and Adjunct Lecturer, Department of Nursing, Asia Eastern University of Science and Technology, New Taipei City, Taiwan

Yao-Lung CHANG
Department of Obstetrics and Gynecology, Linkou Chang Gung Memorial Hospital, Taoyuan City, Taiwan

Chien-Lan CHEN
Department of Nursing, Linkou Chang Gung Memorial Hospital, Taoyuan City, Taiwan

Jui-Chiung SUN
Department of Nursing, Chang Gung University of Science and Technology, Taoyuan City, Taiwan

Oluwamuyiwa Winifred ADEBAYO
College of Nursing, Penn State University, USA

Joseph P. DE SANTIS
School of Nursing and Health Studies, University of Miami, USA

Karina A. GATTAMORTA
School of Nursing and Health Studies, University of Miami, USA

Natalia Andrea VILLEGAS
School of Nursing, University of North Carolina at Chapel Hill, USA

Sultan AYAZ-ALKAYA
Faculty of Health Sciences, Department of Nursing, Gazi University, Ankara, Turkey

Fatma Ozlem OZTURK
Faculty of Nursing, Department of Nursing, Ankara University, Ankara, Turkey

Cheng-Hua NI
Department of Nursing, Center for Nursing and Healthcare Research in Clinical Practice Application, Wan Fang Hospital, Taipei Medical University and School of Nursing, College of Nursing, Taipei Medical University, Taiwan

Li WEI
Graduate Institute of Injury Prevention and Control, College of Public Health, Taipei Medical University and Attending Physician, Division of Neurosurgery, Department of Surgery, Wan Fang Hospital, Taipei Medical University, Taiwan

Chia-Che WU
School of Medicine, College of Medicine, Taipei Medical University and Attending Physician, Department of Otolaryngology, Wan Fang Hospital, Taipei Medical University, Taiwan

Chueh-Ho LIN
Master Program in Long-Term Care, College of Nursing, Taipei Medical University, Taiwan

Pao-Yu CHOU
Department of Nursing and Center for Nursing and Healthcare Research in Clinical Practice Application, Wan Fang Hospital, Taipei Medical University and School of Nursing, College of Nursing, Taipei Medical University, Taiwan

Yeu-Hui CHUANG
School of Nursing, College of Nursing, Taipei Medical University and Center for Nursing and Healthcare Research in Clinical Practice Application, Wan Fang Hospital, Taipei Medical University, Taiwan

Ching-Chiu KAO
Center for Nursing and Healthcare Research in Clinical Practice Application, Wan Fang Hospital, Taipei Medical University and School of Nursing, College of Nursing, Taipei Medical University, Taiwan

Chia-Hui WANG
Department of Nursing, Taipei Medical University Shuang Ho Hospital and School of Nursing, College of Nursing, Taipei Medical University, Taiwan

Shu-Hui YANG
Department of Nursing, Taipei Medical University Shuang Ho Hospital, Taiwan

Hsiu-Ju JEN and Jui-Chen TSAI
Department of Nursing, Taipei Medical University Shuang Ho Hospital and School of Nursing, College of Nursing, Taipei Medical University, Taiwan

Hsi-Kuei LIN
Department of Dentistry, Taipei Medical University Shuang Ho Hospital and School of Dentistry, College of Oral Medicine, Taipei Medical University, Taiwan

El-Wui LOH
Center for Evidence-Based Health Care and Shared Decision Making Resource Center, Department of Medical Research and Department of Dentistry, Taipei Medical University Shuang Ho Hospital; Researcher, Cochrane Taiwan, Taipei Medical University and Graduate Institute of Clinical Medicine, College of Medicine, Taipei Medical University, Taiwan

Zahra FARSI
Faculty of Nursing, Research Department and Community Health Department, Aja University of Medical Sciences, Tehran, Iran

Maa'soumeh KAMALI
Faculty of Nursing, Aja University of Medical Sciences, Tehran, Iran

Samantha BUTLER
Harvard Medical School and Boston Children's Hospital, Boston, Massachusetts, USA

Armin ZAREIYAN
Faculty of Nursing, Community Health Department, Aja University of Medical Sciences, Tehran, Iran

Li Sze CHAI, Lily LIM, Azylina GUNGGU, Sidiah SIOP and Zabidah PUTIT
Faculty of Medicine and Health Sciences, Department of Nursing, Universiti Malaysia Sarawak, Malaysia

Suk Fong TIE
Matron, Sarawak Heart Centre, Malaysia

Jiyun KIM
School of Nursing, Gachon University, Incheon, Republic of Korea

Hyang KIM
College of Nursing, Seoul National University, Seoul, Republic of Korea

Hae-Ra HAN
School of Nursing, Johns Hopkins University, Baltimore, Maryland, USA

Xiaomeng DONG
Huzhou University, Huzhou Central Hospital, Huzhou, China

Jianying PENG
Department of Nursing, Xiangyang No. 1 People's Hospital, Hubei University of Medicine, Hubei, China

Xingxing LI, Qiyuan ZHAO and Xiuwei ZHANG
School of Medicine, Huzhou University, Huzhou Central Hospital, Huzhou, China

Abedalmajeed SHAJRAWI
Faculty of Nursing, Applied Science Private University, Amman, Jordan

Malcolm GRANAT
Health and Rehabilitation Sciences, School of Health Sciences, University of Salford, Manchester, UK

Ian JONES
School of Nursing and Allied Health, Liverpool John Moores University, UK

Felicity ASTIN
Centre for Applied Research in Health, University of Huddersfield and Research and Development, Huddersfield Royal Infirmary, Acre Street, Huddersfield, UK

Shuo-Shin TSAI
College of Nursing, Kaohsiung Medical University and Lecturer, Department of Nursing, Chung-Jen Junior College of Nursing, Health Sciences and Management

Hsiu-Hung WANG and Fan-Hao CHOU
College of Nursing, Kaohsiung Medical University

Tajmohammad ARAZI
Department of Nursing and Operating Room, Neyshabur University of Medical Sciences, Neyshabur, Iran

Mansooreh ALIASGHARPOUR
Faculty of Nursing and Midwifery, Department of Medical Surgical Nursing, Tehran University of Medical Sciences, Tehran, Iran

Sepideh MOHAMMADI
Department of Nursing, Nursing Care Research Center, Health Research Institute, Babol University of Medical Sciences, Babol, Iran

Nooredin MOHAMMADI
Department of Nursing, School of Nursing and Midwifery, Iran University of Medical Sciences, Tehran, Iran

Anoushirvan KAZEMNEJAD
Department of Biostatistics, School of Medicine, Tarbiat Modares University, Tehran, Iran

Shinae AHN
Department of Nursing, Wonkwang University, Jeonbuk, Republic of Korea

Nam-Ju LEE
College of Nursing, The Research Institute of Nursing Science, Seoul National University, Seoul, Republic of Korea

Sevcan FATA and Merlinda ALUŞ TOKAT
Gynecology & Obstetrics Nursing Department, Nursing Faculty, Dokuz Eylul University, Izmir, Turkey

Melyza PERDANA
Department of Medical Surgical Nursing, Universitas Gadjah Mada, Yogyakarta, Indonesia

Miaofen YEN
Department of Nursing, National Cheng Kung University, Tainan City, Taiwan

Young Eun AHN
College of Nursing, Seoul National University, Seoul, Republic of Korea

Chin Kang KOH
College of Nursing, The Research Institute of Nursing Research, Seoul National University, Seoul, Republic of Korea

Mei-Yu LIN
School of Nursing, College of Nursing, Taipei Medical University, Taiwan

Wei-Shih WENG
Department of Nursing, Tri-Service General Hospital, Taiwan

Renny Wulan APRILIYASARI
School of Nursing, College of Nursing, Taipei Medical University, Taiwan and Nursing Lecturer, Sekolah Tinggi Ilmu Kesehatan Cendekia Utama Kudus, Indonesia

Pham VAN TRUONG
School of Nursing, College of Nursing, Taipei Medical University, Taiwan

Pei-Shan TSAI
College of Nursing, Taipei Medical University; Department of Nursing & Center for Nursing and Healthcare Research in Clinical Practice Application, Wan Fang Hospital, Taipei Medical University; and Sleep Research Center, Taipei Medical University Hospital, Taiwan

Eun Sook JUNG
Graduate School, Kyung Hee University, Seoul, Republic of Korea

Ae Kyung CHANG
College of Nursing Science & East-West Nursing Research Institute, Kyung Hee University, Seoul, Republic of Korea

Hao-Yuan CHANG
School of Nursing, College of Medicine, National Taiwan University and Department of Nursing, National Taiwan University Hospital, Taiwan

Chih-Chao YANG
Department of Neurology, National Taiwan University Hospital, Taiwan, ROC

Mark P. JENSEN
Department of Rehabilitation Medicine, University of Washington, Seattle, WA, USA

Yeur-Hur LAI
School of Nursing, College of Medicine, National Taiwan University and Department of Nursing, National Taiwan University Cancer Center, Taipei, Taiwan

SookBin IM
College of Nursing, Eulji University, Daejeon

MiKyoung CHO
Department of Nursing Science, College of Medicine, Chungbuk National University, Cheongju

MyoungLyun HEO
Jeonju University, Jeonju

Henik Tri RAHAYU
International Doctoral Program in Nursing, College of Medicine, National Cheng Kung University, Taiwan and Department of Nursing, Health Sciences Faculty, University of Muhammadiyah Malang, Malang, Indonesia

Ching-Min CHEN
Department of Nursing, Institute of Gerontology and Institute of Allied Health Sciences, National Cheng Kung University, Taiwan

Evanthia ASIMAKOPOULOU, Vaso STYLIANOU and Ioannis DIMITRAKOPOULOS
School of Health Sciences, Frederick University, Nicosia, Cyprus

Alexandros ARGYRIADIS
School of Health Sciences and School of Education and Social Sciences, Frederick University, Nicosia, Cyprus

Panagiota BELLOU–MYLONA
School of Health Sciences, Frederick University, Nicosia, Cyprus

Index

Printed in the USA
CPSIA information can be obtained
at www.ICGtesting.com
JSHW051625061123
51533JS00005B/108

9 781646 466160